NAPLEX®
Prep
2018

NAPLEX®
Prep
2018

Amie D. Brooks, PharmD, FCCP, BCACP
Cynthia Sanoski, BS, PharmD, FCCP, BCPS
Emily R. Hajjar, PharmD, BCPS, BCACP, BCGP
Brian R. Overholser, PharmD, FCCP

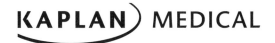

NAPLEX® is a registered trademark and service mark of the National Association of Boards of Pharmacy (NABP), which neither sponsors nor endorses this product.

This publication is designed to provide accurate information in regard to the subject matter covered as of its publication date, with the understanding that knowledge and best practice constantly evolve. The publisher is not engaged in rendering medical, legal, accounting, or other professional service. If medical or legal advice or other expert assistance is required, the services of a competent professional should be sought. This publication is not intended for use in clinical practice or the delivery of medical care. To the fullest extent of the law, neither the Publisher nor the Editors assume any liability for any injury and/or damage to persons or property arising out of or related to any use of the material contained in this book.

© 2018 Kaplan

Published by Kaplan Publishing, a division of Kaplan, Inc.
750 Third Avenue
New York, NY 10017

Printed in the United States of America

Retail ISBN: 978-1-5062-2365-0
10 9 8 7 6 5 4 3 2 1

Course ISBN: 978-1-5062-2367-4
10 9 8 7 6 5 4 3 2 1

Kaplan Publishing books are available at special quantity discounts to use for sales promotions, employee premiums, or educational purposes. For more information or to purchase books, please call the Simon & Schuster special sales department at 866-506-1949.

About the Authors

Amie D. Brooks, PharmD, FCCP, BCACP, is a professor of pharmacy practice, director for the division of ambulatory care at the St. Louis College of Pharmacy, and a clinical pharmacy specialist in ambulatory care at St. Louis County Department of Health. Dr. Brooks is a fellow of the American College of Clinical Pharmacy. She received her Doctor of Pharmacy degree from the St. Louis College of Pharmacy and completed her pharmacy residency training at the Jefferson Barracks VA Medical Center in St. Louis, Missouri. Her research interests include clinical pharmacy services, diabetes, resistant hypertension, and collaborative practice.

Cynthia Sanoski, BS, PharmD, FCCP, BCPS, is the chair of the department of pharmacy practice at the Jefferson College of Pharmacy at Thomas Jefferson University. Dr. Sanoski received her Doctor of Pharmacy degree from Ohio State University, and subsequently completed a 2-year fellowship in cardiovascular pharmacotherapy at the University of Illinois at Chicago. She is also a board-certified pharmacotherapy specialist and a fellow of the American College of Clinical Pharmacy. Dr. Sanoski serves as an instructor with Kaplan Medical, teaching NAPLEX review courses for graduating pharmacy students across the country.

Emily R. Hajjar, PharmD, BCPS, BCACP, BCGP, is associate professor in the Jefferson College of Pharmacy at Thomas Jefferson University in Philadelphia, Pennsylvania. Dr. Hajjar earned her PharmD at Duquesne University. She completed a pharmacy practice residency at the University of Rochester Medical Center in Rochester, New York, a geriatric pharmacy specialty residency at the Minneapolis Veteran's Affairs Medical Center, and a geriatric pharmacotherapy-epidemiology fellowship at the University of Minnesota, College of Pharmacy. Dr. Hajjar provides clinical services to the Jefferson Family and Community Medicine Senior Center Practice and the Kimmel Cancer Center Senior Adult Oncology and Outpatient Palliative Care clinics. Her research interests include geriatric pharmacotherapy and polypharmacy.

Brian R. Overholser, PharmD, FCCP, is associate professor of pharmacy practice in the College of Pharmacy at Purdue University and Adjunct Associate Professor in the Division of Clinical Pharmacology at the Indiana University School of Medicine in Indianapolis, Indiana. Dr. Overholser earned his PharmD and conducted his postdoctoral research in pharmacokinetics and pharmacodynamics at Purdue University. His primary teaching responsibilities include courses in pharmacokinetics, pharmacodynamics, and pharmacogenetics at both Purdue and Indiana University. Dr. Overholser's research program is focused on elucidating the pathological regulation that increases the susceptibility of arrhythmias in patients with heart failure.

The authors wish to thank the following expert reviewers:

Lauren Biehle, PharmD, BCPS
Clinical Assistant Professor of Pharmacy Practice
University of Wyoming School of Pharmacy
Denver, Colorado

Sarah Fowler Braga, PharmD, RPh
Associate Professor Pharmacy Practice and Director of
  Drug Information
South University School of Pharmacy
Columbia, South Carolina

Rebecca Bragg, PharmD, BCPS
Assistant Professor
St. Louis College of Pharmacy
St. Louis, Missouri

Ashley Castleberry, PharmD, MAEd
Assistant Professor
University of Arkansas for Medical Sciences College of
  Pharmacy
Little Rock, Arkansas

Jamie Cavanaugh, PharmD, CPP, BCPS
Assistant Professor of Medicine
University of North Carolina
Chapel Hill, NC

Jill Chao, PharmD
Class of 2017
University of Houston College of Pharmacy
Houston, Texas

Kelly Clark, PharmD
Assistant Professor Pharmacy Practice
Coordinator—Integrated Pharmacy Skills Lab
South University School of Pharmacy
Columbia, South Carolina

Robert Clegg, PhD, MPH, MCHES
Associate Professor of Administrative Sciences
California Health Sciences University, College of Pharmacy
Clovis, California

Kimberly Ference, PharmD
Associate Professor
Wilkes University School of Pharmacy
Wilkes-Barre, Pennsylvania

Patrick R. Finley, PharmD, BCPP
Professor of Clinical Pharmacy
University of California San Francisco
San Francisco, California

Eric Z. Kao, PharmD
Class of 2017
University of Houston College of Pharmacy
Houston, Texas

Sonia Kothari, PharmD
PGY-2 Cardiology Pharmacy Resident
UMass Memorial Medical Center
Worcester, Massachusetts

Kelly C. Lee, PharmD, MAS, BCPP, FCCP
Professor of Clinical Pharmacy
UCSD Skaggs School of Pharmacy and Pharmaceutical
  Sciences
La Jolla, California

Megan Maroney, PharmD, BCPP
Clinical Associate Professor
Ernest Mario School of Pharmacy
Rutgers, The State University of New Jersey
Psychiatric Clinical Pharmacist
Monmouth Medical Center
Long Branch, New Jersey

Santhi Masilamani, PharmD, CDE, MBA
Director, Ambulatory APPE
University of Houston College of Pharmacy
Houston, Texas

Quamrun N. Masuda, PhD, RPh
Associate Professor (Pharmaceutics) & Assistant
  Director of the Center for Compounding Practice &
  Research
Virginia Commonwealth University, School of
  Pharmacy
Richmond, Virginia

James A. Trovato, PharmD, MBA, BCOP, FASHP
Associate Professor and Vice Chair for Academic
  Affairs
Department of Pharmacy Practice and Science
University of Maryland School of Pharmacy
Baltimore, Maryland

Ashley H. Vincent, PharmD, BCACP, BCPS
Clinical Assistant Professor, Purdue University College
  of Pharmacy
Indiana University School of Medicine
Indianapolis, Indiana

The authors also wish to thank the following test item writers: LeAnn C. Boyd, PharmD, BCPS, CDE; Elizabeth Langan, MD; Amy Egras, PharmD, BCPS; Stacey Thacker, PharmD; and Arneka Tillman, PharmD candidate, Xavier College of Pharmacy.

The authors would also like to acknowledge the contributions of Karen Nagel, BS Pharm, PhD, and Steven T. Boyd, PharmD, PCPS, CDE.

Table of Contents

NOTE: Sections in gray appear in the digital version of this book only. See the "How to Use This Book" section for more details.

PART ONE: Overview

PART TWO: Review of Therapeutics

Part One

Overview

How to Use This Book

Congratulations! You've taken the first step to prepare yourself for the NAPLEX®. The content of this book is designed to provide a concentrated and concise review of the competency areas tested on the NAPLEX. This book is not intended to replace standard textbooks in pharmacy. Rather, it should serve as a primary tool in the weeks and months prior to taking the exam. Our intention—and our hope—is that this book will be an integral part of your preparation for the NAPLEX.

Step 1: Access Your Online Center

The 2018 edition of this NAPLEX review is delivered both in print and online. Log on to *kaptest.com/NAPLEX2018* to access your online center. You will be asked for a password derived from the text to access the online center, so have your book handy when you log on.

Your online center resources include the following:

- The **digital version** of the book, including all 31 content review chapters *plus* an exam overview and Kaplan's exclusive test-taking strategies.
- Chapter **quizzes** to assess your strengths and weaknesses as you complete each content area. These quizzes also appear in the printed version of the book.
- **2 full-length practice tests**, each with 250 unique questions.

Step 2: Familiarize Yourself with the Digital Book

The digital version of *NAPLEX Prep 2018* covers all of the areas tested on the NAPLEX in 31 chapters, arranged by disease state (such as pulmonary disorders) or concept discipline (such as pharmaceutics or biostatistics). The digital book is the master version of *NAPLEX Prep 2018*.

Each disease state chapter in the digital version of the book focuses on the following:

- Definitions of the disease
- Diagnosis
- Signs and symptoms
- Guidelines
- Guidelines summary
- Drug tables (*author-determined "Top 200" drugs are indicated with a star*)
- Storage and administration pearls
- Patient education pearls

Step 3: Familiarize Yourself with the Print Book

The printed version of *NAPLEX Prep 2018* is a subset of the digital book. This smaller guide highlights content areas that the authors regard as high-yield—that is, content areas that are especially likely to be tested. For example, Chapter 2: Infectious Diseases, appears in both the digital book and the print book, while Chapter 19: Special Populations, appears in the digital book only.

Within the chapters, the print book focuses on types of information that can be studied on-the-go. For instance, all drug tables appear in the print book, because they are ideal for piecemeal study. Each disease state chapter in the print book presents only the following:

- Disease state
- Guidelines summary
- Summary of treatment recommendations
- Overview of treatment (if applicable)
- Treatment algorithm (if applicable)
- Drug tables

Step 4: Take the First Online Practice Test

You should take Practice Test 1 before the beginning of your study period. Take the exam in a quiet area with a good internet connection, and dedicate 6 hours to the test. This is the same per-question allotment as on the current 250-question NAPLEX exam. The goal is to simulate exam conditions, so eliminate distractions like your cell phone.

When the test is completed, you will receive immediate feedback on your performance as the software analyzes your strengths and weaknesses in various content areas. Use the results to identify your areas of strength and weakness and tailor an individualized study plan for yourself. For example, if you score below average on questions related to oncology therapeutics, plan to spend additional time studying this subject, whereas if cardiovascular therapeutics was the area in which you scored the highest, you might opt to leave this section for last when studying.

As you review the results of Practice Test 1, pay particular attention to the answer explanations. Studying the answer explanations is often one of the most valuable study methods. Note that explanations provide the reasoning for *not* choosing the incorrect answer choices. Use this information to understand the rationale behind eliminating each distracter.

Step 5: Start Your Content Review

Kaplan recommends that you begin your study in the areas that you have determined are your weakest; in this way, you can spend additional review time on difficult concepts. Each chapter in the digital book gives a suggested study time, prepared by the authors. Adjust these times based on the results of Practice Test 1 and the overall amount of time in your study-time "budget." Be sure to take each end-of-chapter practice quiz to assess how well you have retained the material.

Step 6: Take the Second Online Practice Test

You should take Practice Test 2 once you have completed the majority of your study—a week or two prior to your exam date. It is also a full-length online exam with 250 unique questions. Take Practice Test 2 in a quiet, distraction-free area with a good internet connection, and dedicate 6 hours to the test.

Best of luck to you on your journey toward a successful career as a pharmacist!

TEST CHANGES OR LATE-BREAKING DEVELOPMENTS

kaptest.com/publishing

The material in this book is up-to-date at the time of publication. However, the NABP® may have instituted changes in the test after this book was published. Be sure to carefully read the materials you receive when you register for the test. If there are any important late-breaking developments—or any changes or corrections to the Kaplan test preparation materials in this book—we will post that information online at kaptest.com/publishing.

Part Two

Review of Therapeutics

Cardiovascular Disorders

1

This chapter covers the following topics:

- **Hypertension**
- **Dyslipidemia**
- **Heart failure**
- **Antiarrhythmic drugs**
- **Antithrombotic drugs**
- **Ischemic heart disease**
- **Acute pharmacologic management of UA/NSTEMI**
- **Acute pharmacologic management of STEMI**
- **Secondary prevention of MI**

HYPERTENSION

Guidelines Summary

- General population <60 yr: <140/90 mmHg (JNC 8 guidelines)
- General population ≥60 yr: <150/90 mmHg (JNC 8 guidelines)
- CKD
  - BP goal <140/90 mmHg (JNC 8 guidelines)
  - Urine albumin excretion <30 mg/day: BP goal <140/90 mmHg (KDIGO guidelines)
  - Urine albumin excretion ≥30 mg/day: BP goal <130/80 mmHg (KDIGO guidelines)
- Diabetes mellitus (DM)
  - BP goal <140/90 mmHg (JNC 8 guidelines and American Diabetes Association guidelines)

- Heart failure (Stage C HFrEF or Stage C heart failure with preserved ejection fraction)
  - SBP goal <130 mmHg (American College of Cardiology/American Heart Association/Heart Failure Society of America focused update)
- Patients with coronary artery disease (CAD) for secondary prevention of cardiovascular events:
  - BP goal <140/90 mmHg (American Heart Association/American College of Cardiology/American Society of Hypertension guidelines)
- Lifestyle modifications: weight loss (goal body mass index [BMI] 18.5–24.9 kg/m^2), diet rich in fruits, vegetables, and low-fat dairy products with ↓ saturated and total fat, ↓ sodium (Na$^+$) intake (≤2.4 g/day), ↑ physical activity (30 minutes most days of the week), moderation of alcohol use (≤1 ounce of ethanol/day), smoking cessation
- Pharmacologic therapy:
  - Initial antihypertensive drug selection (JNC8 guidelines):
    » Nonblack patients (with or without DM): Thiazide diuretic, angiotensin-converting enzyme inhibitor (ACEI), angiotensin II receptor blocker (ARB), and/or calcium channel blocker (CCB)
    » Black patients (with or without DM): Thiazide diuretic and/or CCB
    » CKD (regardless of race or presence of DM): ACEI or ARB (alone or in combination with other drug class)
    » NOTE: β-blockers are no longer considered first-line therapy for patients with HTN without specific comorbidities (see below)
  - Presence of other comorbidities may warrant selection of other agents as first-line antihypertensive therapy (based on guidelines for each of these conditions):
    » HFrEF: Diuretic, ACEI, β-blocker (carvedilol, metoprolol succinate, or bisoprolol), ARB, aldosterone receptor antagonist (ARA), hydralazine/isosorbide dinitrate (for black patients)
    » Post-MI: β-blocker, ACEI (or ARB)
    » High coronary disease risk: ACEI (or ARB), thiazide diuretic, CCB
    » Recurrent stroke prevention: ACEI, diuretic
  - Three approaches for initiation and titration of antihypertensive therapy:
    » Initiate one antihypertensive drug → Titrate to maximum dose to achieve goal BP → If goal BP not achieved, add second antihypertensive drug → Titrate dose of second drug to maximum → If goal BP still not achieved, add third antihypertensive drug
      – Avoid concomitant use of ACEI and ARB
    » Initiate one antihypertensive drug → If goal BP not achieved, add second antihypertensive drug before maximum dose of initial drug achieved → If

goal BP not achieved, titrate doses of both drugs up to maximum → If goal BP still not achieved, add third antihypertensive drug

- Avoid concomitant use of ACEI and ARB

» Initiate two antihypertensive drugs at same time (avoid concomitant use of ACEI and ARB) → If goal BP not achieved, titrate doses of both drugs up to maximum → If goal BP still not achieved, add third antihypertensive drug

- Initial two-drug approach should be considered when: BP >160 mmHg and/or DBP >100 mmHg **OR** SBP is >20 mmHg and/or DBP is >10 mmHg above goal

Diuretics

Generic • Brand • Dose	Contra-indications	Primary Side Effects	Key Monitoring	Pertinent Drug Interactions	Med Pearl
Thiazide Diuretics – inhibit Na$^+$ reabsorption in the distal convoluted tubule					
Chlorothiazide • Diuril • 500–2,000 mg/day Chlorthalidone☆ • Only available generically • 12.5–100 mg/day Hydrochlorothiazide☆ • Microzide • 12.5–50 mg/day Indapamide • Only available generically • 1.25–5 mg/day Metolazone☆ • Zaroxolyn • 2.5–5 mg/day	Sulfa allergy	• Hypokalemia • Hypomagnesemia • Hyponatremia • Hypercalcemia • Hyperglycemia • Hyperuricemia • Photosensitivity	• BP • Electrolytes • Blood urea nitrogen (BUN)/serum creatinine (SCr) • Blood glucose • Uric acid	• May ↑ risk of lithium toxicity • May ↓ effect of antidiabetic agents • NSAIDs ↓ antihypertensive effects	• Often used as first-line therapy for HTN • Synergistic effect with other antihypertensives • Not effective (except metolazone) when creatinine clearance (CrCl) <30 mL/min; use loop diuretics • Have ceiling dose (unlike loop diuretics) • Chlorothiazide also available as injection
Loop Diuretics – inhibit Na$^+$ reabsorption in the ascending limb of loop of Henle (should only be used for HTN in patients with renal impairment [maintain efficacy when CrCl <30 mL/min], severe edema, or HF) (see HF section for further details)					
Potassium-Sparing Diuretics – inhibit Na$^+$ reabsorption in the collecting ducts					
Amiloride • Only available generically • 5–10 mg/day Triamterene • Dyrenium • 50–100 mg/day	• Hyperkalemia • CKD	Hyperkalemia	• BP • Potassium (K$^+$) • BUN/SCr	Use with K$^+$ supplements, ACEIs, ARBs, ARAs, or NSAIDs may ↑ risk of hyperkalemia	• Not used often as monotherapy (weak antihypertensives) • Often used with hydrochlorothiazide to ↓ K$^+$ loss

Combination products:
    Triamterene/hydrochlorothiazide (Dyazide, Maxzide)
    Amiloride/hydrochlorothiazide (only available generically)					

Diuretics   *(cont'd)*

Generic • Brand • Dose	Contra-indications	Primary Side Effects	Key Monitoring	Pertinent Drug Interactions	Med Pearl
Aldosterone Receptor Antagonists – have similar mechanism of action to K+-sparing diuretics (also block the effects of aldosterone) (not used often for HTN) (see HF section for further details)					
Combination product: Spironolactone/hydrochlorothiazide (Aldactazide)					

β-Blockers

Generic • Brand • Dose	Contra-indications	Primary Side Effects	Key Monitoring	Pertinent Drug Interactions	Med Pearl

Mechanism of action – ↓ cardiac output (CO) by negative inotropic (↓ contractility) and negative chronotropic (↓ heart rate [HR]) effects
• Cardioselective – bind more to β_1 than β_2 receptors (at low doses); less likely to cause bronchoconstriction or vasoconstriction at low doses (safer to use in patients with asthma, chronic obstructive pulmonary disease [COPD], PAD, or DM); cardioselectivity may be lost at higher doses
    – Bisoprolol, atenolol, metoprolol, betaxolol, acebutolol, nebivolol (BAMBAN)
• Intrinsic sympathomimetic activity (ISA) – have partial β-receptor agonist activity
    – Carteolol, acebutolol, pindolol, penbutolol (CAPP)
• Lipophilic vs. hydrophilic – lipophilic (propranolol, metoprolol, carvedilol, labetalol, pindolol, nebivolol) more likely to cause central nervous system (CNS) side effects (e.g., depression, fatigue) than hydrophilic (atenolol)					

Cardioselective:					
Acebutolol • Sectral • 200–1,200 mg/day Atenolol☆ • Tenormin • 25–100 mg/day Betaxolol • Only available generically • 5–20 mg/day Bisoprolol • Zebeta • 2.5–20 mg/day Metoprolol☆ • Tartrate: Lopressor (2 × daily), Succinate: Toprol XL (1 × daily) • 25–400 mg/day Nebivolol☆ • Bystolic • 5–40 mg/day	• ≥2nd degree heart block (in absence of pacemaker) • HF (except metoprolol succinate or bisoprolol)	• Bradycardia/heart block • HF exacerbation • Bronchospasm • Cold extremities • Fatigue • ↓ exercise tolerance • Depression • Glucose intolerance • Mask hypoglycemia (in patients with DM)	• BP • HR • S/S of HF • Blood glucose (in patients with DM)	Use with other negative chronotropes (e.g., digoxin, verapamil, diltiazem, clonidine, or ivabradine) may ↑ risk of bradycardia	• Abrupt discontinuation may cause angina, MI, or hypertensive emergency; need to taper over 2 wk • Metoprolol tartrate also available as injection

β-Blockers *(cont'd)*

Generic • Brand • Dose	Contra-indications	Primary Side Effects	Key Monitoring	Pertinent Drug Interactions	Med Pearl
Nonselective:					
Carvedilol☆ • Coreg, Coreg CR • Immediate-release (IR): 12.5–50 mg/day (in two divided doses) • Controlled-release (CR): 20–80 mg/day (1 × daily)	• ≥2nd degree heart block (in absence of pacemaker) • HF (except carvedilol)	Same as with cardioselective β-blockers	Same as with cardioselective β-blockers	Same as with cardioselective β-blockers	• Same as with cardioselective β-blockers • Labetalol and carvedilol also have α_1-blocking properties • Labetalol and propranolol also available as injection
Labetalol • Trandate • 200–2,400 mg/day					
Nadolol • Corgard • 20–320 mg/day					
Pindolol • Only available generically • 5–60 mg/day					
Propranolol☆ • Inderal, Inderal LA, In-noPran XL • 80–640 mg/day (IR given 2–3 × daily; extended-release [ER] given 1 × daily)					
Timolol • Only available generically • 20–60 mg/day					

Combination products:

Atenolol/chlorthalidone (Tenoretic) Bisoprolol/hydrochlorothiazide (Ziac)	Metoprolol tartrate/hydrochlorothiazide (Lopressor HCT) Metoprolol succinate/hydrochlorothiazide (Dutoprol)	Nadolol/bendroflumethiazide (Corzide) Nebivolol/valsartan (Byvalson) Propranolol/hydrochlorothiazide (only available generically)

Angiotensin-Converting Enzyme Inhibitors

Generic • Brand • Dose	Contra-indications	Primary Side Effects	Key Monitoring	Pertinent Drug Interactions	Med Pearl
Mechanism of action – inhibit angiotensin-converting enzyme and prevent the conversion of angiotensin I to angiotensin II → vasodilation, ↓ aldosterone production; also inhibit degradation of bradykinin					
Benazepril☆ • Lotensin • 5–40 mg/day Captopril • Only available generically • 12.5–450 mg/day Enalapril☆ • Epaned, Vasotec • 2.5–40 mg/day Fosinopril☆ • Only available generically • 5–80 mg/day Lisinopril☆ • Prinivil, Qbrelis, Zestril • 2.5–40 mg/day Moexipril • Univasc • 3.75–30 mg/day Perindopril • Aceon • 4–16 mg/day Quinapril☆ • Accupril • 10–80 mg/day Ramipril☆ • Altace • 1.25–20 mg/day Trandolapril☆ • Mavik • 0.5–4 mg/day	• Pregnancy • History of angioedema or renal failure with prior use • Hyperkalemia • Bilateral renal artery stenosis • Concurrent use with aliskiren in DM	• Hyperkalemia • Renal impairment • Cough (dry) • Angioedema	• BP • BUN/SCr • K^+	• Use with K^+ supplements, K^+-sparing diuretics, ARAs, or NSAIDs may ↑ risk of hyperkalemia • Use with ARBs or aliskiren may ↑ risk of hyperkalemia and renal impairment (avoid concurrent use with aliskiren in DM and CrCl <60 mL/min) • May ↑ risk of lithium toxicity • Use with sirolimus, temsirolimus, or everolimus may ↑ risk of angioedema	• Captopril has shortest duration of action • Enalapril also available as oral solution (Epaned) and injection (enalaprilat) • Lisinopril also available as oral solution (Qbrelis) • If patient has intolerable dry cough, may switch to ARB • Hyperkalemia and renal impairment also likely to occur with ARBs (risk of angioedema cross-sensitivity with ARBs controversial)

Combination products:

Benazepril/amlodipine (Lotrel)
Benazepril/hydrochlorothiazide (Lotensin HCT)
Captopril/hydrochlorothiazide (only available generically)

Enalapril/hydrochlorothiazide (Vaseretic)
Fosinopril/hydrochlorothiazide (only available generically)
Lisinopril/hydrochlorothiazide (Zestoretic)

Moexipril/hydrochlorothiazide (Uniretic)
Perindopril/amlodipine (Prestalia)
Quinapril/hydrochlorothiazide (Accuretic)
Trandolapril/verapamil (Tarka)

Angiotensin II Receptor Blockers

Generic • Brand • Dose	Contra-indications	Primary Side Effects	Key Monitoring	Pertinent Drug Interactions	Med Pearl
Mechanism of action – inhibit the binding of angiotensin II to the angiotensin type 1 (AT$_1$) receptor → vasodilation, ↓ aldosterone production; no effect on bradykinin					
Azilsartan • Edarbi • 40–80 mg/day Candesartan • Atacand • 4–32 mg/day Eprosartan • Teveten • 400–800 mg/day Irbesartan☆ • Avapro • 75–300 mg/day Losartan☆ • Cozaar • 25–100 mg/day Olmesartan☆ • Benicar • 20–40 mg/day Telmisartan☆ • Micardis • 20–80 mg/day Valsartan☆ • Diovan • 80–320 mg/day	Same as for ACEIs	• Same as for ACEIs (except no cough) • Sprue-like enteropathy (olmesartan)	Same as for ACEIs	• Use with K$^+$ supplements, K$^+$-sparing diuretics, ARAs, or NSAIDs may ↑ risk of hyperkalemia • Use with ACEIs or aliskiren may ↑ risk of hyperkalemia or renal impairment (avoid concurrent use with aliskiren in DM and CrCl <60 mL/min) • May ↑ risk of lithium toxicity	Hyperkalemia and renal impairment also likely to occur with ACEIs (risk of angioedema cross-sensitivity with ACEIs is controversial)

Combination products:

Azilsartan/chlorthalidone (Edarbyclor)
Candesartan/hydrochlorothiazide (Atacand HCT)
Eprosartan/hydrochlorothiazide (Teveten HCT)
Irbesartan/hydrochlorothiazide (Avalide)
Losartan/hydrochlorothiazide (Hyzaar)

Olmesartan/amlodipine (Azor)
Olmesartan/amlodipine/hydrochlorothiazide (Tribenzor)
Olmesartan/hydrochlorothiazide (Benicar HCT)
Telmisartan/amlodipine (Twynsta)

Telmisartan/hydrochlorothiazide (Micardis HCT)
Valsartan/amlodipine (Exforge)
Valsartan/hydrochlorothiazide (Diovan HCT)
Valsartan/amlodipine/hydrochlorothiazide (Exforge HCT)

Renin Inhibitor

Generic • Brand • Dose	Contra-indications	Primary Side Effects	Key Monitoring	Pertinent Drug Interactions	Med Pearl
Mechanism of action – inhibits renin and prevents the conversion of angiotensinogen to angiotensin I, which then ↓ production of angiotensin II					
Aliskiren☆ • Tekturna • 150–300 mg/day	• Pregnancy • History of ACEI- or ARB-induced angioedema • Hyperkalemia • Bilateral renal artery stenosis • Use with ACEIs or ARBs in DM	• Headache • Dizziness • Diarrhea • Hyperkalemia • Renal impairment	• BP • BUN/SCr • K^+	• Use with K^+ supplements, K^+-sparing diuretics, ARAs, or NSAIDs may ↑ risk of hyperkalemia • Use with ACEIs or ARBs may ↑ risk of hyperkalemia or renal impairment (avoid concurrent use in DM and CrCl <60 ml/min) • Itraconazole or cyclosporine may ↑ effects; avoid concurrent use • May ↓ effects of furosemide	• Use with caution in patients with CrCl <30 mL/min • Avoid taking with high-fat meals
Combination products: Aliskiren/hydrochlorothiazide (Tekturna HCT)					

Calcium Channel Blockers

Generic • Brand • Dose	Contra-indications	Primary Side Effects	Key Monitoring	Pertinent Drug Interactions	Med Pearl
Mechanism of action – bind to L-type channels in heart and coronary/peripheral arteries to block inward movement of calcium (Ca^{2+}) → vascular smooth-muscle relaxation (vasodilation); all (except for amlodipine and felodipine) have negative inotropic effects (↓ contractility) • Dihydropyridines (DHPs) – more selective to vasculature; more potent vasodilators; have no effect on cardiac conduction • Non-DHPs – cause less peripheral vasodilation than DHPs; have negative chronotropic properties (↓ HR)					
DHPs:					
Amlodipine ☆ • Norvasc • 2.5–10 mg/day Felodipine ☆ • Only available generically • 2.5–20 mg/day Isradipine • Only available generically • 5–10 mg/day Nicardipine • Cardene • 60–120 mg/day Nifedipine ☆ • Adalat CC, Afeditab CR, Procardia XL • 30–180 mg/day Nisoldipine • Sular • ER: 10–40 mg/day • Geomatrix: 17–34 mg/day	None	• Reflex tachycardia • Headache • Flushing • Peripheral edema • Gingival hyperplasia • HF exacerbation (except amlodipine and felodipine)	• BP • HR • S/S of HF	• Cytochrome P450 (CYP) 3A4 substrates • CYP3A4 inhibitors may ↑ effects • CYP3A4 inducers may ↓ effects	• Sublingual nifedipine should not be used → may ↑ risk of MI, death • Do not use grapefruit juice • Nicardipine also available as injection
Non-DHPs:					
Diltiazem ☆ • Cardizem, Cardizem CD, Cardizem LA, Cartia XT, Taztia XT, Tiazac • 120–540 mg/day Verapamil ☆ • Calan, Calan SR, Isoptin SR, Verelan, Verelan PM • 120–360 mg/day (IR given 2–3 × daily, sustained-release [SR] given 1–2 × daily)	• ≥2nd degree heart block (in absence of pacemaker) • HFrEF	• Bradycardia/heart block • Constipation • Peripheral edema • Gingival hyperplasia • HF exacerbation	Same as for DHPs	• CYP3A4 substrates and inhibitors • CYP3A4 inhibitors may ↑ effects • CYP3A4 inducers may ↓ effects • May ↑ effect/toxicity of CYP3A4 substrates • Use with other negative chronotropes (e.g., digoxin, β-blockers, clonidine, or ivabradine) may ↑ risk of bradycardia • May ↑ risk of digoxin toxicity	• Do not use grapefruit juice • Verapamil and diltiazem also available as injection

α_1-Receptor Antagonists

Generic • Brand • Dose	Contra-indications	Primary Side Effects	Key Monitoring	Pertinent Drug Interactions	Med Pearl
Mechanism of action – block the α_1 receptor on peripheral blood vessels → arterial and venous vasodilation					
Doxazosin☆ • Cardura • 1–16 mg/day Prazosin • Minipress • 1–20 mg/day Terazosin☆ • Only available generically • 1–20 mg/day	Should not be used with phosphodiesterase (PDE)-5 inhibitors (e.g., avanafil, sildenafil, tadalafil, vardenafil) → ↑ risk of hypotension	• Orthostatic hypotension • Reflex tachycardia • Peripheral edema • Headache • Drowsiness • Priapism	• BP • HR	↑ risk of hypotension with PDE-5 inhibitors (avoid concurrent use)	• Take dose at bedtime to minimize risk of orthostatic hypotension • ALLHAT trial → 25% ↑ in cardiovascular events with doxazosin • ↑ risk of intraoperative floppy iris syndrome in patients undergoing cataract surgery • Also used for benign prostatic hyperplasia

Central α_2-Receptor Agonists

Generic • Brand • Dose	Contra-indications	Primary Side Effects	Key Monitoring	Pertinent Drug Interactions	Med Pearl
Mechanism of action – stimulate α_2 receptors in brain → ↓ sympathetic outflow (release of norepinephrine) → ↓ BP and HR					
Clonidine☆ • Catapres, Catapres-TTS • Oral: 0.2–2.4 mg/day • Transdermal: 0.1–0.3 mg weekly Methyldopa • Only available generically • 250–1,000 mg/day	Methyldopa: Liver disease	• Sedation • Orthostatic hypotension • Depression • Peripheral edema • Dry mouth • Bradycardia • Hepatitis (methyldopa)	• BP • HR • Liver function tests (LFTs) (methyldopa)	Use with other negative chronotropes (e.g., digoxin, verapamil, diltiazem, β-blockers, or ivabradine) may ↑ risk of bradycardia	• Clonidine patch should be applied once weekly • Abrupt discontinuation (especially in presence of β-blockers) may cause angina, MI, or hypertensive emergency; need to taper over 2 wk • When starting clonidine patch, overlap with oral for 2–3 days, then discontinue oral • Should not be used as first-line therapy • Clonidine also available as epidural injection (for pain) • Clonidine also used to treat attention-deficit/hyperactivity disorder • Methyldopa also available as injection • Methyldopa safe to use in pregnant women with HTN

Direct Vasodilators

Generic • Brand • Dose	Contra-indications	Primary Side Effects	Key Monitoring	Pertinent Drug Interactions	Med Pearl
Mechanism of action – ↑ cyclic GMP → arterial vasodilation					
Hydralazine • Only available generically • 25–300 mg/day Minoxidil • Only available generically • 2.5–100 mg/day	• Acute MI • Aortic dissection	• Reflex tachycardia • Orthostatic hypotension • Peripheral edema • Lupus-like syndrome (hydralazine) • Hirsutism (minoxidil)	• BP • HR • S/S of lupus (e.g., stabbing chest pain, joint pain, fever, rash)	None	• Should not be used as first-line therapy • Minoxidil is usually absolutely last-line therapy (because of side effects) • Hydralazine also available as injection • Minoxidil also available as topical solution/foam to stimulate hair growth

DYSLIPIDEMIA

Guidelines Summary

- Achievement of specific LDL-C goals is *no longer* recommended in the most recent dyslipidemia guidelines.
- Four groups most likely to benefit from statin therapy are:
  - Clinical ASCVD (secondary prevention)
  - LDL-C ≥190 mg/dL (primary prevention)
  - Age 40–75 yr with DM **AND** LDL-C 70–189 mg/dL (primary prevention)
  - Age 40–75 yr without clinical ASCVD or DM, and with LDL-C 70–189 mg/dL and 10-yr ASCVD risk ≥7.5%
- Heart-healthy lifestyle habits should be encouraged for all patients.
- Pharmacologic therapy:
  - Statin therapy recommendations for four major benefit groups:

Major Benefit Groups	Statin Therapy Recommendations
Clinical ASCVD	• Age ≤75 yr → High-intensity statin therapy • Age >75 yr **OR** if not a candidate for high-intensity statin therapy → Moderate-intensity statin therapy
LDL-C ≥190 mg/dL	High-intensity statin therapy (moderate-intensity if not candidate for high-intensity therapy)
Age 40–75 yr with DM **AND** LDL-C 70–189 mg/dL	• 10-yr ASCVD risk <7.5% → Moderate-intensity statin therapy • 10-yr ASCVD risk ≥7.5% → High-intensity statin therapy
Age 40–75 yr without clinical ASCVD or DM, and with LDL-C 70–189 mg/dL and 10-yr ASCVD risk ≥7.5%	Moderate–high intensity statin therapy

- High-intensity versus moderate-intensity statin therapy
  - » High-intensity: ↓ LDL-C by ≥50%
    - Atorvastatin 40–80 mg daily
    - Rosuvastatin 20–40 mg daily
  - » Moderate-intensity: ↓ LDL-C by 30–<50%
    - Atorvastatin 10–20 mg daily
    - Rosuvastatin 5–10 mg daily
    - Simvastatin 20–40 mg daily
    - Pravastatin 40–80 mg daily
    - Lovastatin 40 mg daily
    - Fluvastatin XL 80 mg daily
    - Fluvastatin 40 mg twice daily
    - Pitavastatin 2–4 mg daily
- Nonstatin therapy can be considered in selected high-risk patients (clinical ASCVD, LDL-C ≥190 mg/dL, or age 40–75 yr with DM and LDL-C 70–189 mg/dL) who are/have:
  - » Less than anticipated response to statin therapy
  - » Unable to tolerate a less than recommended intensity of statin therapy
  - » Completely intolerant to statin therapy

Lipid-Lowering Effects of Various Drug Classes

Drug Class	Effect on LDL-C	Effect on HDL-C	Effect on TGs
Bile acid resins	↓ 15–30%	↑ 3–5%	↑ 1–10%
Niacin	↓ 5–25%	↑ 15–35%	↓ 20–50%
Fibric acid derivatives	↓/↑ 5–20%	↑ 10–20%	↓ 20–50%
Statins	↓ 18–55%	↑ 5–15%	↓ 7–30%
Cholesterol absorption inhibitors	↓ 15–20%	↑ 1%	↓ 8%
PCSK9 inhibitors	↓ 40–75%	↑ 4–9%	↓ 2–16%

Bile Acid Resins

Generic • Brand • Dose	Contra-indications	Primary Side Effects	Key Monitoring	Pertinent Drug Interactions	Med Pearl
Mechanism of action – bind bile acids in intestines, forming insoluble complex that is excreted in feces → ↓ in bile acids causes liver to convert cholesterol into bile acids, which then ↓ cholesterol stores → ↑ demand for cholesterol in liver → upregulation of LDL receptors → ↑ LDL-C clearance from bloodstream					
Cholestyramine • Prevalite • 4–24 g/day Colesevelam☆ • Welchol • 3.75 g/day Colestipol • Colestid • Granules: 5–30 g/day • Tablets: 2–16 g/day	Complete biliary obstruction	• Constipation • Bloating • Abdominal pain • Nausea/vomiting (N/V) • Flatulence • ↑ TGs	Lipid panel	Bind to and ↓ absorption of many drugs (e.g., warfarin, digoxin, thiazides, levothyroxine, mycophenolate)	• Used to ↓ LDL-C • Can be used in patients with liver disease • Do not use in patients with ↑ TGs • Colesevelam has fewer gastrointestinal (GI) side effects and drug interactions

Niacin

Generic • Brand • Dose	Contra- indications	Primary Side Effects	Key Monitoring	Pertinent Drug Interactions	Med Pearl
Mechanism of action – ↓ production of very low density lipoproteins (VLDL) in liver → ↓ synthesis of LDL-C					
Niacin☆ • Niaspan; also available as over-the-counter (OTC) product • 500–3,000 mg/day	• Hepatic impairment • Active gout • Active peptic ulcer disease	• Flushing/itching • Nausea • Orthostatic hypotension • ↑ LFTs • Myopathy • Hyperuricemia • Hyperglycemia	• Lipid panel • LFTs • Creatine kinase (CK) (if muscle aches) • Uric acid • Blood glucose (if patient has DM)	None significant	• Used to ↓ LDL-C, ↓ TGs, and ↑ HDL-C • Most effective drug for ↑ HDL-C • Do not ↑ dose by >500 mg in 4 wk period • Avoid use of OTC SR products (↑ risk of hepatotoxicity)

Fibric Acid Derivatives

Generic • Brand • Dose	Contra- indications	Primary Side Effects	Key Monitoring	Pertinent Drug Interactions	Med Pearl
Mechanism of action – ↑ activity of lipoprotein lipase → ↑ catabolism of VLDL → ↓ TGs					
Fenofibrate/fenofibric acid☆ • Antara, Fenoglide, Fibricor, Lipofen, Tricor, Triglide, Trilipix • 30–200 mg/day (depending on brand) Gemfibrozil☆ • Lopid • 1,200 mg/day	• Hepatic impairment • Severe renal impairment • Gallbladder disease • Concurrent use with statins, repaglinide, or dasabuvir (gemfibrozil)	• Nausea/vomiting/diarrhea (N/V/D) • Abdominal pain • ↑ LFTs • Myopathy	• Lipid panel • LFTs • CK (if muscle aches)	• Gemfibrozil is CYP2C8 inhibitor • Avoid using gemfibrozil with statins (↑ risk of myopathy), repaglinide (↑ risk of hypoglycemia), and dasabuvir (↑ risk of QT interval prolongation) • ↑ effects of warfarin and sulfonylureas • ↓ cyclosporine levels	• Used to ↓ TGs and/or ↑ HDL-C • Fenofibrate preferred with statins • Adjust dose in renal impairment

Omega-3 Fatty Acids (Fish Oil)

Generic • Brand • Dose	Contra-indications	Primary Side Effects	Key Monitoring	Pertinent Drug Interactions	Med Pearl
Mechanism of action – ↓ production of TGs in the liver					
Icosapent ethyl • Vascepa • 4 g/day	Fish allergy	Arthralgia	Lipid panel	May ↑ risk of bleeding with antithrombotic agents	• Used to ↓ TGs • Minimal effect on LDL-C • Take with meals
Omega-3-Acid Ethyl Esters☆ • Epanova, Lovaza, Omtryg; also available as OTC product • 2–4 g/day • Omtryg: 4.8 g/day	Fish allergy	• Belching ("fishy taste") • Dyspepsia	Lipid panel	May ↑ risk of bleeding with antithrombotic agents	• Used to ↓ TGs • May ↑ LDL-C • Take Omtryg with meals

HMG-CoA Reductase Inhibitors (Statins)

Generic • Brand • Dose	Contra-indications	Primary Side Effects	Key Monitoring	Pertinent Drug Interactions	Med Pearl
Mechanism of action – inhibit HMG-CoA reductase → prevent the conversion of HMG-CoA to mevalonate (rate-limiting step in cholesterol synthesis)					
Atorvastatin☆ • Lipitor • 10–80 mg/day Fluvastatin • Lescol, Lescol XL • 20–80 mg/day Lovastatin☆ • Altoprev • 20–80 mg/day Pitavastatin • Livalo • 1–4 mg/day Pravastatin☆ • Pravachol • 10–80 mg/day Rosuvastatin☆ • Crestor • 5–40 mg/day Simvastatin☆ • Zocor • 10–40 mg/day	• Hepatic impairment • Pregnancy • Concomitant use with cyclosporine (pitavastatin and atorvastatin) • Concomitant use with strong CYP3A4 inhibitors (lovastatin) • Concomitant use with strong CYP3A4 inhibitors, cyclosporine, or danazol (simvastatin)	• ↑ LFTs • Myopathy • N/V • Constipation	• Lipid panel • LFTs • CK (if muscle aches)	• Atorvastatin, lovastatin, and simvastatin are CYP3A4 substrates; CYP3A4 inhibitors may ↑ risk of side effects; may ↑ effects of warfarin • Fluvastatin and pitavastatin are CYP2C9 substrates; may ↑ effects of warfarin • Pravastatin not metabolized by CYP enzymes	• Most effective drugs for ↓ LDL-C • Lower maximum dosage of atorvastatin when used with clarithromycin, darunavir/ritonavir, fosamprenavir, fosamprenavir/ritonavir, itraconazole, nelfinavir, or saquinavir/ritonavir • Lower maximum dosage of fluvastatin when used with cyclosporine or fluconazole • Lower maximum dosage of lovastatin when used with amiodarone, dronedarone, verapamil, diltiazem, danazol, or lomitapide • Lower maximum dosage of pitavastatin when used with erythromycin or rifampin • Lower maximum dosage of pravastatin when used with clarithromycin • Lower maximum dosage of rosuvastatin when used with cyclosporine, gemfibrozil, lopinavir/ritonavir, atazanavir/ritonavir, or simeprevir • Lower maximum dosage of simvastatin when used with amiodarone, amlodipine, diltiazem, dronedarone, niacin, ranolazine, verapamil, or lomitapide • Adjust dose of pitavastatin and rosuvastatin in renal impairment
Combination products:		Atorvastatin/amlodipine (Caduet)		Simvastatin/ezetimibe (Vytorin)	

Cholesterol Absorption Inhibitor

Generic • Brand • Dose	Contra- indications	Primary Side Effects	Key Monitoring	Pertinent Drug Interactions	Med Pearl
Mechanism of action – prevents absorption of cholesterol from small intestine					
Ezetimibe ☆ • Zetia • 10 mg/day	None	• Headache • Diarrhea	Lipid panel	• Cyclosporine and fibrates may ↑ effects • ↑ cyclosporine levels • ↑ effects of warfarin	• Used to ↓ LDL-C • Can add to statin to further ↓ LDL-C or if dose-limiting side effects occur with statin

Microsomal Triglyceride Transfer Protein (MTP) Inhibitor

Generic • Brand • Dose	Contra- indications	Primary Side Effects	Key Monitoring	Pertinent Drug Interactions	Med Pearl
Mechanism of action – inhibits MTP and prevents the assembly of apo-B containing lipoproteins, which results in ↓ LDL-C					
Lomitapide • Juxtapid • 5–60 mg/day	• Pregnancy • Concomitant use with moderate or strong CYP3A4 inhibitors • Hepatic impairment	• ↑ LFTs • N/V/D	• Lipid panel • LFTs (monitor before every dose ↑)	• CYP3A4 substrate • CYP3A4 inhibitors may ↑ risk of side effects • May ↑ effects of warfarin • May ↑ risk of side effects with simvastatin and lovastatin (limit statin dose) • May ↑ effect/toxicity of P-glycoprotein (P-gp) substrates	• Used to ↓ LDL-C in patients with homozygous familial hypercholesterolemia • Has REMS program • Lower maximum dosage when used with weak CYP3A4 inhibitor (alprazolam, amiodarone, amlodipine, atorvastatin, bicalutamide, cilostazol, cimetidine, cyclosporine, fluoxetine, fluvoxamine, isoniazid, lapatinib, nilotinib, oral contraceptives, pazopanib, ranitidine, ranolazine, ticagrelor, or zileuton) • Take ≥2 hr after evening meal with glass of water (food ↑ GI side effects) • Take daily vitamin supplement (containing 400 IU vitamin E and ≥200 mg linoleic acid, 210 mg alpha-linoleic acid, 110 mg eicosapentaenoic acid, and 80 mg docosahexaenoic acid)

PCSK9 Inhibitors

Generic • Brand • Dose	Contra-indications	Primary Side Effects	Key Monitoring	Pertinent Drug Interactions	Med Pearl
Mechanism of action – inhibit binding of proprotein convertase subtilisin kexin type 9 (PCSK9) to LDL receptors on the surface of the hepatocyte, which ↑ number of LDL receptors available to clear circulating LDL and lowers LDL-C					
Alirocumab • Praluent • 75–150 mg subcut q2wk	None	• Hypersensitivity reactions • ↑ LFTs • Diarrhea	Lipid panel	None	Used to ↓ LDL-C (by up to 60%)
Evolocumab • Repatha • 140 mg subcut q2wk or 420 mg subcut monthly	None	Hypersensitivity reactions	Lipid panel	None	• Used to ↓ LDL-C (by up to 60%) • To administer 420 mg dose, give 3 consecutive injections within 30 min

HEART FAILURE

Guidelines Summary

The goals of therapy are to relieve symptoms, improve quality of life, improve survival, reduce hospitalizations, and slow the progression of disease.

- Nonpharmacologic therapy: Regular low-intensity physical activity, ↓ Na⁺ (≤3 g/day), ↓ fluid intake (<2 L/day), weight loss (if obese), alcohol restriction, and smoking cessation
- Pharmacologic therapy:
  - Stage A: Modify risk factors and control HTN, DM, CAD, and dyslipidemia; ACEI or ARB in patients with risk factors for vascular disease
  - Stage B: ACEI + β-blocker
  - Stage C: ACEI (or ARB or sacubitril/valsartan) + β-blocker + diuretic
    - » Other drugs to be considered:
      - Sacubitril/valsartan: NYHA class II-III patients who tolerate an ACEI or ARB (to be used in place of ACEI or ARB)
      - ARA: NYHA class II-IV patients who are already receiving ACEI (or ARB) and β-blocker; NYHA class II patients should have history of prior cardiovascular hospitalization or ↑ BNP level to be considered for ARA therapy
      - ARBs: Patients who cannot tolerate an ACEI due to intractable cough or angioedema

- Digoxin: Patients who remain symptomatic despite optimal therapy with ACEI (or ARB), β-blocker, and diuretic

- Hydralazine/isosorbide dinitrate (HDZ/ISDN): Patients with intolerance or contraindications (renal insufficiency, hyperkalemia) to ACEI or ARB; African-American patients with NYHA class III or IV symptoms who remain symptomatic despite optimal therapy with ACEI (or ARB) and β-blocker

- Ivabradine: NYHA class II-III patients with stable HFrEF (LVEF ≤35%) and in sinus rhythm who are receiving a β-blocker at a maximally tolerated dose and having a resting heart rate ≥70 bpm

• Stage D: Chronic positive inotrope therapy (e.g., dobutamine, milrinone), mechanical circulatory support (e.g., LV assist device), heart transplant, end-of-life care/hospice

Chronic HFrEF Treatment Summary

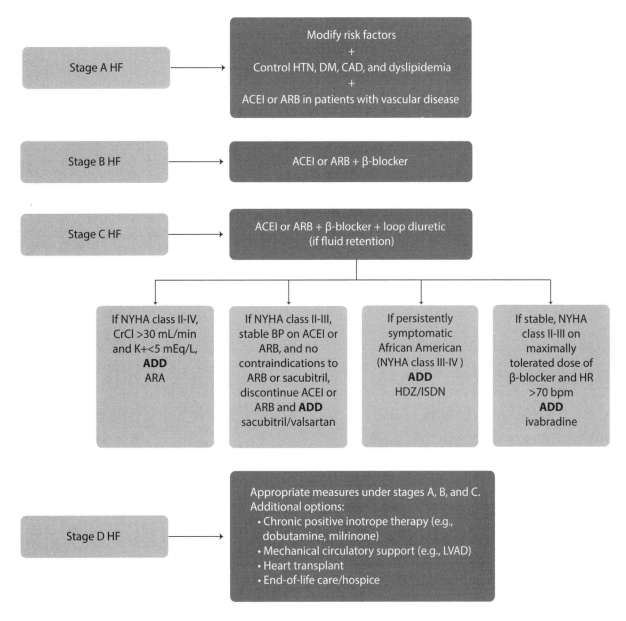

Loop Diuretics

Generic • Brand • Dose	Contra-indications	Primary Side Effects	Key Monitoring	Pertinent Drug Interactions	Med Pearl
Mechanism of action – inhibit Na$^+$ reabsorption in the ascending limb of loop of Henle; ↓ preload					
Bumetanide • Bumex • 0.5–10 mg/day Furosemide☆ • Lasix • 20–600 mg/day Torsemide • Demadex • 10–200 mg/day	Sulfa allergy	• Hypocalcemia • Hypokalemia • Hypomagne-semia • Hyponatremia • Hyperglycemia • Hyperuricemia • Metabolic alkalosis • Azotemia	• BP • Electrolytes • BUN/SCr • Blood glucose • Uric acid • Jugular venous pressure • Urine output • Weight (↓ by 0.5–1 kg/day initially)	• May ↑ risk of lithium toxicity • May ↑ risk of ototoxicity with aminoglycosides • May ↓ effect of antidiabetic agents • NSAIDs ↓ effects	• ↓ symptoms; effect on mortality unknown • Bumetanide and furosemide also available IV • If initial dose inadequate, double dose, dose 2 × daily, add metola-zone, or use IV • Similar side effects as thiazides (except loops cause hypocalce-mia) • BUN/SCr ratio >20:1 → dehydra-tion (prerenal azotemia) • 1 mg bumetanide = 20 mg torse-mide = 40 mg furosemide • Furosemide PO dose = 2 × IV dose • Bumetanide PO dose = IV dose

ACE Inhibitors

- See HTN monograph for further details
- Medication pearls specific to their use in HF:
  - ↓ mortality; ↓ preload and afterload
  - Strive to achieve target dose, if possible (titrate dose to symptoms, not BP)

Drug	Initial Dose	Target Dose
Captopril	6.25 mg TID	50 mg TID
Enalapril	2.5 mg BID	10–20 mg BID
Lisinopril	2.5 mg daily	20–40 mg daily
Ramipril	1.25 mg daily	10 mg daily
Trandolapril	1 mg daily	4 mg daily
Fosinopril	5 mg daily	40 mg daily
Quinapril	5 mg BID	20 mg BID
Perindopril	2 mg daily	8–16 mg daily

β-Blockers

Generic • Brand • Dose	Contra-indications	Primary Side Effects	Key Monitoring	Pertinent Drug Interactions	Med Pearl
Mechanism of action – ↓ activation of the sympathetic nervous system; slow and potentially reverse detrimental effects (e.g., ventricular remodeling) of catecholamines					
Bisoprolol • Zebeta • 1.25–10 mg/day • Target dose: 10 mg daily Carvedilol☆ • Coreg, Coreg CR • IR: 6.25–100 mg/day (in two divided doses) • Target dose: <85 kg = 25 mg BID; >85 kg = 50 mg BID • CR: 10–80 mg/day (1 × daily) • Target dose: 80 mg daily Metoprolol succinate☆ • Toprol XL • 12.5–200 mg/day • Target dose: 200 mg daily	• Symptomatic bradycardia • ≥2nd-degree heart block (in absence of pacemaker) • SBP <85 mmHg • Severe asthma • Decompensated HF	See HTN section	• BP • HR • S/S of HF • Weight	Carvedilol may ↑ digoxin levels	• ↓ mortality • Metoprolol succinate (not tartrate) approved for HF • Patient should be fairly euvolemic before starting • Strive to achieve target dose, if possible • Dose can be doubled every 2–4 wk to achieve target dose (unless side effects) • Manage worsening HF by ↑ diuretic dose • If hypotension occurs, may ↓ dose of ACEI, ARB, or other vasodilator (more common with carvedilol) • If bradycardia occurs, ↓ dose • Abrupt discontinuation may cause worsening HF

Angiotensin II Receptor Blockers

- See HTN monograph for further details
- Medication pearls specific to their use in HF:
  - Only candesartan, losartan, or valsartan recommended for the management of HF (only candesartan and valsartan approved for HF)
  - Should not be considered equivalent or superior to ACEIs

Drug	Initial Dose	Target Dose
Candesartan	4–8 mg daily	32 mg daily
Losartan	25–50 mg daily	25–150 mg daily
Valsartan	20–40 mg BID	160 mg BID

Sacubitril/Valsartan

Generic • Brand • Dose	Contra-indications	Primary Side Effects	Key Monitoring	Pertinent Drug Interactions	Med Pearl
Mechanism of action – sacubitril: prodrug, inhibits neprilysin (neutral endopeptidase) $\rightarrow$ $\uparrow$ levels of peptides (including natriuretic peptides); valsartan: ARB					
Sacubitril/valsartan • Entresto • Sacubitril 49–97 mg/valsartan 51–103 mg BID • New or previously low-dose user of ACEI/ARB: Start with sacubitril 24 mg/valsartan 26 mg BID • Target dose: sacubitril 97 mg/valsartan 103 mg BID	• Pregnancy • History of angioedema with prior ACEI/ARB use • Concurrent use with ACEI • Concurrent use with aliskiren in DM	• Angioedema • Hypotension • Renal impairment • Hyperkalemia	• BP • BUN/SCr • K^+	• Use with K^+ supplements, K^+-sparing diuretics, ARAs, or NSAIDs may $\uparrow$ risk of hyperkalemia • Use with ACEI $\uparrow$ risk of angioedema (contraindicated) • Use with aliskiren may $\uparrow$ risk of hyperkalemia and renal impairment (avoid concurrent use in DM and CrCl <60 mL/min) • May $\uparrow$ risk of lithium toxicity	• $\downarrow$ cardiovascular death and hospitalizations • Do not give within 36 hr of change from/to ACEI • Double dose every 2–4 wk to achieve target dose (unless side effects) • Adjust dose in renal or hepatic impairment

Digoxin

Generic • Brand • Dose	Contra-indications	Primary Side Effects	Key Monitoring	Pertinent Drug Interactions	Med Pearl
Mechanism of action – inhibits Na^+/K^+ ATPase pump $\rightarrow$ $\uparrow$ intracellular Ca^{2+} $\rightarrow$ $\uparrow$ myocardial contractility; also $\downarrow$ neurohormonal activation					
Digoxin ☆ • Lanoxin • 0.125–0.25 mg/day (loading doses not necessary in HF)	≥2nd-degree heart block (in absence of pacemaker)	• Bradycardia/heart block • S/S of digoxin toxicity (visual disturbances, N/V, confusion, anorexia, arrhythmias)	• HR • Electrolytes (predisposed to toxicity if hypokalemia, hypomagnesemia, or hypercalcemia) • BUN/SCr • Digoxin concentrations	• P-gp substrate • Amiodarone, dronedarone, quinidine, verapamil, clarithromycin, lapatinib, propafenone, and ritonavir may $\uparrow$ levels • Antacids may $\downarrow$ levels (separate by 1–2 hours) • Use with other negative chronotropes (e.g., β-blockers, verapamil, diltiazem, clonidine, or ivabradine) may $\uparrow$ risk of bradycardia	• Improves symptoms, $\downarrow$ hospitalizations; no effect on mortality • Used to $\uparrow$ contractility in HFrEF and to $\downarrow$ HR in atrial fibrillation (AF) • Abrupt discontinuation may cause worsening HF • $\downarrow$ dose by 50% when starting amiodarone or dronedarone • Adjust dose renal impairment • Target level: 0.5–0.9 ng/mL ($\uparrow$ mortality if >0.9 ng/mL)

Aldosterone Receptor Antagonists

Generic • Brand • Dose	Contra-indications	Primary Side Effects	Key Monitoring	Pertinent Drug Interactions	Med Pearl
Mechanism of action – inhibit the effects of aldosterone → ↓ remodeling and Na⁺/water retention • Spironolactone is nonselective ARA (also blocks androgen and progesterone receptors → associated with endocrine side effects) • Eplerenone is selective ARA (not associated with endocrinologic side effects)					
Eplerenone • Inspra • 25–50 mg/day Spironolactone • Aldactone • 12.5–25 mg/day	• K⁺ >5 mEq/L • SCr >2.5 mg/dL (men) or >2 mg/dL (women) (or CrCl ≤30 mL/min) • Concomitant ACEI **and** ARB use • Concurrent use of eplerenone with strong CYP3A4 inhibitors (e.g., ritonavir, ketoconazole, itraconazole, nefazodone, clarithromycin, nelfinavir)	• Hyperkalemia • Also for spironolactone: Gynecomastia, breast tenderness, menstrual changes, hirsutism	• BP • K⁺ • BUN/SCr	• Eplerenone is CYP3A4 substrate • CYP3A4 inhibitors may ↑ effects • Use with ACEIs, ARBs, K⁺ supplements, or NSAIDs may ↑ risk of hyperkalemia	• ↓ mortality • Should consider discontinuing or ↓ dose of K⁺ supplements • Eplerenone tends to be used in patients who develop endocrine side effects (e.g., gynecomastia) with spironolactone • Lower maximum dosage of eplerenone when used with erythromycin, saquinavir, verapamil, or fluconazole

Hydralazine/Isosorbide Dinitrate

Generic • Brand • Dose	Contra-indications	Primary Side Effects	Key Monitoring	Pertinent Drug Interactions	Med Pearl
Mechanism of action: • Hydralazine – causes arterial vasodilation (↓ afterload) • Isosorbide dinitrate – causes venous vasodilation (↓ preload)					
Hydralazine • Only available generically • 40–300 mg/day	None	• Headache • Dizziness • Reflex tachycardia • Peripheral edema (hydralazine) • Lupus-like syndrome (hydralazine)	• BP • HR	None	• ↓ mortality (when used together) • Combination often used in patients who cannot tolerate ACEIs or ARBs due to renal impairment, hyperkalemia, or angioedema • Do not use hydralazine alone (↑ mortality)
Isosorbide dinitrate ☆ • Isordil • 30–120 mg/day	None				
Combination product: Hydralazine/isosorbide dinitrate (BiDil) – approved for African-American patients with NYHA class III or IV HF due to LV systolic dysfunction (LVEF ≤40%) who are receiving an ACEI (or ARB) and a β-blocker (can also use individual products together if there are financial concerns)					

I$_f$ Channel Inhibitor

Generic • Brand • Dose	Contra-indications	Primary Side Effects	Key Monitoring	Pertinent Drug Interactions	Med Pearl
Mechanism of action – blocks hyperpolarization-activated cyclic nucleotide-gated channel responsible for cardiac pacemaker I$_f$ current in sinoatrial node, resulting in ↓ in HR					
Ivabradine • Corlanor • 2.5–7.5 mg BID	• ADHF • BP <90/50 mmHg • Sick sinus syndrome or 3rd-degree heart block (in absence of pacemaker) • HR <60 bpm (at baseline) • Severe hepatic impairment • Pacemaker dependence • Concurrent use of strong CYP3A4 inhibitors	• Bradycardia • Heart block • AF • Phosphenes	• HR • Electrocardiogram (ECG)	• CYP3A4 substrate • CYP3A4 inhibitors may ↑ effects • CYP3A4 inducers may ↓ effects (avoid use) • Use with other negative chronotropes (e.g., β-blockers, verapamil, diltiazem, digoxin, or clonidine) may ↑ risk of bradycardia	• ↓ hospitalizations; no effect on mortality • Titrate dose by 2.5 mg BID to achieve target resting HR of 50–60 bpm

Intravenous Drugs for Treatment of ADHF

Drug	Mechanism of Action	Primary Side Effects	Med Pearl
Vasodilators			
Nitroglycerin (NTG)	• Venous vasodilation → ↓ preload • Can cause arterial vasodilation at higher doses	• Hypotension • Tachycardia • Headache • Tolerance	• Especially useful in patients with myocardial ischemia • Tolerance can develop (overcome by ↑ infusion rate)
Nitroprusside	Arterial and venous vasodilation → ↓ preload and afterload	• Hypotension • N/V • Cyanide/thiocyanate toxicity (risk ↑ if infusion >24 hours)	Avoid in patients with renal impairment
Nesiritide (Natrecor)	• BNP • Arterial and venous vasodilation → ↓ preload and afterload	• Hypotension • Headache	Infusion should not be titrated more frequently than every 3 hours

Intravenous Drugs for Treatment of ADHF *(cont'd)*

Drug	Mechanism of Action	Primary Side Effects	Med Pearl
Positive Inotropes			
Dopamine	• 0.5–3 mcg/kg/min → Stimulates dopamine receptors → ↑ urine output • 3–10 mcg/kg/min → Stimulates β_1 receptors → ↑ CO, ↑ HR • >10 mcg/kg/min → Stimulates α_1 receptors → ↑ BP	• Arrhythmias • Tachycardia • Myocardial ischemia • N/V	Avoid in patients with myocardial ischemia
Dobutamine	β_1 and β_2 receptor agonist and weak α_1 receptor agonist → ↑ CO and vasodilation	• Arrhythmias • Tachycardia • Myocardial ischemia • Hypokalemia • Tremor	• Avoid in patients with myocardial ischemia • Should not be used in patients receiving chronic β-blocker therapy • Tolerance can develop
Milrinone	PDE III inhibitor → ↑ CO and vasodilation	• Hypotension • Arrhythmias	• Can be used in patients receiving chronic β-blocker therapy, or in those not responding to or tolerating dobutamine • Tolerance does not develop • Use lower initial dose in patients with renal impairment

ANTIARRHYTHMIC DRUGS

Class IA

Generic • Brand • Dose	Contra-indications	Primary Side Effects	Key Monitoring	Pertinent Drug Interactions	Med Pearl
Mechanism of action – Na$^+$ channel blockers; slow conduction velocity, prolong refractoriness, ↓ automaticity					
Disopyramide • Norpace, Norpace CR • 400–1,600 mg/day	• HF • ≥2nd-degree heart block (in absence of pacemaker) • Long QT syndrome	• Dry mouth • Urinary retention • Blurred vision • Constipation • HF exacerbation • Hypotension • Torsade de pointes (TdP)	• ECG (QTc interval, QRS duration) • BP • S/S of HF • Electrolytes • Disopyramide concentrations	• CYP3A4 substrate • CYP3A4 inhibitors and anticholinergics may ↑ risk of side effects • CYP3A4 inducers may ↓ effects • ↑ risk of TdP with other drugs that prolong QT interval	• Used for atrial and ventricular arrhythmias • Therapeutic range: 2–5 mcg/mL • Adjust dose in renal impairment
Procainamide • Only available generically • IV: • *Loading dose:* 15–17 mg/kg over 25–60 min • *Maintenance dose:* 1–4 mg/min continuous infusion	• ≥2nd-degree heart block (in absence of pacemaker) • Long QT syndrome	• Lupus-like syndrome • TdP • Hypotension • Agranulocytosis	• ECG (QTc interval, QRS duration) • BP • S/S of lupus (e.g., stabbing chest pain, joint pain, rash) • Procainamide/N-acetylprocainamide (NAPA) concentrations • Complete blood count (CBC) with differential • Electrolytes	↑ risk of TdP with other drugs that prolong QT interval	• Used for atrial and ventricular arrhythmias • Therapeutic range: 4–10 mcg/mL (procainamide); 15–25 mcg/mL (NAPA); 10–30 mcg/mL (total) • Use with caution, if at all, in renal impairment
Quinidine • Only available generically • Sulfate: 800–2,400 mg/day • Gluconate: 648–2,916 mg/day	• ≥2nd-degree heart block (in absence of pacemaker) • Long QT syndrome • Concurrent use of ritonavir	• Diarrhea • Stomach cramps • TdP • Hypotension • Cinchonism (tinnitus, blurred vision, headache) • Thrombocytopenia	• ECG (QTc interval, QRS duration) • BP • Quinidine concentrations • CBC with differential • LFTs • Electrolytes	• CYP3A4 substrate and CYP2D6 inhibitor • CYP3A4 inhibitors may ↑ risk of side effects • CYP3A4 inducers may ↓ effects • May ↑ toxicity of CYP2D6 substrates • ↑ risk of digoxin toxicity • ↑ risk of TdP with other drugs that prolong QT interval	• Used for atrial and ventricular arrhythmias • Therapeutic range: 2–5 mcg/mL • Administer with food to minimize GI effects

- Avoid all Class IA antiarrhythmics in patients with structural heart disease (i.e., HF, CAD, left ventricular hypertrophy, valvular disease)

Class IB

Generic • Brand • Dose	Contra-indications	Primary Side Effects	Key Monitoring	Pertinent Drug Interactions	Med Pearl
Mechanism of action – Na⁺ channel blockers; little effect on conduction velocity, shorten refractoriness, ↓ automaticity					

Lidocaine
• Xylocaine
• IV:
  • *Loading dose:* 1–1.5 mg/kg, up to 3 mg/kg (total)
  • *Maintenance dose:* 1–4 mg/min
	≥2nd-degree heart block (in absence of pacemaker)	CNS toxicity (dizziness, blurred vision, slurred speech, confusion, paresthesias, seizures)	• ECG (QRS duration)
			• BP
			• Neurologic exam
			• Lidocaine concentrations (if duration of therapy >24 hours)
				Amiodarone may ↑ risk of toxicity	• Used only for ventricular arrhythmias
					• Therapeutic range: 1.5–5 mcg/mL
					• Use lower infusion rate in elderly, HF or hepatic impairment

Mexiletine • Only available generically • 600–1,200 mg/day	Same as for lidocaine	• CNS toxicity (same as lidocaine) • N/V	• ECG (QRS duration) • BP • LFTs • Neurologic exam	• CYP1A2 and CYP2D6 substrate • ↑ risk of theophylline toxicity • CYP1A2 and CYP2D6 inhibitors may ↑ risk of toxicity	• Used only for ventricular arrhythmias • Take with food to minimize GI effects • ↓ dose in HF or hepatic impairment

- Class IB antiarrhythmics do not cause TdP

Class IC

Generic • Brand • Dose	Contra-indications	Primary Side Effects	Key Monitoring	Pertinent Drug Interactions	Med Pearl
Mechanism of action – Na$^+$ channel blockers (most potent); markedly slow conduction velocity, no effect on refractoriness, ↓ automaticity; propafenone also has nonselective β-blocking properties					
Flecainide • Only available generically • *Loading dose (for AF conversion):* 200–300 mg × 1 dose • *Maintenance dose:* 100–400 mg/day	• ≥2nd-degree heart block (in absence of pacemaker) • History of MI • HF	• Dizziness • Tremor • HF exacerbation • Ventricular tachycardia (VT)	• ECG (QRS duration) • Echocardiogram (at baseline to evaluate LV function) • Electrolytes	↑ risk of digoxin toxicity	• Used for atrial and ventricular arrhythmias • Adjust dose in renal impairment

Propafenone
• Rythmol, Rythmol SR
• IR:
  • *Loading dose (for AF conversion):* 450–600 mg × 1
  • *Maintenance dose:* 450–900 mg/day (in 3 divided doses)
• SR:
  • *Maintenance dose:* 450–950 mg/day (in 2 divided doses)
	• ≥2nd-degree heart block (in absence of pacemaker)
	• Bradycardia
	• Bronchospastic disorders
	• HF
	• History of MI
		• Bradycardia/heart block
		• HF exacerbation
		• Bronchospasm
		• Taste disturbances
		• VT
			• ECG (QRS duration, PR interval)
			• BP
			• HR
			• Echocardiogram (at baseline to evaluate LV function)
			• Electrolytes
				• ↑ risk of digoxin toxicity
				• ↑ effects of warfarin
				• Use with other negative chronotropes (e.g., β-blockers, digoxin, verapamil, diltiazem, clonidine, or ivabradine) may ↑ risk of bradycardia
					Used for atrial and ventricular arrhythmias

- Avoid Class IC antiarrhythmics in patients with structural heart disease
- Class IC antiarrhythmics do not cause TdP

Class II

(See medication chart in HTN section for discussion on β-blockers)

Class III

Generic • Brand • Dose	Contra-indications	Primary Side Effects	Key Monitoring	Pertinent Drug Interactions	Med Pearl
Mechanism of action – K⁺ channel blockers; no effect on conduction velocity or automaticity; amiodarone and dronedarone also have Na⁺-channel blocking, β-blocking, and CCB properties; sotalol also has nonselective β-blocking properties					

Amiodarone☆
• Cordarone, Nexterone, Pacerone
• Loading dose (IV):
  • *Stable VT:* 150 mg over 10 min
  • *Pulseless VT/ventricular fibrillation:* 300 mg IV push
  • *AF:* 5 mg/kg over 30–60 min
• Loading dose (PO):
  • *Ventricular arrhythmias:* 1,200–1,600 mg/day (in 2–3 divided doses)
  • *Atrial arrhythmias:* 800–1,200 mg/day (in 2–3 divided doses) until 10 g total
• Maintenance dose:
  • IV: 1 mg/min × 6 hr, then 0.5 mg/min
  • PO: 100–400 mg/day
	≥2nd-degree heart block (in absence of pacemaker)	IV:
		• Hypotension
		• Bradycardia/heart block
		• Phlebitis
		PO:
		• Hypo-/hyperthyroidism
		• Pulmonary fibrosis
		• Bradycardia/heart block
		• Corneal microdeposits
		• Optic neuritis
		• N/V
		• ↑ LFTs
		• Ataxia
		• Paresthesias
		• Photosensitivity
		• Blue-gray skin discoloration
			• ECG (QTc interval, QRS duration, PR interval)
			• BP
			• HR
			• Chest x-ray (baseline; then every 12 months)
			• Pulmonary function tests (baseline; then if symptoms develop)
			• High-resolution chest CT scan (if symptoms develop)
			• Thyroid function tests (TFTs) (baseline; then every 6 months)
			• LFTs (baseline; then every 6 months)
			• Ophthalmologic exam (baseline if visual impairment present; then if symptoms develop)
				• CYP2C8 and CYP3A4 substrate
				• CYP1A2, CYP2C9, CYP2D6, and CYP3A4 inhibitor
				• CYP3A4 inhibitors may ↑ risk of side effects
				• CYP3A4 inducers may ↓ effects
				• ↑ risk of digoxin toxicity (↓ digoxin dose by 50%)
				• ↑ effects of warfarin (↓ warfarin dose by 30%)
				• Use with other negative chronotropes (e.g. β-blockers, digoxin, verapamil, diltiazem, clonidine, or ivabradine) or sofosbuvir-containing regimens may ↑ risk of bradycardia
				• May ↑ cyclosporine or phenytoin levels
				• May ↑ risk of side effects of simvastatin and lovastatin
					• Used for atrial and ventricular arrhythmias
					• Safe to use in HF
					• Half-life = 40–60 days
					• If pulmonary fibrosis or blurred vision occur, discontinue therapy
					• If TFTs abnormal, treat thyroid disorder
					• If ↑ LFTs occur, ↓ amiodarone dose or discontinue therapy if LFTs >2x upper limit of normal
					• Take with food to minimize GI effects
					• Advise patients to wear sunscreen

Class III *(cont'd)*

Generic • Brand • Dose	Contra-indications	Primary Side Effects	Key Monitoring	Pertinent Drug Interactions	Med Pearl
Dronedarone • Multaq • 400 mg BID with meals	• Permanent AF • NYHA class IV HF or NYHA class II–III HF with recent decompensation requiring hospitalization or referral to specialized HF clinic • ≥2nd-degree heart block (in absence of pacemaker) • Bradycardia • Concurrent use of strong CYP3A4 inhibitors or strong CYP3A4 inducers • Concurrent use of other drugs that prolong QT interval • QTc interval ≥500 msec • PR interval >280 msec • Severe hepatic impairment • Liver or lung toxicity related to previous amiodarone use • Pregnancy	• N/V/D • ↑ SCr/acute renal failure • Bradycardia • ↑ LFTs • New-onset or worsening HF	• ECG (QTc interval, PR interval) • HR • BUN/SCr • S/S of HF • LFTs	• CYP3A4 substrate • CYP2D6 and CYP3A4 inhibitor • May ↑ toxicity of CYP2D6 and CYP3A4 substrates • CYP3A4 inhibitors may ↑ risk of side effects • CYP3A4 inducers may ↓ effects • ↑ risk of digoxin toxicity (↓ digoxin dose by 50% or consider discontinuing) • Use with other negative chronotropes (e.g., β-blockers, digoxin, verapamil, diltiazem, clonidine, or ivabradine) may ↑ risk of bradycardia • ↑ effects of dabigatran (↓ dose of dabigatran to 75 mg BID if CrCl 30–50 mL/min) • May ↑ risk of side effects of simvastatin and lovastatin	• Used only for atrial arrhythmias • Structurally related to amiodarone (does not have iodine component); less likely to cause thyroid toxicity; also has shorter half-life
Dofetilide • Tikosyn • 500 mcg BID	• CrCl <20 mL/min • QTc interval >440 msec • Hypokalemia/hypomagnesemia • Concurrent use of verapamil, ketoconazole, cimetidine, trimethoprim, prochlorperazine, hydrochlorothiazide, dolutegravir, megestrol, or other drugs that prolong QT interval	TdP	• ECG (QTc interval) • SCr • Electrolytes	↑ risk of TdP with other drugs that prolong QT interval	• Used only for atrial arrhythmias • Adjust dose based on renal function and QT interval • Must be initiated in hospital • Safe to use in HF

Class III *(cont'd)*

Generic • Brand • Dose	Contra-indications	Primary Side Effects	Key Monitoring	Pertinent Drug Interactions	Med Pearl
Ibutilide • Corvert • IV: 1 mg over 10 min; repeat × 1, if needed	• QTc interval >440 msec • Hypokalemia/hypomagnesemia • Concurrent use of other drugs that prolong QT interval	TdP	• ECG (QTc interval) • Electrolytes	↑ risk of TdP with other drugs that prolong QT interval	Used only for atrial arrhythmias
Sotalol • Betapace, Betapace AF, Sorine, Sotylize • PO: 160–640 mg/day (in 2 divided doses)	• ≥2nd-degree heart block (in absence of pacemaker) • Concurrent use of other drugs that prolong QT interval • CrCl <40 mL/min (for AF) • Long QT syndrome • HF	• TdP • Bradycardia/heart block • Bronchospasm • HF exacerbation	• ECG (QTc interval, PR interval) • HR • SCr • Electrolytes	• ↑ risk of TdP with other drugs that prolong QT interval • Use with other negative chronotropes (e.g., β-blockers, digoxin, verapamil, diltiazem, clonidine, or iv-abradine) may ↑ risk of bradycardia	• Used for atrial and ventricular arrhythmias • Adjust dosing interval in renal impairment • Also available as oral solution and injection

Class IV Antiarrhythmics

(See medication chart in HTN section for discussion on non-DHP CCBs)

ANTITHROMBOTIC DRUGS

Vitamin K Antagonist

Generic • Brand • Dose	Contra-indications	Primary Side Effects	Key Monitoring	Pertinent Drug Interactions	Med Pearl
Mechanism of action – interferes with synthesis of vitamin-K dependent clotting factors of the liver (II, VII, IX, and X) as well as protein C and S					
Warfarin • Coumadin, Jantoven • Usual initial dose: 5–10 mg daily (2.5–10 mg daily in older adults)	• Pregnancy • Recent surgery	• Bleeding • Skin necrosis (especially in patients with protein C deficiency) • Purple toe syndrome	• Prothrombin time (PT)/international normalized ratio (INR) • Hemoglobin (Hgb)/hematocrit (Hct) • Bleeding	• CYP2C9 and CYP3A4 substrate • CYP2C9 and CYP3A4 inhibitors may ↑ effects and risk of bleeding • CYP3A4 inducers may ↓ effects and ↑ risk of clotting	• Vitamin K is antidote (PO preferred) • Full effect of a particular dose not seen for 3–4 days

Direct Thrombin Inhibitor

Generic • Brand • Dose	Contra-indications	Primary Side Effects	Key Monitoring	Pertinent Drug Interactions	Med Pearl
Mechanism of action – oral direct thrombin inhibitor					

Dabigatran
• Pradaxa
• AF:
  • CrCl >30 mL/min: 150 mg BID
  • CrCl 15–30 mL/min: 75 mg BID
  • CrCl <15 mL/min: Not recommended
• Treatment of deep venous thrombosis (DVT)/pulmonary embolism (PE):
  • CrCl >30 mL/min: 150 mg BID (after 5–10 days of parenteral anticoagulation)
  • CrCl ≤30 mL/min: No dosing recommendations
• Prevention of recurrent DVT/PE:
  • CrCl >30 mL/min: 150 mg BID
  • CrCl ≤30 mL/min: No dosing recommendations
• Prevention of DVT/PE after hip replacement surgery:
  • CrCl >30 mL/min: 110 mg 1–4 hr after surgery, then 220 mg daily × 28–35 days
  • CrCl ≤30 mL/min: No dosing recommendations
	• Active bleeding
	• Mechanical prosthetic heart valve
		• Bleeding
		• Dyspepsia
			• Hgb/Hct
			• Bleeding
				• P-gp substrate
				• P-gp inhibitors may ↑ effects and risk of bleeding
				• Rifampin ↓ effects and ↑ risk of clotting (avoid concurrent use)
				AF:
				• ↓ dabigatran dose to 75 mg BID when used with dronedarone or ketoconazole if CrCl 30–50 mL/min (avoid concurrent use with P-gp inhibitors if CrCl <30 mL/min)
				DVT/PE treatment/prevention (including after hip replacement surgery):
				• Avoid concurrent use with P-gp inhibitors if CrCl <50 mL/min
					• When converting from warfarin, discontinue warfarin and start dabigatran when INR <2
					• When converting to warfarin, adjust starting time of warfarin based on CrCl
					• When converting from parenteral anticoagulant, start dabigatran 0–2 hr before time of next dose of or at time of discontinuation of parenteral anticoagulant
					• When converting to parenteral anticoagulant, wait 12–24 hr (based on CrCl) after last dose of dabigatran before starting therapy with parenteral anticoagulant
					• Antidote = idarucizumab (Praxbind); 2.5 g IV; repeat dose in 15 min

Factor Xa Inhibitors

Generic • Brand • Dose	Contra-indications	Primary Side Effects	Key Monitoring	Pertinent Drug Interactions	Med Pearl
Mechanism of action – oral factor Xa inhibitor					

Apixaban
• Eliquis
• AF:
  • 5 mg BID
  • If patient has ≥2 of the following (age ≥80 yr, weight ≤60 kg, SCr ≥1.5 mg/dL): 2.5 mg BID
• Postoperative DVT/PE prophylaxis:
  • 2.5 mg BID (× 35 days for hip replacement; × 12 days for knee replacement)
• Treatment of DVT/PE:
  • 10 mg BID × 7 days, then 5 mg BID
• Prevention of recurrent DVT/PE:
  • 2.5 mg BID after ≥6 mo of treatment for DVT/PE
	Active bleeding	Bleeding	• Hgb/Hct
			• Bleeding
				• CYP3A4 and P-gp substrate
				• CYP3A4 and P-gp inhibitors may ↑ effects and risk of bleeding (if receiving 5 mg BID or 10 mg BID dose, ↓ apixaban dose by 50% when used with strong dual inhibitors of CYP3A4 and P-gp; if receiving 2.5 mg BID dose, avoid concurrent use with strong dual inhibitors of CYP3A4 and P-gp)
				• CYP3A4 and P-gp inducers ↓ effects and ↑ risk of clotting (avoid concurrent use)
					• When converting from warfarin, discontinue warfarin and start apixaban when INR <2
					• When converting to warfarin, discontinue apixaban and start parenteral anticoagulant and warfarin at the time the next dose of apixaban would have been taken; discontinue parenteral anticoagulant when desired INR achieved
					• When converting from parenteral anticoagulant, discontinue parenteral anticoagulant and start apixaban at the usual time of the next dose of parenteral anticoagulant
					• When converting to parenteral anticoagulant, discontinue apixaban and initiate parenteral anticoagulant at time the next dose of apixaban would have been taken
					• No antidote currently available

Factor Xa Inhibitors   *(cont'd)*

Generic • Brand • Dose	Contra-indications	Primary Side Effects	Key Monitoring	Pertinent Drug Interactions	Med Pearl
Edoxaban • Savaysa • AF: 　• CrCl >95 mL/min: Avoid use 　• CrCl 51–95 mL/min: 60 mg daily 　• CrCl 15–50 mL/min: 30 mg daily • Treatment of DVT/PE: 　• CrCl ≥51 mL/min: 60 mg daily (after 5–10 days of parenteral anticoagulation) 　• CrCl 15-50 mL/min or weight ≤60 kg: 30 mg daily (after 5–10 days of parenteral anticoagulation)	Active bleeding	Bleeding	• Hgb/Hct • Bleeding	• P-gp substrate • P-gp inhibitors may ↑ effects and risk of bleeding • Rifampin may ↓ effects and ↑ risk of clotting (avoid concurrent use) Treatment of DVT/PE: • ↓ edoxaban dose to 30 mg daily when used with verapamil, quinidine, azithromycin, clarithromycin, erythromycin, itraconazole, or ketoconazole	• When converting from warfarin, discontinue warfarin and start edoxaban when INR ≤2.5 • When converting to warfarin, ↓ dose of edoxaban (60 mg to 30 mg daily; 30 mg to 15 mg daily) and begin warfarin concurrently; discontinue edoxaban when desired INR achieved; may also discontinue edoxaban and start parenteral anticoagulant and warfarin at the time the next dose of edoxaban would have been taken; discontinue parenteral anticoagulant when desired INR achieved • When converting from low molecular weight heparin (LMWH), start edoxaban at the time of the next dose of LMWH (and discontinue LMWH); for unfractionated heparin (UFH), discontinue infusion and start edoxaban 4 hr later • When converting to parenteral anticoagulant, discontinue edoxaban and initiate parenteral anticoagulant at time the next dose of edoxaban would have been taken • No antidote currently available

Factor Xa Inhibitors   *(cont'd)*

Generic • Brand • Dose	Contra-indications	Primary Side Effects	Key Monitoring	Pertinent Drug Interactions	Med Pearl

Rivaroxaban
• Xarelto
• AF:
  • CrCl >50 mL/min: 20 mg daily with evening meal
  • CrCl 15–50 mL/min: 15 mg daily with evening meal
• Postoperative DVT/PE prophylaxis:
  • 10 mg daily (× 35 days for hip replacement; × 12 days for knee replacement)
• Treatment of DVT/PE:
  • 15 mg BID with food × 21 days, then 20 mg daily with food
• Prevention of recurrent DVT/PE:
  • 20 mg daily with food
	Active bleeding	Bleeding	• Hgb/Hct
			• Bleeding
				• CYP3A4 and P-gp substrate
				• CYP3A4 and P-gp inhibitors may ↑ effects and risk of bleeding (avoid concurrent use with combined P-gp and strong CYP3A4 inhibitors)
				• CYP3A4 and P-gp inducers ↓ effects and ↑ risk of clotting (avoid concurrent use with combined P-gp and strong CYP3A4 inducers)
					• When converting from warfarin, discontinue warfarin and start rivaroxaban when INR <3
					• When converting to warfarin, discontinue rivaroxaban and start parenteral anticoagulant and warfarin at the time the next dose of rivaroxaban would have been taken; discontinue parenteral anticoagulant when desired INR achieved
					• When converting from parenteral anticoagulant, start rivaroxaban 0–2 hr before time of next dose of parenteral anticoagulant (and discontinue parenteral anticoagulant); for UFH, discontinue infusion and start rivaroxaban
					• When converting to parenteral anticoagulant, discontinue rivaroxaban and initiate parenteral anticoagulant at time the next dose of rivaroxaban would have been taken
					• No antidote currently available

ISCHEMIC HEART DISEASE

Findings	UA	NSTEMI	STEMI
Cardiac enzymes (troponin, CK-MB)	Negative	Positive	Positive
ECG changes	ST-segment depression, T-wave inversion, or no ECG changes (any changes are usually transient)	ST-segment depression, T-wave inversion, or no ECG changes	ST-segment elevation

ACUTE PHARMACOLOGIC MANAGEMENT OF UA/NSTEMI

Anti-Ischemic and Analgesic Therapy

Morphine

- May be reasonable for patients who continue to have chest discomfort despite maximally tolerated anti-ischemic medications
- Dose: 1–5 mg IV every 5–30 minutes as needed for pain

NTG

- Can be given to patients with ongoing chest discomfort (0.4 mg sublingually every 5 min × 3 doses); following these doses, give IV NTG within the initial 48 hours if patients continue to have ischemia, or if they present with HF or are hypertensive
- Dose: 5–10 mcg/min continuous infusion; can be titrated up to 100 mcg/min for relief of symptoms
- Adverse effects: Reflex tachycardia, hypotension, headache

β-Blockers

- Oral β-blockers: Given within the first 24 hours to patients who **do not** have signs/symptoms of HF, risk factors for developing cardiogenic shock (age >70 years, SBP <120 mmHg, HR >110 bpm, or prolonged duration since presenting with UA/NSTEMI), PR interval >0.24 sec, ≥2nd-degree heart block, or severe reactive airway disease
- IV β-blockers no longer recommended

CCBs

- A non-DHP CCB (verapamil or diltiazem) can be used alternatively if the patient has a contraindication to β-blocker therapy and does not have evidence of LV dysfunction
- A long-acting non-DHP CCB can be used in patients who have recurrent ischemia despite being on a β-blocker and nitrate therapy

ACEIs

- Should be given to all patients with LVEF ≤40% and in those with HTN, DM, or stable CKD, provided they have no contraindications
- May be reasonable in all other patients with cardiac or other vascular disease
- An ARB can be used alternatively in patients who cannot tolerate ACEIs

Antiplatelet Therapy

Aspirin

- All patients should receive 162–325 mg (non–enteric-coated) at the onset of chest pain (should be chewed and swallowed).
- Patients should continue to receive 81–325 mg daily indefinitely (regardless of whether the patient undergoes PCI)

Clopidogrel (Plavix)

- Prodrug; must be converted via CYP2C19 to active drug
- Avoid concurrent use of omeprazole or esomeprazole (use pantoprazole if PPI needed)
- The following loading and maintenance doses should be given (**with** aspirin):
  - Early invasive strategy (PCI ± stent)
    - » Loading dose = 600 mg × 1
    - » Maintenance dose = 75 mg daily
    - » Continue for ≥12 months
  - Ischemia-guided strategy
    - » Loading dose = 300 mg × 1
    - » Maintenance dose = 75 mg daily
    - » Continue for up to 12 months
- Can also be used as an alternative to aspirin in patients who are allergic or have a major GI intolerance to aspirin
- Discontinue ≥5 days before CABG

Prasugrel (Effient)

- Prodrug
- Alternative to clopidogrel in patients with ACS managed with early invasive strategy
- Initiate only in patients with known coronary artery anatomy (after angiography, but before PCI)
- Achieves faster inhibition of platelet aggregation than clopidogrel
- Administered as a loading dose of 60 mg prior to PCI, followed by maintenance dose of 10 mg daily (↓ dose to 5 mg daily in patients <60 kg)
- Not recommended for patients ≥75 years unless they have DM or history of MI (↑ risk of bleeding), in patients with prior history of stroke or TIA, or in patients requiring triple antithrombotic therapy
- Continue for ≥12 months
- Discontinue ≥7 days before CABG

Ticagrelor (Brilinta)

- NOT a thienopyridine
  - Reversibly binds to the P2Y12 receptor
  - Does not require conversion to an active metabolite (NOT a prodrug)
- Alternative to clopidogrel in patients with ACS managed with early invasive or ischemia-guided strategy
- Contraindicated in severe hepatic impairment
- Drug interactions
  - CYP3A4 substrate; CYP3A4 and P-gp inhibitor
  - Avoid concurrent use with strong CYP3A4 inhibitors or inducers
  - Avoid simvastatin or lovastatin doses >40 mg/day
  - May ↑ digoxin levels
- Administered as a loading dose of 180 mg prior to PCI, followed by maintenance dose of 90 mg BID (dose of aspirin during maintenance therapy should not exceed 100 mg/day); if continued >12 months, ↓ dose to 60 mg BID
- Continue for
  - ≥12 months (early invasive strategy) or up to 12 months (ischemia-guided strategy)
- Discontinue ≥5 days before CABG

Glycoprotein IIb/IIIa Receptor Blockers (GPBs)

- PCI planned: Clopidogrel (or ticagrelor) and/or GPB (eptifibatide or tirofiban) can be initiated prior to angiography. Do not need GPB if bivalirudin + 300 mg loading dose of clopidogrel (given ≥6 hours before angiography) are used.
- Conservative strategy: Adding eptifibatide or tirofiban to clopidogrel or ticagrelor can be considered (especially if patient has recurrent ischemia and requires angiography).

Anticoagulant Therapy

- Early invasive strategy: UFH, enoxaparin, fondaparinux, or bivalirudin should be added to antiplatelet therapy.
- Ischemia-guided strategy: UFH, enoxaparin, or fondaparinux should be added to antiplatelet therapy.

ACUTE PHARMACOLOGIC MANAGEMENT OF STEMI

Anti-Ischemic and Analgesic Therapy

Morphine, NTG, β-Blockers, ACEIs

- Same recommendations as for UA/NSTEMI

Antiplatelet Therapy

Aspirin

- Same recommendations as for UA/NSTEMI

Clopidogrel

- The following loading and maintenance doses should be given:
  - Patients undergoing primary PCI:
    - » Loading dose = 600 mg × 1
    - » Maintenance dose = 75 mg daily
  - Patients receiving fibrinolytic therapy and patients who do not receive reperfusion therapy:
    - » Loading dose = 300 mg × 1 (no loading dose in patients age ≥75 years)
    - » Maintenance dose = 75 mg daily
- Can also be used as an alternative to aspirin in patients who are allergic or have a major GI intolerance to aspirin.
- Clopidogrel should be continued (**with** aspirin) for the following durations of time:
  - Bare metal stent (BMS) or drug-eluting stent (DES): 12 months
  - No stent: At least 14 days (can be considered for up to 1 year)
- Discontinue ≥ 5 days before CABG

Prasugrel

- Same recommendations as for UA/NSTEMI

Ticagrelor

- Same recommendations as for UA/NSTEMI

GPBs

- Can be used if patient undergoing primary PCI

Fibrinolytic Therapy

- Should be used in patients presenting to a hospital without the capability to perform PCI or cannot perform PCI within 120 minutes of first medical contact ("door-to-balloon" time)
- Should be initiated within 30 minutes of presenting to the hospital ("door-to-needle" time)

Anticoagulant Therapy

- Fibrinolytic administered: UFH, enoxaparin, or fondaparinux can be used; should be continued for up to 8 days; UFH should only be used if the treatment duration is <48 hours because of risk for heparin-induced thrombocytopenia (HIT) with prolonged therapy.
- Primary PCI: UFH or bivalirudin can be used.

SECONDARY PREVENTION OF MI

- **Aspirin:** See recommendation above regarding dosing and duration of therapy.
- **Clopidogrel, prasugrel, or ticagrelor:** See recommendations in respective NSTEMI and STEMI sections regarding dosing and duration of therapy.
- **β-blockers:** Continue indefinitely.
- **ACEIs:** Should be given and continued indefinitely in all patients; ARB can be used in patients intolerant of ACEIs.
- **ARAs:** Should be given to patients with LVEF ≤40% receiving optimal ACEI and β-blocker therapy who have DM or HF.
- **Statins:** Should be given and continued indefinitely in all patients.

Glycoprotein IIb/IIIa Receptor Blockers

Generic • Brand • Dose	Contra-indications	Primary Side Effects	Key Monitoring	Pertinent Drug Interactions	Med Pearl
Mechanism of action – block the glycoprotein IIb/IIIa receptor on platelets to prevent the binding of fibrinogen → Inhibit platelet aggregation					

Abciximab
• ReoPro
• *Loading dose:* 0.25 mg/kg IV bolus
• *Maintenance dose:* 0.125 mcg/kg/min (max of 10 mcg/min); continue for 12 hr after PCI
 	
Eptifibatide
• Integrilin
• *Loading dose:* 180 mcg/kg (max of 22.6 mg) IV bolus × 2 (given 10 min apart)
• *Maintenance dose:* 2 mcg/kg/min (max of 15 mg/hr); continue for 18–24 hr after PCI
 	
Tirofiban
• Aggrastat
• NSTEMI:
  • *Loading dose:* 25 mcg/kg IV over ≤5 min
  • *Maintenance dose:* 0.15 mcg/kg/min; continue for up to 18 hr after PCI
• STEMI (with PCI):
  • *Loading dose:* 25 mcg/kg IV bolus
  • *Maintenance dose:* 0.15 mcg/kg/min; continue for 18–24 hr after PCI
	• Active bleeding
	• Prior stroke within past 30 days or any hemorrhagic stroke
	• History of intracranial neoplasms or aneurysm
	• Thrombocytopenia
	• BP >180/110 mmHg
	• Dialysis-dependent (for eptifibatide)
		• Bleeding
		• Thrombocytopenia
			• CBC
			• PT/activated partial thromboplastin time (aPTT)
			• Activated clotting time (ACT) (with PCI)
			• S/S bleeding
			• SCr (baseline)
				Anticoagulants and other anti-platelets may ↑ risk of bleeding	Adjust dose of maintenance infusion of tirofiban and eptifibatide in renal impairment

Anticoagulants

Generic • Brand • Dose	Contra-indications	Primary Side Effects	Key Monitoring	Pertinent Drug Interactions	Med Pearl
Mechanism of action: • UFH: Potentiates the action of antithrombin III, which inactivates the clotting factors, IIa (thrombin), IXa, Xa, XIa, and XIIa, and ultimately prevents the conversion of fibrinogen to fibrin • Enoxaparin: LMWH; similar mechanism as UFH, but primarily inhibits factor Xa • Fondparinux: Selective inhibitor of factor Xa • Bivalirudin: Direct thrombin inhibitor					
UFH • Only available generically • *Loading dose:* 60 units/kg IV bolus (max = 4,000 units) • *Maintenance dose:* 12 units/kg/hr (max = 1,000 units/hr)	• Active bleeding • History of HIT • Recent stroke	• Bleeding • Thrombocytopenia (UFH and LMWH)	• PT/aPTT (only for UFH) • CBC • Anti-Xa levels (for enoxaparin) (consider in obese or renal impairment) • S/S bleeding	Antiplatelets and other anticoagulants may ↑ risk of bleeding	• If platelets <100,000 or ↓ by >50% from baseline, test for HIT; discontinue UFH and start direct thrombin inhibitor (e.g., argatroban, bivalirudin) • Protamine can be used to reverse effects
Enoxaparin • Lovenox • *Loading dose:* 30 mg IV × 1 (for STEMI only) • *Maintenance dose:* 1 mg/kg subcut every 12 hr					• ↓ enoxaparin dose to 1 mg/kg every 24 hr if CrCl <30 mL/min • Should not use in patients with suspected HIT • Protamine only partially reverses effects
Fondaparinux • Arixtra • 2.5 mg subcut daily	• Active bleeding • CrCl <30 mL/min				For STEMI, can give initial dose IV
Bivalirudin • Angiomax • *Loading dose:* 0.75 mg/kg IV bolus • *Maintenance dose:* 1.75 mg/kg/hr	Active bleeding		• PT/aPTT • ACT		Can also be used during PCI in patients with HIT

Fibrinolytic Agents

Generic • Brand • Dose	Contra-indications	Primary Side Effects	Key Monitoring	Pertinent Drug Interactions	Med Pearl
Mechanism of action – activate and convert plasminogen into plasmin, which then degrades fibrin (lyses the clot) to form fibrin degradation products					
Alteplase • Activase • 15 mg IV bolus, then 0.75 mg/kg (max = 50 mg) over 30 min, then 0.5 mg/kg (max = 35 mg) over 60 min Reteplase (rPA) • Retavase • 10 units IV × 2 doses (separated by 30 min) Tenecteplase (TNK) • TNKase • All doses given as IV bolus: • <60 kg: 30 mg • 60–69.9 kg: 35 mg • 70–79.9 kg: 40 mg • 80–89.9 kg: 45 mg • ≥90 kg: 50 mg	• Active bleeding • Any history of intracranial hemorrhage • Known intracranial neoplasm or arteriovenous malformation • Suspected aortic dissection • Significant closed head or facial trauma within 3 months	Bleeding	• CBC • ECG (for signs of reperfusion) • S/S bleeding	Antiplatelets and other anticoagulants may ↑ risk of bleeding	Alteplase also approved for treatment of acute ischemic stroke and pulmonary embolism

PRACTICE QUESTIONS

1. Which of the following drugs may be associated with bradycardia? (Select ALL that apply.)

    (A) Amlodipine
    (B) Bisoprolol
    (C) Clonidine
    (D) Enalapril
    (E) Ivabradine

2. A patient has been taking simvastatin 80 mg PO at bedtime for 3 weeks and is now complaining of muscle pain. Which of the following laboratory tests should be obtained?

    (A) Blood glucose
    (B) Creatine kinase
    (C) Complete blood count
    (D) Simvastatin blood concentration
    (E) Thyroid function tests

3. Which of the following is a common side effect of nitroglycerin?

    (A) Arrhythmias
    (B) Bleeding
    (C) Headache
    (D) Hyperkalemia
    (E) Stevens-Johnson syndrome

4. Which of the following drugs is considered a positive inotrope?

    (A) Dobutamine
    (B) Hydralazine
    (C) Nesiritide
    (D) Nitroglycerin
    (E) Verapamil

5. Which of the following drugs antagonize both β_1 and β_2 receptors at low doses?

    (A) Atenolol
    (B) Bisoprolol
    (C) Carvedilol
    (D) Metoprolol
    (E) Nebivolol

6. Which of the following statements regarding niacin is TRUE?

   (A) It is also available over-the-counter.
   (B) Patients should be advised to take acetaminophen 30 minutes before each dose.
   (C) It can increase a patient's risk for developing hypoglycemia.
   (D) It is contraindicated in patients with hypertriglyceridemia.
   (E) The dose should be titrated up on a weekly basis until a daily dose of 3,000 mg is achieved.

7. Which of the following drugs has been shown to improve survival in patients with heart failure with reduced ejection fraction (HFrEF)? (Select ALL that apply.)

   (A) Carvedilol
   (B) Digoxin
   (C) Enalapril
   (D) Ivabradine
   (E) Spironolactone

8. Which of the following oral antithrombotic agents is/are approved for the treatment of deep venous thrombosis (DVT) and pulmonary embolism (PE)? (Select ALL that apply.)

   (A) Apixaban
   (B) Aspirin
   (C) Dabigatran
   (D) Rivaroxaban
   (E) Ticagrelor

9. Nitroglycerin is available in which of the following formulations? (Select ALL that apply.)

   (A) Injection
   (B) Nasal spray
   (C) Sublingual tablets
   (D) Topical ointment
   (E) Transdermal patch

10. Which of the following drugs is considered a class IV antiarrhythmic?

    (A) Dofetilide
    (B) Diltiazem
    (C) Flecainide
    (D) Metoprolol
    (E) Procainamide

ANSWERS AND EXPLANATIONS

1. **B, C, E**

Bisoprolol (B), clonidine (C), and ivabradine (E) may cause bradycardia and/or heart block. The nondihydropyridine (non-DHP) calcium channel blockers (CCBs) (i.e., verapamil, diltiazem) also decrease atrioventricular (AV) nodal conduction and can cause bradycardia. However, the DHP CCBs, including amlodipine (A), have no effect on AV nodal conduction. Instead, these drugs can actually cause reflex tachycardia. Angiotensin-converting enzyme inhibitors (ACEIs), such as enalapril (D), have no effect on cardiac conduction.

2. **B**

For a patient on a statin who complains of muscle pain, a creatine kinase should be obtained. Therefore, choice (B) is correct.

3. **C**

Nitroglycerin could potentially cause headaches, so choice (C) is correct. Nitroglycerin does not cause cardiac arrhythmias (A), bleeding (B), hyperkalemia (D), or Stevens-Johnson syndrome (E).

4. **A**

Dobutamine (A) stimulates β_1 receptors in the heart and increases myocardial contractility and is therefore considered a positive inotrope. Hydralazine (B) is a direct arterial vasodilator. Nesiritide (C) is an arterial and venous vasodilator. While both of these drugs may increase cardiac output (CO), they do so by decreasing afterload and not by increasing myocardial contractility. Nitroglycerin (D) is a venous vasodilator and is used to reduce preload; it has no effect on CO. Verapamil (E) is a negative inotrope.

5. **C**

Carvedilol (C) is a nonselective β-blocker, antagonizing both the β_1 and β_2 receptors. Atenolol (A), bisoprolol (B), metoprolol (D), and nebivolol (E) are all considered cardioselective β-blockers (i.e., selectively block β_1 receptors), especially at low doses.

6. **A**

Niacin is available as a prescription product as well as an over-the-counter product (A). To prevent niacin-induced flushing, patients should be counseled to take either an aspirin or a nonsteroidal anti-inflammatory drug 30 minutes before each dose because this adverse reaction is mediated by prostaglandins. Acetaminophen (B) does not antagonize the effects of prostaglandins and would not reduce the incidence of niacin-induced flushing. Niacin has been associated with hyperglycemia, not hypoglycemia (C). Niacin is effective in lowering triglycerides and can be used in patients with hypertriglyceridemia (D). To minimize the flushing reactions, the dose of niacin should not be increased by more than 500 mg every 4 weeks (E).

7. **A, C, E**

ACEIs (C), certain β-blockers (carvedilol, metoprolol succinate, and bisoprolol) (A), aldosterone receptor antagonists (E), and isosorbide/dinitrate have all been associated with a reduction in mortality in patients with HFrEF. Although the use of digoxin (B) has been shown to reduce symptoms in patients with HFrEF, it has not been associated with a reduction in mortality. Although the use of ivabradine (D) has been associated with a reduction in hospitalizations in patients with HFrEF, it also has not been associated with a reduction in mortality.

8. **A, C, D**

All three of the novel oral anticoagulants—apixaban, dabigatran, and rivaroxaban—are currently approved by the FDA for the treatment of DVT and PE. Antiplatelet medications such as aspirin (B) or ticagrelor (E) would not be useful for the treatment of DVT or PE.

9. **A, C, D, E**

Nitroglycerin is currently available as an intravenous injection (A), sublingual tablet (C), topical ointment (D), and a transdermal patch (E). This drug is also available as a sublingual spray and rectal ointment (for chronic anal fissures). It is not available as a nasal spray (B).

10. **B**

The non-DHP CCBs—verapamil and diltiazem (B)—are considered class IV antiarrhythmics. Dofetilide (A) is primarily a K^+ channel blocker and is considered a class III antiarrhythmic. Flecainide (C) and procainamide (E) are Na^+ channel blockers and are considered class I antiarrhythmics, with flecainide designated a class Ic antiarrhythmic and procainamide a class Ia antiarrhythmic. β-blockers such as metoprolol (D) are considered class II antiarrhythmics.

Infectious Diseases

2

This chapter reviews various antibiotic agents, including antibacterial, antifungal, and antiviral agents. A brief overview of the recommended pharmacologic treatments of the following infections is also provided:

- **Urinary tract infections**
- **Pneumonia**
- **Meningitis**
- **Infective endocarditis**
- **Infectious diarrhea**
- **Otitis media**
- **Sexually transmitted diseases**
- **Skin and soft tissue infections**
- **Invasive fungal infections**
- **Human immunodeficiency virus**
- **Tuberculosis**

PRINCIPLES OF ANTIBIOTIC THERAPY

Factors to Consider When Selecting Antibiotic Therapy

- Identity/susceptibility of bacteria
  - Important to know which bacteria may be causing the infection
    - » Can begin empiric antibiotic therapy without knowing the actual identity (or sensitivities) of the organism; select antibiotic(s) (usually broad-spectrum) based on the organism(s) *most* likely to cause a particular infection
    - » Once organism (and sensitivities) identified, adjust/narrow antibiotic therapy, as needed, to cover this organism

- Site of infection
  - Especially important for meningitis, urinary tract infections (UTIs), prostatitis, and osteomyelitis
    - » Only certain antibiotics can penetrate into these areas to target the infection; these drugs may need to be used at higher doses, especially for meningitis, prostatitis, and osteomyelitis
- Patient allergies
- Concomitant medications
  - May need to be concerned with potential drug interactions when selecting an antibiotic
- Hepatic and renal function
  - May need to adjust antibiotic dosages if hepatic or renal dysfunction present
- Past medical history
  - Certain antibiotics may need to be avoided in particular disease states (e.g., seizure disorders)
- Patient age
  - Some antibiotics are contraindicated in pediatric patients
- Pregnancy/breastfeeding
  - Some antibiotics are contraindicated in these patients

URINARY TRACT INFECTIONS

Guidelines Summary

Acute Uncomplicated Cystitis

First-line therapy	Nitrofurantoin 100 mg PO BID × 5 days
Second-line therapy	Trimethoprim/sulfamethoxazole (TMP/SMX) 160/800 mg (double-strength [DS]) PO BID × 3 days
Third-line therapy	Fosfomycin 3 g PO × 1 dose

- *Alternative agents:*
  - Fluoroquinolone (FQ) × 3 days
    - » Only use when other agents cannot be used
  - β-lactams (i.e., amoxicillin-clavulanate, cefdinir, cefaclor, cefpodoxime) × 3–7 days
    - » Avoid unless other agents are not appropriate

Acute Pyelonephritis (Outpatient Therapy)

- First-line therapy:
  - Ciprofloxacin 500 mg PO BID × 7 days
  - Cipro XR 1 g PO daily × 7 days
  - Levofloxacin 750 mg PO daily × 5 days
  - May be combined with either of the following:
    - Ceftriaxone 1 g IV × 1 day **OR**
    - Gentamicin 5–7 mg/kg IV × 1 day
- Second-line therapy: TMP/SMX DS PO BID × 14 days
  - May be combined with either of the following:
    - Ceftriaxone 1 g IV × 1 day **OR**
    - Gentamicin 5–7 mg/kg IV × 1 day
- Third-line therapy: Oral β-lactam (i.e., amoxicillin-clavulanate) × 10–14 days **AND** one-time dose of ceftriaxone 1 g IV or gentamicin 5–7 mg/kg IV

Acute Pyelonephritis (Inpatient Therapy)

- IV FQ
- Aminoglycoside +/– IV ampicillin
- IV extended-spectrum cephalosporin or penicillin +/– aminoglycoside
- IV carbapenem (e.g., imipenem/cilastatin)

Complicated UTIs

- Duration of therapy: 10–14 days

PNEUMONIA

Guidelines Summary

Diagnosis	Treatment	Duration
Community-acquired (ambulatory)	*Previously healthy and no antibiotic therapy in past 3 months:* Macrolide (clarithromycin or azithromycin) **OR** Doxycycline	≥5 days
	With comorbidities (see table notes)[1] that place patient at risk for drug-resistant Streptococcus pneumoniae or antibiotic use in past 3 months: FQ (moxifloxacin, gemifloxacin, or levofloxacin) **OR** Macrolide (or doxycycline) *plus* one of the following: • High-dose amoxicillin • Amoxicillin/clavulanate • Cephalosporin (ceftriaxone, cefuroxime, or cefpodoxime)	
Community-acquired (hospitalized)	*Not in Intensive Care Unit (ICU):* FQ (moxifloxacin, gemifloxacin, or levofloxacin) **OR** Macrolide (or doxycycline) *plus* one of the following: • Ampicillin • Ceftriaxone • Cefotaxime	
	In ICU: FQ (moxifloxacin, gemifloxacin, or levofloxacin) *plus* one of the following: • Ampicillin/sulbactam • Ceftriaxone • Cefotaxime **OR** Azithromycin *plus* one of the following: • Ampicillin/sulbactam • Ceftriaxone • Cefotaxime	

Guidelines Summary *(cont'd)*

Diagnosis	Treatment	Duration
Hospital-acquired	*Not at high risk for mortality (see below)[2] AND no factors increasing likelihood of methicillin-resistant S. aureus (MRSA) (see below)[3] (select one of the following drugs):* • Piperacillin/tazobactam • Cefepime • Levofloxacin • Imipenem/cilastatin or meropenem	7 days
	Not at high risk for mortality (see below)[2] but WITH factors increasing the likelihood of MRSA (see below)[3]: Vancomycin **OR** Linezolid **PLUS** one of the following: • Piperacillin/tazobactam • Ceftazidime • Cefepime • Levofloxacin or ciprofloxacin • Imipenem/cilastatin or meropenem • Aztreonam	
	High risk for mortality (see below)[2] or receipt of IV antibiotics in the past 90 days: Vancomycin **OR** Linezolid **PLUS** 2 of the following (avoid 2 β-lactams): • Piperacillin/tazobactam • Ceftazidime • Cefepime • Levofloxacin or ciprofloxacin • Imipenem/cilastatin or meropenem • Aztreonam • Amikacin, or gentamicin, or tobramycin	

[1] *Comorbidities: Chronic obstructive pulmonary disease (COPD), diabetes, chronic renal failure, chronic liver failure, heart failure (HF), cancer, asplenia, immunosuppressed*

[2] *Risk factors for mortality: Need for ventilatory support due to pneumonia and septic shock.*

[3] *Risk factors for MRSA infection: Prior IV antibiotic use in past 90 days, hospitalization in a unit where >20% of S. aureus isolates are methicillin-resistant or the prevalence of MRSA is unknown.*

MENINGITIS

Guidelines Summary

Empiric Treatment

Age Group	Treatment
<1 mo	Ampicillin + aminoglycoside **OR** Ampicillin + cefotaxime
1–23 mo	Third-generation cephalosporin (cefotaxime or ceftriaxone) + vancomycin
2–50 yr	Third-generation cephalosporin (cefotaxime or ceftriaxone) + vancomycin
>50 yr	Third-generation cephalosporin (cefotaxime or ceftriaxone) + vancomycin + ampicillin

- Dexamethasone may be considered as adjunctive therapy for the following:
  - Infants and children: *H. influenzae* meningitis
  - Adults: *Streptococcus pneumoniae* meningitis

INFECTIVE ENDOCARDITIS

Modified Duke Criteria

Major Criteria	Minor Criteria
Blood culture positive for IE (one of the following): • Typical microorganisms consistent with IE from 2 separate blood cultures • Persistently positive cultures defined as: ≥2 positive cultures of blood samples drawn >12 hr apart or all 3 or a majority of ≥4 separate blood cultures (with 1st and last sample drawn ≥1 hr apart	Predisposition, predisposing heart condition, or injection drug use
Evidence of endocardial involvement	Fever (temperature >38°C)
Echocardiogram positive for IE (vegetation, abscess, or new partial dehiscence of prosthetic valve or new valvular regurgitation)	Vascular phenomena, major arterial emboli, septic pulmonary infarcts, mycotic aneurysm, intracranial hemorrhage, conjunctival hemorrhages, and Janeway lesions
	Immunological phenomena (e.g., glomerulonephritis, Osler nodes, Roth spots, rheumatoid factor)
	Microbiological evidence (positive blood culture but does not meet a major criterion) or serological evidence of active infection with organism consistent with IE

Guidelines Summary, Empiric Treatment

Viridans Group Streptococci and *Streptococcus bovis* Highly Susceptible to Penicillin (MIC ≤0.12 mcg/mL): Native Valve IE

Treatment Regimen	Duration	Clinical Pearls
Penicillin G 12–18 million units/day IV in 4–6 divided doses **OR** Ceftriaxone 2 g IV/IM q24h	4 wk 4 wk	If patient has NO β-lactam allergy
Penicillin G 12–18 million units/day IV in 6 divided doses **OR** ceftriaxone 2 g IV/IM q24h **PLUS** Gentamicin 3 mg/kg IV q24h or 1 mg/kg IV q8h	2 wk 2 wk	Should not be used if patients have: • Cardiac or extracardiac abscess • Creatinine clearance <20 mL/min For gentamicin q8h dosing: • Target peak concentration = 3–4 mcg/mL • Target trough concentration <1 mcg/mL
Vancomycin 15 mg/kg IV q12h	4 wk	• For patients with β-lactam allergy • Target trough concentration = 10–15 mcg/mL

Viridans Group Streptococci and *Streptococcus bovis* Relatively Resistant to Penicillin (MIC >0.12 and <0.5 mcg/mL): Native Valve IE

Treatment Regimen	Duration	Clinical Pearls
Penicillin G 24 million units/day IV in 4–6 divided doses **PLUS** Gentamicin 3 mg/kg IV q24h or 1 mg/kg IV q8h	4 wk 2 wk	If organism susceptible to ceftriaxone, may use ceftriaxone monotherapy For gentamicin q8h dosing: • Target peak concentration = 3–4 mcg/mL • Target trough concentration <1 mcg/mL
Vancomycin 15 mg/kg IV q12h	4 wk	• For patients with β-lactam allergy • Target trough concentration = 10–15 mcg/mL

Viridans Group Streptococci and *Streptococcus bovis* Resistant to Penicillin (MIC ≥0.5 mcg/mL): Native Valve IE

- Treat as enterococcal IE

Viridans Group Streptococci and *Streptococcus bovis* Susceptible to Penicillin (MIC ≤0.12 mcg/mL): Prosthetic Valve IE

Treatment Regimen	Duration	Clinical Pearls
Penicillin G 24 million units/day IV in 4–6 divided doses **OR** ceftriaxone 2 g IV/IM q24h **WITH OR WITHOUT** Gentamicin 3 mg/kg IV q24h or 1 mg/kg IV q8h	6 wk 2 wk	Do NOT give gentamicin if patient's CrCl <30 mL/min For gentamicin q8h dosing: • Target peak concentration = 3–4 mcg/mL • Target trough concentration <1 mcg/mL
Vancomycin 15 mg/kg IV q12h	6 wk	• For patients with β-lactam allergy • Target trough concentration = 10–15 mcg/mL

Viridans Group Streptococci and Streptococcus bovis Relatively or Fully Resistant to Penicillin (MIC >0.12 mcg/mL): Prosthetic Valve IE

Treatment Regimen	Duration	Clinical Pearls
Penicillin G 24 million units/day IV in 4–6 divided doses **OR** ceftriaxone 2 g IV/IM q24h **PLUS** Gentamicin 3 mg/kg IV q24h or 1 mg/kg IV q8h	6 wk 6 wk	For gentamicin q8h dosing: • Target peak concentration = 3–4 mcg/mL • Target trough concentration <1 mcg/mL
Vancomycin 15 mg/kg IV q12h	6 wk	• For patients with β-lactam allergy • Target trough concentration = 10–15 mcg/mL

Staphylococci: Native Valve IE

Treatment Regimen	Duration	Clinical Pearls
Oxacillin-susceptible strains:		
Nafcillin or oxacillin 12 g/day IV in 4–6 divided doses	6 wk (complicated, right-sided IE and uncomplicated, left-sided IE); ≥6 wk (complicated, left-sided IE); 2 wk (uncomplicated, right-sided IE)	
Cefazolin 2 g IV q8h	6 wk	For patients with non-anaphylactoid-type β-lactam allergy
Vancomycin 15 mg/kg IV q12h	6 wk	• For patients with anaphylactoid-type β-lactam allergy • Target trough concentration = 10–20 mcg/mL
Oxacillin-resistant strains:		
Vancomycin 15 mg/kg IV q12h	6 wk	Target trough concentration = 10–20 mcg/mL
Daptomycin ≥8 mg/kg/dose	6 wk	

Staphylococci: Prosthetic Valve IE

Treatment Regimen	Duration	Clinical Pearls
Oxacillin-susceptible strains:		
Nafcillin or oxacillin 2 g IV q4h **PLUS** Rifampin 300 mg IV/PO q8h **PLUS** Gentamicin 3 mg/kg/day IV in 2–3 divided doses	≥6 wk ≥6 wk 2 wk	Cefazolin may be substituted for nafcillin/oxacillin in patients with non-anaphylactoid-type β-lactam allergy Vancomycin may be substituted for nafcillin/oxacillin in patients with anaphylactoid-type β-lactam allergy For gentamicin: • Target peak concentration = 3–4 mcg/mL • Target trough concentration <1 mcg/mL
Oxacillin-resistant strains:		
Vancomycin 15 mg/kg IV q12h **PLUS** Rifampin 300 mg IV/PO q8h **PLUS** Gentamicin 3 mg/kg/day IV in 2–3 divided doses	≥6 wk ≥6 wk 2 wk	Target vancomycin trough concentration = 10–20 mcg/mL For gentamicin: • Target peak concentration = 3–4 mcg/mL • Target trough concentration <1 mcg/mL

Enterococcus Species Susceptible to Penicillin and Gentamicin in Patients Who Can Tolerate β-Lactam Therapy: Native or Prosthetic Valve IE

Treatment Regimen	Duration	Clinical Pearls
Ampicillin 2 g IV q4h **OR** penicillin G 18–30 million units IV in 6 divided doses **PLUS** Gentamicin 3 mg/kg/day IV in 2–3 divided doses	4–6 wk 4–6 wk	Recommended for patients with CrCl >50 mL/min 4 wk of therapy recommended for patients with native valve IE with symptoms <3 mo 6 wk of therapy recommended for patients with native valve IE with symptoms >3 mo **OR** prosthetic valve IE For gentamicin: • Target peak concentration = 3–4 mcg/mL • Target trough concentration <1 mcg/mL
Ampicillin 2 g IV q4h **PLUS** Ceftriaxone 2 g IV q12h	6 wk 6 wk	Recommended for patients with CrCl <50 mL/min

Enterococcus Species Susceptible to Vancomycin and Gentamicin and Resistant to Penicillin in Patients Who Cannot Tolerate β-Lactam Therapy: Native or Prosthetic Valve IE

Treatment Regimen	Duration	Clinical Pearls
Vancomycin 15 mg/kg IV q12h **PLUS** Gentamicin 1 mg/kg IV q8h	6 wk 6 wk	Target vancomycin trough concentration = 10–20 mcg/mL For gentamicin: • Target peak concentration = 3–4 mcg/mL • Target trough concentration <1 mcg/mL

Enterococcus Species Resistant to Penicillin, Aminoglycosides, and Vancomycin: Native or Prosthetic Valve IE

Treatment Regimen	Duration
Linezolid 600 mg IV/PO q12h **OR** Daptomycin 10–12 mg/kg per dose	>6 wk >6 wk

INFECTIOUS DIARRHEA

Guidelines Summary

Organism	First-Line Treatment
Shigella	TMP/SMX or FQ
Salmonella	TMP/SMX or FQ
Campylobacter	Erythromycin
E. coli, enterotoxigenic	TMP/SMX or FQ
E.coli, enterohemorrhagic (STEC)	Avoid antimotility drugs and antibiotics
C. difficile	• Discontinue antibiotics and avoid antimotility agents • Mild-to-moderate: Metronidazole 500 mg PO TID × 10–14 days • Severe: Vancomycin 125 mg PO 4 times daily × 10–14 days • Bezlotoxumab (Zinplava), a monoclonal antibody that binds *C. difficile* toxin B, can be used in patients who are receiving antibacterial therapy for *C. difficile* infection and are at risk for recurrence of disease (age ≥65 years, history of *C. difficile* infection in previous 6 mo, immunocompromised, severe *C. difficile* infection, or *C. difficile* ribotype 027)
Giardia	Metronidazole
Cryptosporidium	Paromomycin (if severe)
Isospora	TMP/SMX
Cyclospora	TMP/SMX

OTITIS MEDIA

Guidelines Summary

Initial Management of Uncomplicated AOM

Age	Otorrhea with AOM	Unilateral or Bilateral AOM with Severe Symptoms	Bilateral AOM without Otorrhea	Unilateral AOM without Otorrhea
6 months–2 years	Antibiotic therapy	Antibiotic therapy	Antibiotic therapy	Antibiotic therapy **OR** additional observation
≥2 years	Antibiotic therapy	Antibiotic therapy	Antibiotic therapy **OR** additional observation	Antibiotic therapy **OR** additional observation

Recommended Antibiotic Therapy for Management of Uncomplicated AOM

	First-Line Therapy	**Alternative Therapy**
Initial Immediate or Delayed Treatment	Amoxicillin (high-dose) 80–90 mg/kg/day PO in 2 divided doses **OR** *If history of amoxicillin use in past 90 days, concurrent purulent conjunctivitis, or history of recurrent AOM unresponsive to amoxicillin:* Amoxicillin-clavulanate (high-dose) 90 mg/kg/day of amoxicillin + 6.4 mg/kg/day of clavulanate PO in 2 divided doses	*If penicillin allergy:* Cefdinir **OR** Cefuroxime **OR** Cefpodoxime **OR** Ceftriaxone × 1 or 3 days
Treatment After 48–72 Hours of Failure of Initial Antibiotic Treatment	Amoxicillin-clavulanate (high-dose) 90 mg/kg/day of amoxicillin + 6.4 mg/kg/day of clavulanate PO in 2 divided doses **OR** Ceftriaxone 50 mg IM or IV for 3 days	Clindamycin

Duration of Therapy

Age/Characteristic of Symptoms	**Duration**
<2 yr or severe symptoms	10 days
2–5 yr with mild–moderate symptoms	7 days
≥6 yr with mild–moderate symptoms	5–7 days

SEXUALLY TRANSMITTED DISEASES

Guidelines Summary

Disease	Treatment
Chlamydia	Azithromycin 1 g PO × 1 dose **OR** Doxycycline 100 mg PO q12h × 7 days
Gonorrhea	Ceftriaxone 250 mg IM × 1 dose **PLUS** Azithromycin 1 g PO × 1 dose
Syphilis	*Primary, secondary, or early latent syphilis (<1 yr in duration):* • Benzathine penicillin G 2.4 million units IM × 1 dose *Late latent syphilis (>1 yr in duration), latent syphilis of unknown duration, or tertiary syphilis (not neurosyphilis):* • Benzathine penicillin G 2.4 million units IM once weekly × 3 weeks *Neurosyphilis:* • Aqueous penicillin G 3–4 million units IV q4h or as continuous infusion × 10–14 days

SKIN AND SOFT TISSUE INFECTIONS

Guidelines Summary

Infection	Empiric Treatment
Purulent SSTIs	
Mild	Incision and drainage; no antibiotics
Moderate (with systemic signs of infection*)	Incision and drainage **PLUS** antibiotics: TMP/SMX **OR** Doxycycline
Severe (failed incision and drainage plus PO antibiotics **OR** have systemic signs of infection*, **OR** are immunocompromised)	Incision and drainage **PLUS** antibiotics: Vancomycin **OR** Daptomycin / **OR** Dalbavancin **OR** Linezolid / **OR** Oritavancin **OR** Telavancin / **OR** Tedizolid **OR** Ceftaroline
Nonpurulent SSTIs	
Mild	Penicillin VK **OR** Cephalosporin (PO) **OR** Dicloxacillin **OR** Clindamycin (PO)
Moderate (with systemic signs of infection*)	Penicillin (IV) **OR** Ceftriaxone **OR** Cefazolin **OR** Clindamycin (IV)
Severe (failed PO antibiotics **OR** signs of systemic infection,* **OR** immunocompromised **OR** signs of deeper infection [e.g., bullae, skin sloughing, hypotension, evidence of organ dysfunction])	Emergent surgical inspection/debridement **PLUS** antibiotics: Vancomycin **AND** Piperacillin/tazobactam

* Signs of systemic infection: Temperature >38°C, heart rate >90 beats/minute, respiratory rate >24 breaths/minute, WBCs >12,000 cells/μL or <400 cells/μL

INVASIVE FUNGAL INFECTIONS

Drugs of Choice for Selected Invasive Fungal Infections

Organism	Disease	First-Line Therapy	Duration
Candida albicans, C. glabrata, C. krusei, C. tropicalis	Candidemia	*Nonneutropenic:* Echinocandin **OR** Fluconazole (if not critically ill) *Neutropenic:* Echinocandin **OR** Lipid amphotericin B **OR** Fluconazole (if not critically ill and no prior azole exposure) If *C. krusei*: Echinocandin, lipid amphotericin B, or voriconazole	14 days after first negative blood culture
	Urinary candidiasis	*Asymptomatic:* Eliminate predisposing factor (i.e., remove urinary catheter) Treat only if high-risk for dissemination: • Neutropenic: Treat as for candidemia (see above) • Undergoing urologic manipulation: Fluconazole (PO) **OR** amphotericin B *Symptomatic:* • Fluconazole-susceptible organism: Fluconazole (PO) • Fluconazole-resistant *C. glabrata*: Amphotericin B **OR** flucytosine • *C. krusei*: Amphotericin B	*Asymptomatic:* Treatment for urologic manipulation: Several days before and after procedure *Symptomatic:* • Fluconazole-susceptible organisms: 14 days • Fluconazole-resistant *C. glabrata*: 7–10 days • *C. krusei*: 1–7 days

Drugs of Choice for Selected Invasive Fungal Infections *(cont'd)*

Organism	Disease	First-Line Therapy	Duration
Blastomyces dermatitidis	Pulmonary blastomycosis	*Mild to moderate:* Itraconazole *Moderately severe to severe:* Amphotericin B × 1–2 wk, then itraconazole × 6–12 mo	6–12 mo
	Disseminated blastomycosis	*Mild to moderate:* Itraconazole *Moderately severe to severe:* Amphotericin B × 1–2 wk, then itraconazole × 12 mo	*Mild to moderate:* 6–12 mo *Moderately severe to severe:* 12 mo
	Immunosuppressed	Amphotericin B × 1–2 wk, then itraconazole × 12 mo	12 mo
Aspergillus fumigatus, A. flavus, A. niger	Pulmonary aspergillosis	Voriconazole	6–12 wk
Coccidioides immitis	Pulmonary coccidioidomycosis	High-dose fluconazole	3–6 mo
	Disseminated (nonmeningeal) coccidioidomycosis	Fluconazole or itraconazole	≥6–12 mo
	Disseminated (meningeal) coccidioidomycosis	Fluconazole	Lifelong
Histoplasma capsulatum	Pulmonary histoplasmosis	*Mild to moderate:* Symptoms <4 wk: No treatment Symptoms >4 wk: Itraconazole *Moderately severe to severe:* Amphotericin B × 1–2 wk, then itraconazole × total of 12 wk	*Mild to moderate:* 6–12 wk *Moderately severe to severe:* 12 wk
Cryptococcus neoformans	Cryptococcal meningoencephalitis (in HIV-infected patients)	*Induction:* Amphotericin B + flucytosine *Consolidation:* Fluconazole	*Induction:* ≥2 wk *Consolidation:* ≥8 wk

Antibacterial Agents

Penicillins (β-Lactams)

Generic • Brand • Dose/Dosage Forms	Spectrum of Activity	Contraindications	Primary Side Effects	Pertinent Drug Interactions	Med Pearl
Mechanism of action – inhibit bacterial cell wall synthesis; bactericidal					
Natural Penicillins					
Penicillin G • Only available generically • 2–4 million units IV q4–6h • Injection Penicillin G benzathine • Bicillin LA • 1.2–2.4 million units IM at specified intervals • Injection Penicillin G procaine • Only available generically • 1.2–4.8 million units IM/day at specified intervals • Injection Penicillin VK☆ • Only available generically • 250–500 mg PO q6h • Solution, tabs	• *Strep. viridans* • *Strep. pyogenes* • *Strep. pneumoniae* (↑ resistance) • Mouth anaerobes	Allergy to penicillins, cephalosporins, or carbapenems	• Hypersensitivity reaction (rash, hives, dyspnea, throat swelling) • Nausea/vomiting/diarrhea (N/V/D) • Interstitial nephritis • Hemolytic anemia (with prolonged administration) • Stevens-Johnson syndrome, toxic epidermal necrolysis	• Probenecid may ↑ effects (may be used for this purpose) • May ↓ effects of oral contraceptives	• Adjust dose in renal impairment • Penicillin G benzathine or procaine used for syphilis; benzathine also used for Strep throat • Take penicillin VK 1 hour before or 2 hours after meals
Penicillinase-Resistant Penicillins					
Dicloxacillin • Only available generically • 125–500 mg PO q6h • Caps Nafcillin • Only available generically • 500 mg–2 g IV q4–6h • Injection Oxacillin • Bactocill • 250 mg–2 g IV q4–6h • Injection	• *Staph aureus* (methicillin-sensitive, MSSA) • *Streptococcus*	Same as natural penicillins	Same as natural penicillins	Same as natural penicillins	• No need to adjust dose in renal impairment (cleared by biliary excretion) • Take dicloxacillin 1 hour before or 2 hours after meals • Patients on nafcillin (IV) or oxacillin (IV) can be switched to dicloxacillin (PO)

Penicillins (β-Lactams) *(cont'd)*

Generic • Brand • Dose/Dosage Forms	Spectrum of Activity	Contraindications	Primary Side Effects	Pertinent Drug Interactions	Med Pearl
Aminopenicillins					
Amoxicillin ☆ • Moxatag • Immediate-release (IR): 250–500 mg PO q8h or 500–875 mg PO q12h • Extended release (ER): 775 mg PO daily • Caps, chewable tabs, suspension, tabs (ER and IR)	• *Strep pneumoniae* • *H. influenzae* • *E. coli* • *Proteus mirabilis* • *Salmonella* • *Shigella*	Same as natural penicillins	Same as natural penicillins	Same as natural penicillins	• Amoxicillin can be used in 3-drug regimen for *H. pylori* • Adjust dose in renal impairment • Take ampicillin 1 hour before or 2 hours after meals
Ampicillin • Only available generically • 250–500 mg PO q6h • 250 mg–2 g IV q4–6h • Caps, injection, suspension					
Aminopenicillins + β-Lactamase Inhibitors					
Amoxicillin-clavulanate ☆ • Augmentin • IR: 250–500 mg PO q8h or 500–875 mg PO q12h • ER: 2,000 mg PO q12h • Chewable tabs, suspension, tabs (ER and IR)	• β-lactamase producing *Staph. aureus* (MSSA), *H. influenzae*, *M. catarrhalis*, *E. coli*, and *K. pneumoniae* • Anaerobes	Same as natural penicillins	Same as natural penicillins	Same as natural penicillins	• Adjust dose in renal impairment • Patients on ampicillin sulbactam (IV) can be switched to amoxicillin-clavulanate (PO) • Good anaerobic coverage
Ampicillin-sulbactam • Unasyn • 1.5–3 g IV q6h • Injection					
Antipseudomonal Penicillin + β-Lactamase Inhibitor					
Piperacillin-tazobactam • Zosyn • 3.375 IV q6h or 4.5 g IV q6–8h • Injection	• Same as amoxicillin-clavulanate and ampicillin-sulbactam • *Pseudomonas aeruginosa*	Same as natural penicillins	Same as natural penicillins	Same as natural penicillins	• Adjust dose in renal impairment • Primarily used for *Pseudomonas* infections • Good anaerobic coverage • Contains Na+ (use with caution in volume-overloaded patients) • ↑ risk of nephrotoxicity when used with vancomycin

Cephalosporins (β-Lactams)

Generic • Brand • Dose/Dosage Forms	Spectrum of Activity	Contraindications	Primary Side Effects	Pertinent Drug Interactions	Med Pearl
Mechanism of action – inhibit bacterial cell wall synthesis; bactericidal • As drugs move from 1st through 4th generation, ↑ activity against Gram (−) organisms and ↓ activity against Gram (+) organisms					
First-Generation					
Cefadroxil • Only available generically • 500 mg–1 g PO q12h • Caps, suspension, tabs Cefazolin • Ancef • 250 mg–1 g IV q8h • Injection Cephalexin☆ • Keflex • 250–500 mg PO q6h • Caps, suspension, tabs	• *Staph. aureus* (MSSA) • *Staph. epidermidis* • *Strep. pyogenes* • *Strep. pneumoniae* • *E. coli* • *P. mirabilis* • *K. pneumoniae*	Allergy to penicillins, cephalosporins, or carbapenems (up to 10% risk of cross-sensitivity)	Same as natural penicillins	Same as natural penicillins	• Adjust dose in renal impairment • Patients on cefazolin (IV) can be switched to cephalexin (PO) • Cefazolin often used for surgical prophylaxis
Second-Generation					
Cefaclor • Only available generically • 250–500 mg PO q8h • Caps, ER tabs, suspension Cefotetan • Cefotan • 1–2 g IV q12h • Injection Cefoxitin • Mefoxin • 1–2 g IV q6–8h • Injection Cefprozil • Only available generically • 250–500 mg q12–24h • Suspension, tabs Cefuroxime • Ceftin, Zinacef • 250–500 mg PO q12h • 500 mg–1.5 g IV q8h • Injection, suspension, tabs	• Gram (+) activity similar to 1st-generation agents • Same Gram (−) activity as 1st-generation agents, but with added activity against *Acinetobacter, Citrobacter, Enterobacter, Neisseria, Serratia,* and *H. influenzae* • Anaerobes (cefotetan and cefoxitin only)	Same as 1st-generation agents	• Same as natural penicillins • Bleeding/bruising (with cefotetan and cefoxitin)	• Same as natural penicillins • Disulfiram-like reaction may occur if alcohol is used during treatment with cefotetan • Cefotetan and cefoxitin may ↑ risk of bleeding with warfarin	• Adjust dose in renal impairment • Take cefaclor ER tabs and cefuroxime suspension with food to ↑ absorption

Cephalosporins (β-Lactams) *(cont'd)*

Generic • Brand • Dose/Dosage Forms	Spectrum of Activity	Contraindications	Primary Side Effects	Pertinent Drug Interactions	Med Pearl
Third-Generation					
Cefdinir☆ • Only available generically • 300 mg PO q12h or 600 mg PO daily • Caps, suspension Cefixime • Suprax • 400 mg PO daily • Caps, chewable tabs, suspension, tabs Cefotaxime • Claforan • 1–2 g IV q8h • Injection Cefpodoxime • Only available generically • 100-400 mg PO q12h • Suspension, tabs Ceftazidime • Fortaz, Tazicef • 1–2 g IV q8–12h • Injection Ceftazidime-avibactam • Avycaz • 2.5 g IV q8h • Injection Ceftriaxone • Only available generically • 1–2 g IV daily • Injection	• Limited Gram (+) activity • More extensive Gram (−) activity vs. 2nd-generation agents • *Pseudomonas aeruginosa* (ceftazidime and ceftazidime-avibactam only)	• Same as 1st-generation agents • Ceftriaxone should be avoided in neonates ($\uparrow$ risk of hyperbilirubinemia, kernicterus)	Same as natural penicillins	• Same as natural penicillins • Antacids and iron may $\downarrow$ absorption of cefdinir • Antacids and H_2 antagonists may $\downarrow$ absorption of cefpodoxime • Ceftriaxone may cause precipitation if given with Ca^{2+}-containing solutions	• Adjust dose for all, except cefoperazone and ceftriaxone, in renal impairment • Take cefpodoxime tabs with food to $\uparrow$ absorption • Ceftriaxone often used for meningitis and sexually transmitted diseases (STDs) • Ceftazidime-avibactam indicated for complicated intra-abdominal infections (with metronidazole) and complicated UTIs • $\downarrow$ efficacy of ceftazidime-avibactam in patients with CrCl 30–50 mL/min

Cephalosporins (β-Lactams) *(cont'd)*

Generic • Brand • Dose/Dosage Forms	Spectrum of Activity	Contraindications	Primary Side Effects	Pertinent Drug Interactions	Med Pearl
Fourth-Generation					
Cefepime • Maxipime • 1–2 g IV q8–12h • Injection	• Gram (+) activity better than 3rd-generation agents • More extensive Gram (−) activity vs. 3rd-generation agents • *Pseudomonas aeruginosa*	Same as 1st-generation agents	Same as natural penicillins	Same as natural penicillins	Adjust dose in renal impairment
Fifth-Generation					
Ceftaroline • Teflaro • 600 mg IV q12h • Injection	• *Staph. aureus* (MSSA and MRSA [for skin infections only]) • *Strep. pyogenes* • *Strep. pneumoniae* • *Klebsiella* • *E. coli* • *H. influenzae*	Same as 1st-generation agents	Same as natural penicillins	Same as natural penicillins	• Indicated for SSTIs and community-acquired pneumonia • Adjust dose in renal impairment
Ceftolozane-tazobactam • Zerbaxa • 1.5 g IV q8h • Injection	• Active against Gram (+) and Gram (−) organisms, including drug-resistant organisms • *Pseudomonas aeruginosa* • Some activity against anaerobes (*Bacteroides fragilis*) • No activity against *Staph. aureus*				• Indicated for complicated intra-abdominal infections (with metronidazole) and complicated UTIs • Adjust dose in renal impairment • ↓ efficacy in patients with CrCl 30–50 mL/min

Carbapenems (β-Lactams)

Generic • Brand • Dose/Dosage Forms	Spectrum of Activity	Contraindications	Primary Side Effects	Pertinent Drug Interactions	Med Pearl
Mechanism of action – inhibit bacterial cell wall synthesis; bactericidal					
Doripenem • Doribax • 500 mg IV q8h • Injection Ertapenem • Invanz • 1 g IV daily • Injection Imipenem-cilastatin • Primaxin • 250 mg–1 g IV q6–12h • Injection Meropenem • Merrem • 500 mg–1 g IV q8h • Injection	• Broad-spectrum (active against Gram [+], Gram [−], and anaerobic organisms) • All, except ertapenem, are active against *Pseudomonas aeruginosa*	Allergy to penicillins, cephalosporins, or carbapenems	• Same as natural penicillins • Seizures (esp. in patients with renal impairment or history of seizure disorder)	• Same as natural penicillins • May ↓ valproic acid levels	• Adjust dose in renal impairment • Risk of seizures is highest with imipenem/cilastatin

Monobactam (β-Lactam)

Generic • Brand • Dose/Dosage Forms	Spectrum of Activity	Contraindications	Primary Side Effects	Pertinent Drug Interactions	Med Pearl
Mechanism of action – inhibits bacterial cell wall synthesis; bactericidal					
Aztreonam • Azactam, Cayston • IV: 500 mg–2 g IV q6–12h • Nebs: 75 mg via nebulization 3× daily (at least 4 hr apart) × 28 days • Injection, nebulizer solution	Only effective against Gram (−) organisms, including *Pseudomonas aeruginosa*	None	Same as natural penicillins	None	• Can be used in patients allergic to penicillins, cephalosporins, or carbapenems • Adjust dose for IV in renal impairment • Cayston used for patients with cystic fibrosis (*Pseudomonas*); do not repeat for 28 days after completion

Aminoglycosides

Generic • Brand • Dose/Dosage Forms	Spectrum of Activity	Contra indications	Primary Side Effects	Pertinent Drug Interactions	Med Pearl
Mechanism of action – inhibit bacterial protein synthesis by binding to the 30S subunit of the bacterial ribosome; bactericidal					
Amikacin • Only available generically • 15 mg/kg IV q24h or 5–7.5 mg/kg IV q8h • Injection Gentamicin • Gentak • 5–7 mg/kg IV q24h or 1–2.5 mg/kg IV q8–12h • Injection, ophthalmic ointment/solution, topical cream/ointment Neomycin • Only available generically • 500 mg–2 g PO q6–8h • Tabs Streptomycin • Only available generically • 15 mg/kg/day IM • Injection Tobramycin • Bethkis, Kitabis Pak, TOBI, Tobrex • 5–7 mg/kg IV q24h or 1–2.5 mg/kg IV q8–12h • Caps for inhalation, injection, nebulizer solution, ophthalmic ointment/solution	• Primarily used for Gram (−) organisms (*E.coli, Klebsiella, P. mirabilis, Enterobacter, Acinetobacter, Serratia, Pseudomonas aeruginosa*) • Provide synergistic activity against *Staph., Strep.,* or *Enterococcus* when used with penicillins or vancomycin • Streptomycin and amikacin active against *Mycobacteria* • Neomycin used as prep for bowel surgery or for hepatic encephalopathy	None	• Nephrotoxicity • Ototoxicity (both related to dose and duration of therapy; may be reversible) • Bronchospasm (inhalation only)	• May ↑ effects of neuromuscular blocking agents • ↑ risk of nephrotoxicity when used with amphotericin B, loop diuretics, tacrolimus, cyclosporine, or cisplatin	• Bactericidal effect is concentration-dependent • Target serum concentrations (for traditional dosing): *Amikacin:* Peak = Life-threatening infections: 25–40 mcg/mL; serious infections: 20–25 mcg/mL, UTIs: 15–20 mcg/mL; Trough <8 mcg/mL (The American Thoracic Society [ATS] recommends trough levels of <4–5 mcg/mL for patients with hospital-acquired pneumonia) *Tobramycin and gentamicin:* Peak = 4–10 mcg/mL, depending on the infection; Trough = 0.5–2 mcg/mL for serious infections; <1 mcg/mL for hospital-acquired pneumonia • Target serum concentrations (for extended-interval dosing) (peaks not routinely monitored): *Amikacin:* Trough <8 mcg/mL (The ATS recommends trough levels of <4–5 mcg/mL for patients with hospital-acquired pneumonia) *Tobramycin and gentamicin:* Trough = 0.5–2 mcg/mL for serious infections, <1 mcg/mL for hospital-acquired pneumonia • Bethkis, Kitabis Pak, and TOBI used for patients with cystic fibrosis (*Pseudomonas*)

Macrolides

Generic • Brand • Dose/Dosage Forms	Spectrum of Activity	Contraindications	Primary Side Effects	Pertinent Drug Interactions	Med Pearl
Mechanism of action – inhibit bacterial protein synthesis by binding to the 50S subunit of the bacterial ribosome; bacteriostatic					
Macrolides					
Azithromycin ☆ • AzaSite, Zithromax, Zmax • 250–500 mg PO/IV q24h • Zmax: 2 g PO × 1 • Injection, ophthalmic solution, suspension (IR and ER), tabs Clarithromycin ☆ • Biaxin • IR: 250–500 mg PO q12h • ER: 1,000 mg PO q24h • Suspension, tabs (IR and ER) Erythromycin • E.E.S, Erygel, EryPed, Ery-Tab, Erythrocin, PCE • 250–500 mg PO q6h • 500 mg–1 g IV q6h • Caps, injection, ophthalmic ointment, suspension, tabs, topical gel/ointment/solution Fidaxomicin • Dificid • 200 mg PO q12h • Tabs	• Gram (+) organisms (esp. *Streptococcus*); azithromycin and clarithromycin have better activity against *Streptococcus* than erythromycin • Gram (−) organisms • Atypical organisms (e.g., *Chlamydia pneumoniae, Legionella, Mycoplasma pneumoniae*) • Azithromycin and clarithromycin active against *Mycobacteria* • Fidaxomicin active against *Clostridium difficile*	QT interval prolongation or concurrent use with other drugs that prolong QT interval (azithromycin, clarithromycin, and erythromycin)	• Prolonged QT interval (azithromycin, clarithromycin, and erythromycin) • N/V/D • Phlebitis (erythromycin IV) • Stevens-Johnson syndrome, toxic epidermal necrolysis	• Clarithromycin and erythromycin are major substrates and inhibitors of CYP3A4 (azithromycin less affected by CYP interactions) • CYP3A4 inhibitors may ↑ risk of side effects of clarithromycin and erythromycin • CYP3A4 inducers may ↓ effects of clarithromycin and erythromycin • Clarithromycin and erythromycin may ↑ effect/toxicity of CYP3A4 substrates • ↑ risk of torsade de pointes (TdP) with other drugs that prolong QT interval (azithromycin, clarithromycin, and erythromycin) • Azithromycin, clarithromycin, and erythromycin may ↑ risk of bleeding of warfarin • Azithromycin, clarithromycin, and erythromycin may ↑ risk of digoxin toxicity	• Azithromycin ER suspension is not interchangeable with IR formulations • 400 mg erythromycin ethylsuccinate (EES) = 250 mg erythromycin base or stearate • Azithromycin, clarithromycin, and erythromycin are good alternatives for patients allergic to penicillin • Take with food to ↓ gastrointestinal (GI) effect • Clarithromycin can be used in three-drug regimen for *H. pylori* • Erythromycin can be used for diabetic gastroparesis and acne • Take ER azithromycin suspension 1 hour before or 2 hours after meals • Take ER clarithromycin tabs with food to ↑ absorption • Azithromycin or erythromycin preferred in pregnancy • Use clarithromycin with caution in patients with coronary artery disease (↑ mortality) • Fidaxomicin used to treat *Clostridium difficile*

Tetracyclines

Generic • Brand • Dose/Dosage Forms	Spectrum of Activity	Contraindications	Primary Side Effects	Pertinent Drug Interactions	Med Pearl
Mechanism of action – inhibit bacterial protein synthesis by binding to the 30S subunit of the bacterial ribosome; bacteriostatic					
Demeclocycline • Only available generically • 150 mg PO q6h or 300 mg PO q12h • Tabs Doxycycline☆ • Acticlate, Doryx, Monodox, Oracea, Vibramycin • 100 mg IV/PO q12h • Caps, delayed-release caps/tabs, injection, suspension, syrup, tabs Minocycline☆ • Minocin, Minolira, Solodyn • 100 mg PO q12h • Caps, injection, tabs (IR and ER) Tetracycline • Only available generically • 250–500 mg PO q6–12h • Caps	• Gram (+) organisms • Gram (−) organisms • Atypical organisms	Children ≤8 yr and pregnant/breast-feeding women (may cause permanent teeth discoloration and impaired teeth/bone growth)	• N/V/D • Photosensitivity • Phlebitis (IV) • Vertigo (minocycline) • Intracranial hypertension (pseudotumor cerebri)	• Absorption ↓ with antacids, dairy products, and products containing iron, magnesium, aluminum, calcium, or zinc (separate by 2 hr) • Tetracycline is a CYP3A4 substrate • CYP3A4 inhibitors may ↑ risk of side effects of tetracycline • CYP3A4 inducers may ↓ effects • May ↑ risk of bleeding with warfarin • May ↓ effects of oral contraceptives • Use with isotretinoin may ↑ risk of intracranial hypertension	• Good alternative for patients allergic to penicillin • Demeclocycline also used to treat syndrome of inappropriate antidiuretic hormone secretion (SIADH) • Tetracycline can be used in four-drug regimen for *H. pylori* • All except demeclocycline can be used for acne • Doxycycline is drug of choice for Lyme disease • Take demeclocycline and tetracycline 1 hour before or 2 hours after meals • Do not use after expiration date (can cause Fanconi syndrome) • Adjust dose for all, except doxycycline, in renal impairment

Glycylcyclines

Generic • Brand • Dose/Dosage Forms	Spectrum of Activity	Contraindications	Primary Side Effects	Pertinent Drug Interactions	Med Pearl
Mechanism of action – inhibits bacterial protein synthesis by binding to the 30S subunit of the bacterial ribosome (mechanism similar to tetracyclines); bacteriostatic					
Tigecycline • Tygacil • 100 mg IV × 1, then 50 mg IV q12h • Injection	• Gram (+) organisms (MSSA, MRSA, vancomycin-sensitive *Enterococcus faecalis*) • Gram (−) organisms (*E. coli, Enterobacter, H. influenzae, Klebsiella, Legionella*)	Children ≤8 yr and pregnant/breast-feeding women (may cause permanent teeth discoloration and impaired teeth/bone growth)	• N/V/D • Infusion site reaction • Photosensitivity • Hepatotoxicity • Pancreatitis	May ↑ risk of bleeding with warfarin	• Indicated for complicated SSTIs, complicated intra-abdominal infections, and community-acquired pneumonia • Structurally similar to tetracyclines

Oxazolidinones

Generic • Brand • Dose/Dosage Forms	Spectrum of Activity	Contraindications	Primary Side Effects	Pertinent Drug Interactions	Med Pearl
Mechanism of action – inhibit bacterial protein synthesis by binding to the 50S subunit of the bacterial ribosome; bacteriostatic					
Linezolid☆ • Zyvox • 400–600 mg IV/PO q12h • Injection, suspension, tabs	Gram (+) organisms (vancomycin-resistant *Enterococcus faecium* [VRE], MRSA, resistant *Strep. pneumoniae*)	• Concurrent or recent (within 2 wk) use of MAO inhibitors (MAOI) • Patients with uncontrolled hypertension, pheochromocytoma, thyrotoxicosis, and/or taking sympathomimetic agents (e.g., pseudoephedrine), vasopressor agents (e.g., epinephrine), or dopaminergic agents (e.g., dopamine) • Concurrent use of selective serotonin reuptake inhibitors, tricyclic antidepressants, 5-HT$_1$ receptor agonists (triptans), meperidine or buspirone	• N/V/D • Headache • Myelosuppression (more common if therapy >2 wk) • Peripheral/optic neuropathy (more common if therapy >4 wk) • Seizures	• Avoid taking with foods or beverages with high tyramine content (may ↑ risk of hypertensive crises) • Use with serotonergic agents may ↑ risk of serotonin syndrome; avoid concurrent use • Use with adrenergic agents (e.g., dopamine, epinephrine) may ↑ risk of hypertensive crises • Use with tramadol may ↑ risk of seizures • Use with insulin or oral hypoglycemic agents may ↑ risk of hypoglycemia	• Indicated for nosocomial/community-acquired pneumonia, SSTIs, and VRE • Weak MAOI • Monitor complete blood count (CBC) weekly if therapy >2 wk
Tedizolid • Sivextro • 200 mg IV/PO q24h × 6 days • Injection, tabs	Gram (+) organisms (MSSA, MRSA, *Enterococcus faecalis, Streptococcus*)	None	• N/V/D • Headache • Dizziness	None	• Indicated for SSTIs • Weak MAOI

Streptogramin

Generic • Brand • Dose/Dosage Forms	Spectrum of Activity	Contraindications	Primary Side Effects	Pertinent Drug Interactions	Med Pearl
Mechanism of action – inhibits bacterial protein synthesis by binding to the 50S subunit of the bacterial ribosome; bactericidal					
Quinupristin-dalfopristin • Synercid • 7.5 mg/kg IV q8–12h • Injection	Gram (+) organisms (MSSA and *Strep. pyogenes*)	None	• N/V/D • Infusion site reactions (pain, phlebitis) • Muscle/joint pain • ↑ bilirubin	• CYP3A4 inhibitor • May ↑ effect/toxicity of CYP3A4 substrates	• Indicated for complicated SSTIs • Flush line with D5W before and after infusion • If infusion reaction occurs, can ↑ volume of diluent or administer via central line

Fluoroquinolones

Generic • Brand • Dose/Dosage Forms	Spectrum of Activity	Contraindications	Primary Side Effects	Pertinent Drug Interactions	Med Pearl
Mechanism of action – inhibit bacterial DNA topoisomerase and gyrase → inhibit bacterial DNA replication; bactericidal					
Besifloxacin • Besivance • 1 drop TID • Ophthalmic solution Ciprofloxacin☆ • Cetraxal, Ciloxan, Cipro, Cipro XR, Otipro • IR: 250–750 mg PO q12h • ER: 500 mg–1 g PO q24h • IV: 200–400 mg IV q8–12h • Injection, ophthalmic ointment/solution, suspension, otic solution/suspension, tabs (ER and IR) Gatifloxacin • Zymaxid • 1 drop q2h while awake on day 1, then 1 drop 2–4 times/day while awake • Ophthalmic solution Gemifloxacin • Factive • 320 mg PO q24h • Tabs Levofloxacin☆ • Levaquin • 250–750 mg IV/PO q24h • Injection, ophthalmic solution, solution, tabs Moxifloxacin☆ • Avelox, Moxeza, Vigamox • 400 mg IV/PO q24h • Injection, ophthalmic solution, tabs Ofloxacin • Ocuflox • 200–400 mg PO q12h • Ophthalmic solution, otic solution, tabs	• Gram (+) organisms (levofloxacin, gemifloxacin, and moxifloxacin have greatest activity against *Streptococcus*) • Gram (–) organisms • Ciprofloxacin active against *Pseudomonas aeruginosa* • Atypical organisms	• Children <18 yr and pregnant/breastfeeding women (may cause impaired bone growth) • Concurrent use with other drugs that prolong QT interval • Myasthenia gravis	• N/D • Photosensitivity • Tendinitis/tendon rupture • Hyper-/hypoglycemia • Peripheral neuropathy • Seizures • Prolonged QT interval	• Absorption ↓ with antacids, dairy products, and products containing iron, magnesium, aluminum, calcium, or zinc (separate by 2 hr) • Use with corticosteroids may ↑ risk of tendon rupture • Use with nonsteroidal anti-inflammatory drugs (NSAIDs) may ↑ risk of seizures • Ciprofloxacin and ofloxacin are strong CYP1A2 inhibitors • Ciprofloxacin and ofloxacin may ↑ effects of CYP1A2 substrates • Ciprofloxacin may ↓ phenytoin levels • May ↑ risk of bleeding with warfarin • Use with antidiabetic agents may ↑ risk of hypoglycemia • ↑ risk of TdP with other drugs that prolong QT interval	• Should only be used when patients have no other alternative treatment options for chronic bronchitis, uncomplicated UTI, and acute sinusitis • Ciprofloxacin ER and IR tabs are not interchangeable • Adjust dose for all, except moxifloxacin, in renal impairment • Take levofloxacin oral solution 1 hr before or 2 hr after meals • Patients with diabetes should monitor their blood glucose more frequently • Ciprofloxacin, levofloxacin, and moxifloxacin can be used to treat plague (*Yersinia pestis*) • Ophthalmic preparations used to treat bacterial conjunctivitis

Sulfonamide

Generic • Brand • Dose/Dosage Forms	Spectrum of Activity	Contraindications	Primary Side Effects	Pertinent Drug Interactions	Med Pearl
Mechanism of action – inhibits incorporation of para-aminobenzoic acid (PABA) into DNA → inhibits folic acid production and bacterial growth; bacteriostatic					
Trimethoprim/sulfa-methoxazole☆ • Bactrim, Septra, Sulfatrim • 1 double-strength tab PO q12h • 10–20 mg/kg/day of TMP IV in divided doses • Injection, suspension, tabs	• Gram (+) organisms (including MSSA, MRSA) • Gram (−) organisms • TMP/SMX is 1st-line drug to treat/prevent *Pneumocystis jiroveci* pneumonia (PJP)	• Sulfa allergy • Porphyria • Megaloblastic anemia • Infants and pregnant/breast-feeding women (↑ risk of kernicterus) • Glucose-6-phosphate dehydrogenase (G6PD) deficiency	• N/V/D • Rash • Stevens-Johnson syndrome • Photosensitivity • Folate deficiency • Hypoglycemia (in patients with diabetes)	• May ↑ effects/toxicity of methotrexate • May ↑ risk of bleeding with warfarin • Use with antidiabetic agents may ↑ risk of hypoglycemia	• Instruct patients to take with a full glass of water (to prevent crystalluria) • Adjust dose in renal impairment

Cyclic Lipopeptide

Generic • Brand • Dose/Dosage Forms	Spectrum of Activity	Contraindications	Primary Side Effects	Pertinent Drug Interactions	Med Pearl
Mechanism of action – binds to bacterial cell membranes and causes rapid depolarization → inhibits protein, DNA, and RNA synthesis; bactericidal					
Daptomycin • Cubicin • 4–6 mg/kg IV q24h • Injection	Gram (+) organisms (MSSA, MRSA, vancomycin-sensitive *Enterococcus faecalis*)	Children <1 yr (↑ risk of muscular, neuromuscular, and/or central nervous system [CNS] toxicity)	• N/D • Infusion site reactions • Myopathy/rhabdomyolysis • Peripheral neuropathy • Eosinophilic pneumonia	Use with statins may ↑ risk of myopathy; consider discontinuing statin therapy throughout treatment	• Monitor creatine kinase levels weekly • Adjust dose in renal impairment • Indicated for complicated SSTIs and *Staph. aureus* bloodstream infections

Glycopeptides

Generic • Brand • Dose/Dosage Forms	Spectrum of Activity	Contraindications	Primary Side Effects	Pertinent Drug Interactions	Med Pearl
Mechanism of action – inhibit bacterial cell wall synthesis; bactericidal					
Dalbavancin • Dalvance • 1,000 mg IV × 1, then 500 mg IV 1 wk later **OR** 1,500 mg IV × 1 • Injection	Gram (+) organisms (MSSA, MRSA, *Streptococcus*, vancomycin-sensitive *Enterococcus faecalis*)	None	• Hypersensitivity reactions • Headache • N/D • Red-man syndrome (flushing, hypotension, erythema, pruritus)	None	• Indicated for SSTIs • Adjust dose in renal impairment • If red-man syndrome occurs, ↓ infusion rate
Oritavancin • Orbactiv • 1,200 mg IV × 1 • Injection	Gram (+) organisms (MSSA, MRSA, *Streptococcus*, vancomycin-sensitive *Enterococcus faecalis*)	Use of IV unfractionated heparin × 5 days after administration	• Hypersensitivity reactions • Headache • N/V/D • Red-man syndrome	May ↑ risk of bleeding with warfarin	• Indicated for SSTIs • If red-man syndrome occurs, ↓ infusion rate • May falsely ↑ prothrombin time (PT), international normalized ratio (INR), activated partial thromboplastin time (aPTT), and activated clotting time (ACT) (PT/INR effects can last up to 12 hr after discontinuation; aPTT effects can last up to 5 days after discontinuation; ACT effects can last up to 24 hr after discontinuation)

Glycopeptides *(cont'd)*

Generic • Brand • Dose/Dosage Forms	Spectrum of Activity	Contraindications	Primary Side Effects	Pertinent Drug Interactions	Med Pearl
Telavancin • Vibativ • 10 mg/kg IV q24h • Injection	Gram (+) organisms (MSSA, MRSA, *Streptococcus*, vancomycin-sensitive *Enterococcus faecalis*)	• Pregnancy • Concurrent use of IV unfractionated heparin	• Hypersensitivity reactions • Insomnia • Headache • Nephrotoxicity • Red-man syndrome • Metallic taste • N/V/D • QT interval prolongation	• ↑ risk of nephrotoxicity when used with amphotericin B, loop diuretics, tacrolimus, cyclosporine, or cisplatin • ↑ risk of TdP with other drugs that prolong QT interval	• Indicated for complicated SSTIs and hospital-acquired and ventilator-associated pneumonia • ↑ risk of mortality in hospital-acquired and ventilator-associated pneumonia in patients with CrCl ≤50 mL/min • Adjust dose in renal impairment • Monitor renal function • If red-man syndrome occurs, ↓ infusion rate • May falsely ↑ PT, INR, aPTT, and ACT (can last up to 18 hr after discontinuation) • Has REMS program
Vancomycin • Vancocin • 125–250 mg PO q6h • 500 mg–1 g IV q12h • Caps, injection	• Gram (+) organisms (MSSA, MRSA) • *Clostridium difficile*	None	• Red-man syndrome • Nephrotoxicity • Ototoxicity	↑ risk of nephrotoxicity when used with amphotericin B, loop diuretics, tacrolimus, cyclosporine, or cisplatin	• Bactericidal effect is time-dependent • Adjust dose in renal impairment • Often used in patients with penicillin allergy • Use PO (NOT IV) to treat *Clostridium difficile* (PO not effective for any other type of infection) • If red-man syndrome occurs, ↓ infusion rate • Target serum concentrations (peaks not routinely monitored); trough ≥10 mcg/mL (15–20 mcg/mL for complicated infections)

Miscellaneous Antibacterial Agents

Generic • Brand • Dose/Dosage Forms	Spectrum of Activity	Contraindications	Primary Side Effects	Pertinent Drug Interactions	Med Pearl
Mechanism of action – inhibits bacterial protein synthesis by binding to the 50S subunit of the bacterial ribosome; bacteriostatic					
Chloramphenicol • Only available generically • 12.5–25 mg/kg IV q6h • Injection	• Gram (+) organisms (VRE) • Gram (−) organisms	Neonates (↑ risk of gray-baby syndrome)	• N/V/D • Myelosuppression (anemia, leukopenia, thrombocytopenia, aplastic anemia) • Gray-baby syndrome (vomiting, lethargy, respiratory depression, death) • Optic neuritis	• Phenobarbital and rifampin may ↓ effects • May ↑ effects of warfarin and phenytoin	• Only used for life-threatening infections • Monitor CBC frequently • Target serum concentrations: Peak = 15–25 mcg/mL; Trough = 5–10 mcg/mL
Mechanism of action – inhibits bacterial protein synthesis by binding to the 50S subunit of the bacterial ribosome; bacteriostatic					
Clindamycin☆ • Cleocin, Clindagel, Clindesse, Evoclin • 150–450 mg PO q6h • 300–900 mg IV q8h • Caps, injection, solution, topical foam/gel/lotion/pledgets/solution, vaginal cream/suppository	• Gram (+) organisms • Anaerobes	History of pseudomembranous colitis or ulcerative colitis	• N/V/D • Pseudomembranous colitis (*Clostridium difficile*) (highest incidence) • Metallic taste	• CYP3A4 substrate • CYP3A4 inhibitors may ↑ risk of side effects • CYP3A4 inducers may ↓ effects	• Also used for acne (topical) • Patients using intravaginally should avoid intercourse (↓ efficacy of condoms and diaphragms)
Mechanism of action – interferes with bacterial DNA synthesis; bactericidal					
Metronidazole☆ • Flagyl, Flagyl ER, Metro, Metrocream, Metrogel, Metrolotion, Noritate, Nuvessa, Vandazole • 250–500 mg PO q8–12h • 500 mg IV q8–12h • Caps, injection, tabs (ER and IR), topical cream/gel/lotion, vaginal gel	• Anaerobes • *Clostridium difficile*	Pregnancy (1st trimester)	• N/D • Confusion • Dizziness • Peripheral neuropathy • Metallic taste	• Disulfiram-like reaction may occur if alcohol is used during treatment • May ↑ effects of warfarin and lithium • Phenobarbital and phenytoin may ↓ effects • Cimetidine may ↑ effects	• Can be used in four-drug regimen for *H. pylori* • Drug of choice for *Clostridium difficile* • Take ER tabs 1 hour before or 2 hours after meals

Antifungal Agents

Azole Antifungals

Generic • Brand • Dose/Dosage Forms	Spectrum of Activity	Contraindications	Primary Side Effects	Pertinent Drug Interactions	Med Pearl
Mechanism of action – inhibit synthesis of ergosterol (essential component of fungal cell membrane) • Imidazoles: butoconazole, clotrimazole, econazole, efinaconazole, ketoconazole, luliconazole, miconazole, oxiconazole, sulconazole, tioconazole • Triazoles: fluconazole, itraconazole, isavuconazonium terconazole, posaconazole, voriconazole					
Fluconazole ☆ • Diflucan • 100–800 mg IV/PO q24h • Injection, suspension, tabs	• *Candida* spp. • *Coccidioides* spp. • *Histoplasma* spp. • *Cryptococcus* spp.	None	• Headache • N/V/D • Abdominal pain • Rash • ↑ liver function tests (LFTs) • Prolonged QT interval	• CYP2C9, CYP2C19, and CYP3A4 inhibitor • May ↑ effect/toxicity of CYP2C9, CYP2C19, and CYP3A4 substrates • Rifampin may ↓ effects • ↑ risk of TdP with other drugs that prolong QT interval	• Adjust dose in renal impairment • Conversion from IV to PO is 1:1 • Monitor LFTs
Isavuconazonium • Cresemba • 372 mg IV/PO q8h × 6 doses (48 hr), then 372 mg IV/PO q24h • Caps, injection	• *Aspergillus* spp. • *Mucormycetes* spp.	• Concurrent use of strong CYP3A4 inhibitors or inducers • Familial short QT syndrome	• ↑ LFTs • Infusion reactions • Rash • N/V/D • Headache • Shortened QT interval	• CYP3A4 substrate and inhibitor • CYP3A4 inhibitors may ↑ risk of side effects • CYP3A4 inducers may ↓ effects • May ↑ effect/toxicity of CYP3A4 substrates • ↑ risk of digoxin toxicity	Monitor LFTs
Itraconazole • Onmel, Sporanox • 100–400 mg/day PO • Caps, solution, tabs	• *Candida* spp. • *Coccidioides* spp. • *Histoplasma* spp. • *Cryptococcus* spp. • *Aspergillus* spp.	• Concurrent use of disopyramide, dofetilide, dronedarone, eplerenone, ergot alkaloids, felodipine, irinotecan, ivabradine, lovastatin, lurasidone, methadone, midazolam, nisoldipine, pimozide, ranolazine, quinidine, simvastatin, ticagrelor, or triazolam • HF	• Nausea • Abdominal pain • Rash • ↑ LFTs • Prolonged QT interval	• CYP3A4 substrate and inhibitor • CYP3A4 inhibitors may ↑ risk of side effects • CYP3A4 inducers may ↓ effects • May ↑ effect/toxicity of CYP3A4 substrates • ↑ risk of digoxin toxicity • Absorption ↓ with antacids, H₂ antagonists, and proton pump inhibitors (PPIs) (acidic environment required for absorption) (separate by 2 hr) • ↑ risk of TdP with other drugs that prolong QT interval	• Caps and solution cannot be used interchangeably (bioavailability of solution > caps) • Potent negative inotrope • Monitor LFTs
Ketoconazole ☆ • Extina, Nizoral, Xolegel • 200–400 mg PO q24h • Rx: Tabs, topical cream/foam/gel/shampoo • OTC: Shampoo	• *Candida* spp. • *Coccidioides* spp. • *Histoplasma* spp. • *Cryptococcus* spp.	• Concurrent use of ergot alkaloids • Hepatic impairment	• N/V • Gynecomastia • Sexual dysfunction • ↑ LFTs • Prolonged QT interval	Same as itraconazole	• May ↓ testosterone levels • Monitor LFTs

Azole Antifungals *(cont'd)*

Generic • Brand • Dose/Dosage Forms	Spectrum of Activity	Contraindications	Primary Side Effects	Pertinent Drug Interactions	Med Pearl
Posaconazole • Noxafil • 300 mg IV/PO (tabs) q12h × 1 day, then 300 mg IV/PO (tabs) q24h • 200 mg PO TID (suspension) (for prophylaxis); 100 mg PO BID × 1 day, then 100 mg PO q24h × 13 days (suspension) (for treatment) • Injection, suspension, tabs	• *Candida* spp. • *Aspergillus* spp.	Concurrent use of ergot alkaloids, quinidine, pimozide, sirolimus, atorvastatin, lovastatin, or simvastatin	• Headache • N/V • Rash • ↑ LFTs • Prolonged QT interval	• CYP3A4 inhibitor • May ↑ effect/toxicity of CYP3A4 substrates • Absorption of suspension ↓ with cimetidine and esomeprazole (avoid concurrent use) • Metoclopramide may ↓ effects of suspension • Efavirenz, fosamprenavir, rifabutin, and phenytoin may ↓ effects • ↑ risk of TdP with other drugs that prolong QT interval	• Tabs and suspension cannot be used interchangeably • Take tabs with food to ↑ absorption • Suspension must be taken with full meal (or liquid nutritional supplement or acidic carbonated beverage) to ↑ absorption • IV and tabs ONLY used for prophylaxis of invasive *Aspergillus* or *Candida* infections • Use PO when CrCl <50 mL/min (diluent in IV can accumulate) • Monitor LFTs
Voriconazole • Vfend • 6 mg/kg IV q12h × 24 hr, then 3–4 mg/kg IV q12h or 100–300 mg PO q12h • Injection, suspension, tabs	• *Candida* spp. • *Aspergillus* spp.	Concurrent use of pimozide, quinidine, long-acting barbiturates, carbamazepine, ergot alkaloids, rifampin, rifabutin, ritonavir (≥ 800 mg/day), efavirenz (≥ 800 mg/day), St. John's wort, or sirolimus	• Visual disturbances (transient) (blurred vision, photophobia, altered perception of color) • Rash • Photosensitivity • ↑ LFTs • Hallucinations • N/V • Prolonged QT interval	• CYP2C9 and CYP2C19 substrate • CYP2C9, CYP2C19, and CYP3A4 inhibitor • May ↑ effect/toxicity of CYP2C9, CYP2C19, and CYP3A4 substrates • CYP2C9 and CYP2C19 inhibitors may ↑ risks of side effects • CYP2C9 and CYP2C19 inducers may ↓ effects • May ↑ efavirenz levels • Efavirenz may ↓ effects • ↑ risk of TdP with other drugs that prolong QT interval	• ↓ dose of cyclosporine by 50% • When using with efavirenz, ↑ voriconazole dose and ↓ efavirenz dose • ↑ dose of voriconazole when using with phenytoin • Use PO when CrCl <50 mL/min (diluent in IV can accumulate) • Take PO 1 hour before or after meals • Monitor LFTs and vision

Echinocandins

Generic • Brand • Dose/Dosage Forms	Spectrum of Activity	Contraindications	Primary Side Effects	Pertinent Drug Interactions	Med Pearl
Mechanism of action – inhibit synthesis of 1,3-β-d-glucan (essential component of fungal cell wall)					
Anidulafungin • Eraxis • 100–200 mg IV on day 1, then 50–100 mg IV q24h • Injection	• *Candida* spp. • *Aspergillus* spp. (caspofungin only)	None	• N/V • Headache • Hypokalemia • Rash • Fever • ↑ LFTs • Phlebitis	None	Monitor LFTs
Caspofungin • Cancidas • 70 mg IV on day 1, then 50 mg IV q24h • Injection				• Rifampin, carbamazepine, dexamethasone, efavirenz, nevirapine, and phenytoin may ↓ effects • May ↓ tacrolimus levels • Cyclosporine may ↑ risk of side effects	• ↑ dose of caspofungin to 70 mg/day when used with rifampin, carbamazepine, dexamethasone, efavirenz, nevirapine, or phenytoin • Adjust dose in moderate hepatic impairment • Monitor LFTs
Micafungin • Mycamine • 50–150 mg IV q24h • Injection				None	Monitor LFTs

Amphotericin B

Generic • Brand • Dose/Dosage Forms	Spectrum of Activity	Contraindications	Primary Side Effects	Pertinent Drug Interactions	Med Pearl
Mechanism of action – bind to ergosterol in cell membrane $\rightarrow$ produce a channel in cell membrane ($\uparrow$ permeability) $\rightarrow$ allow K^+ and Mg^{2+} to leak out of cell ("leaky membrane") $\rightarrow$ cell death					
Amphotericin B desoxycholate • Only available generically • Test dose of 1 mg IV should be given over 20–30 min (monitor patient for 2–4 hr before starting infusion) • 0.5–1.5 mg/kg/ day IV • Injection Amphotericin B lipid complex (ABLC) • Abelcet • 5 mg/kg IV q24h • Injection Liposomal ampho- tericin B (L-AmB) • AmBisome • 3–6 mg/kg IV q24h • Injection	• *Candida* spp. • *Coccidioides* spp. • *Blastomyces* spp. • *Histoplasma* spp. • *Cryptococcus* spp. • *Aspergillus* spp.	None	• Nephrotoxicity (less common with lipid-based formulations) • Infusion reactions (fever, chills, hypoten- sion, nausea, tachypnea) • Phlebitis • Electrolyte disturbances (i.e., hypokalemia, hypomagnese- mia)	$\uparrow$ risk of nephrotoxic- ity when used with amino- glycosides, loop diuretics, tacrolimus, cyclosporine, or cisplatin	• May premedicate with acetaminophen, NSAIDs, diphenhydramine, and/or corticosteroid to prevent infusion reactions (give 30–60 min before infusion); meperidine may be used for rigors • Infusion reactions less common with lipid-based formulations (amphotericin B deoxycholate > ABLC > L-Amb) • Infusion reactions $\downarrow$ after first few doses • Sodium loading (500 mL of 0.9% NaCl IV before and after infusion) may $\downarrow$ risk of nephrotoxicity with amphotericin B desoxycholate • Monitor blood urea nitrogen (BUN)/serum creatinine (SCr), potassium, and magnesium

Other Antifungals

Generic • Brand • Dose/Dosage Forms	Spectrum of Activity	Contraindications	Primary Side Effects	Pertinent Drug Interactions	Med Pearl
Mechanism of action – similar to amphotericin B					
Nystatin ☆ • Nystop • Suspension: 400,000–600,000 units 4 times/day • Topical: Apply 2–3 times daily • Suspension, tabs, topical cream/ointment/powder	*Candida* spp.	None	• N/V/D • Abdominal pain	None	Suspension should be swished and swallowed
Mechanism of action – inhibits squalene epoxidase → inhibits synthesis of ergosterol					
Terbinafine ☆ • Lamisil • PO: 250 mg q24h • Topical: Apply 1–2 times daily • Rx: Granules, tabs, topical solution • OTC: Topical cream/gel/solution	*Trichophyton* spp.	• Hepatic impairment • CrCl <50 mL/min	• Headache • N/V/D • ↑ LFTs	• CYP2D6 inhibitor • May ↑ effect/toxicity of CYP2D6 substrates • May ↓ cyclosporine levels	• Oral used for onychomycosis or tinea capitis (scalp ringworm); topical used for tinea pedis (athlete's foot), tinea corporis (ringworm), or tinea cruris (jock itch) • Give for 6 wk for fingernail infection; 12 wk for toenail infection • Monitor LFTs
Mechanism of action – inhibits fungal protein synthesis					
Tavaborole • Kerydin • Apply once daily × 48 wk • Topical solution	*Trichophyton* spp.	None	Application reactions	None	Indicated for onychomycosis

Other Antifungals *(cont'd)*

Generic • Brand • Dose/Dosage Forms	Spectrum of Activity	Contraindications	Primary Side Effects	Pertinent Drug Interactions	Med Pearl
Mechanism of action – enters fungal cell wall → converted into 5-fluorouracil, which interferes with fungal RNA and protein synthesis					
Flucytosine • Ancobon • 25–37.5 mg/kg PO q6h (administered with amphotericin B) • Caps	• *Candida* spp. • *Cryptococcus* spp.	None	• Confusion • Hallucinations • Ataxia • Headache • N/V/D • ↑ LFTs • Renal impairment • Bone marrow depression	None	• Should not be used as monotherapy • Adjust dose in renal impairment • Monitor LFTs, BUN/SCr, and CBC • Flucytosine concentrations: Peak: 50–100 mcg/mL; Trough: 25–50 mcg/mL
Mechanism of action – inhibits fungal cell mitosis					
Griseofulvin • Gris-PEG • Microsize: 500–1,000 mg/day PO • Ultramicrosize: 375 mg/day PO • Microsize: Suspension, tabs • Ultramicrosize: Tabs	*Trichophyton* spp.	• Hepatic impairment • Porphyria	• Rash/hives • N/V/D • Headache • Confusion • Photosensitivity	• Barbiturates may ↓ effects • May ↓ effects of cyclosporine and warfarin • Disulfiram-like reaction may occur if alcohol is used during treatment	• Monitor LFTs • Administer with high-fat meal to ↑ absorption

Antiviral Agents

Drugs for Treatment of Herpes Simplex Virus and Varicella-Zoster Virus

Generic • Brand • Dose/Dosage Forms	Spectrum of Activity	Contraindications	Primary Side Effects	Pertinent Drug Interactions	Med Pearl
Mechanism of action – inhibit viral DNA polymerase → inhibit replication of viral DNA					
Acyclovir☆ • Sitavig, Zovirax • *Genital herpes (initial episode):* 200 mg PO 5 times/day × 7–10 days **OR** 5 mg/kg IV q8h × 5–7 days • *Herpes labialis (cold sores):* 400 mg PO 5 times/day × 5 days • *Varicella (chickenpox):* 800 mg PO q6h × 5 days **OR** 10 mg/kg IV q8h × 7 days • *Herpes zoster (shingles):* 800 mg PO 5 times/day × 7–10 days **OR** 10 mg/kg IV q8h × 7 days • Buccal tabs, caps injection, suspension, tabs, topical cream/ointment	• Herpes simplex virus (HSV)-1 (herpes labialis) and HSV-2 (genital herpes) • Varicella zoster virus (causes chickenpox and shingles)	None	• N/V/D • Headache • Phlebitis (IV acyclovir) • Renal impairment (IV acyclovir) • Seizures (esp. in patients with renal impairment)	None	• Adjust dose for all, except penciclovir, in renal impairment • To avoid renal damage with IV acyclovir (can crystallize), infuse slowly and keep patient hydrated • Sitavig is a buccal tab for treatment of recurrent cold sores
Famciclovir☆ (prodrug of penciclovir) • Only available generically • *Genital herpes (initial episode):* 250 mg PO q8h × 7–10 days • *Cold sores:* 1,500 mg PO × 1 • *Herpes zoster:* 500 mg PO q8h × 7 days • Tabs					
Penciclovir • Denavir • *Cold sores:* Apply q2h while awake × 4 days • Topical cream					
Valacyclovir☆ (prodrug of acyclovir) • Valtrex • *Genital herpes (initial episode):* 1 g PO q12h × 10 days • *Genital herpes (recurrence):* 500 mg PO q12h × 3 days • *Cold sores:* 2 g PO q12h × 1 day • *Herpes zoster:* 1 g PO q8h × 7 days • Tabs					

Drugs for Treatment of Cytomegalovirus

Generic • Brand • Dose/Dosage Forms	Spectrum of Activity	Contraindications	Primary Side Effects	Pertinent Drug Interactions	Med Pearl
Mechanism of action – inhibit replication of viral DNA					
Cidofovir • Only available generically • 5 mg/kg IV once weekly × 2 wk, then q2 wk • Injection	• Cytomegalovirus • HSV (foscarnet) • Acute herpetic keratitis (ophthalmic gangiclovir)	• SCr >1.5 mg/dL, CrCl ≤55 mL/min, or proteinuria • Use of other nephrotoxic drugs within 7 days	• Nephrotoxicity • Neutropenia • Metabolic acidosis • ↓ intraocular pressure • Uveitis/iritis	Use of antiretroviral drugs may ↑ risk of side effects	• Monitor BUN/SCr • To minimize renal damage, administer 1 L of 0.9% NaCl before and after each infusion; also give 2 g of probenecid 3 hr before each infusion and then 1 g at 2 hr and 8 hr after each infusion • If SCr ↑ by 0.3–0.4 mg/dL above baseline, ↓ dose to 3 mg/kg; if SCr ↑ by ≥0.5 mg/dL, discontinue • Advise patients to use effective contraception
Foscarnet • Foscavir • 60 mg/kg IV q8h **OR** 90 mg/kg IV q12h × 14–21 days, then 90–120 mg/kg IV q24h • Injection		None	• Nephrotoxicity • N/V • Anemia • Electrolyte disturbances • Genital sores • Seizures	• ↑ risk of nephrotoxicity when used with amphotericin B, aminoglycosides, loop diuretics, tacrolimus, cyclosporine, or cisplatin • Zidovudine may ↑ risk of anemia	• Adjust dose in renal impairment • Monitor BUN/SCr • To minimize renal damage, administer 1 L of 0.9% NaCl IV with each infusion • Rapid infusion associated with seizures and arrhythmias
Ganciclovir • Cytovene, Zirgan • IV: 5 mg/kg q12h × 14–21 days, then either 5 mg/kg/day 7 times/wk or 6 mg/kg/day 5 times/wk • Ophth: 1 drop 5 times/day until ulcer heals, then 1 drop 3 times/day × 7 days • Injection, ophthalmic gel		• Neutropenia • Thrombocytopenia • Anemia	• Myelosuppression • Fever • Rash • Phlebitis (IV ganciclovir) • ↑ LFTs • Nephrotoxicity • Seizures • N/V/D	• ↑ risk of myelosuppression when used with other immunosuppressive drugs • ↑ risk of nephrotoxicity when used with amphotericin B, aminoglycosides, loop diuretics, tacrolimus, cyclosporine, or cisplatin • May ↑ effects/toxicity of zidovudine	• Adjust dose in renal impairment • Advise patients to use effective contraception during treatment and for at least 90 days after treatment • Take valganciclovir with food
Valganciclovir (prodrug of ganciclovir) • Valcyte • 900 mg PO q12h × 21 days, then 900 mg PO q24h • Solution, tabs					

Drugs for Treatment of Influenza

Generic • Brand • Dose/Dosage Forms	Spectrum of Activity	Contraindications	Primary Side Effects	Pertinent Drug Interactions	Med Pearl
Mechanism of action – inhibit the enzyme (neuraminidase) responsible for releasing the newly formed mature virus from the host cell					
Oseltamivir • Tamiflu • *Prophylaxis:* 75 mg PO q24h × ≥10 days (6 wk for community outbreak) • *Treatment:* 75 mg PO q12h × 5 days • Caps, suspension	• Influenza A and B • H1N1 influenza	None	• N/V/D • Headache • Rash • Neuropsychiatric events (e.g., confusion, delirium, hallucinations, self-injury)	None	• For prophylaxis, initiate therapy within 2 days of contact with infected person • For treatment, initiate therapy within 2 days of onset of symptoms • Adjust dose in renal impairment • ↓ flu severity and duration by ~ 1 day • Can be used in children ≥1 yr (prophylaxis) or ≥2 wk (treatment)
Peramivir • Rapivab • *Treatment:* 600 mg IV × 1 • Injection			• Rash • Neuropsychiatric events (e.g., confusion, delirium, hallucinations, self-injury)		• Initiate therapy within 2 days of onset of symptoms • For adults only • Adjust dose in renal impairment
Zanamivir • Relenza • *Prophylaxis:* 2 inhalations q24h × 10 days (28 days for community outbreak) • *Treatment:* 2 inhalations q12h × 5 days • Powder for oral inhalation		Asthma/COPD	• Bronchospasm • Cough • Headache • N/D • Rash • Neuropsychiatric events (e.g., confusion, delirium, hallucinations, self-injury)		• For prophylaxis, initiate therapy within 1.5 days (5 days in community setting) of contact with infected person • For treatment, initiate therapy within 2 days of onset of symptoms • ↓ flu severity and duration by ~ 1 day • Can be used in children ≥5 yr (prophylaxis) or ≥7 yr (treatment)

HUMAN IMMUNODEFICIENCY VIRUS

Guidelines Summary

For the NAPLEX, make learning the names of the medications and their respective classes a priority.

- Memorize the non-nucleoside reverse transcriptase inhibitors (NNRTIs)
  - Efavirenz, nevirapine, etravirine, rilpivirine
- All protease inhibitors (PIs) end in "-navir"
  - Examples: Darunavir, atazanavir, ritonavir
- There are only three integrase inhibitors: Dolutegravir, raltegravir, elvitegravir
- There is only one fusion inhibitor: Enfuvirtide
- There is only one CCR5 inhibitor: Maraviroc
- The remaining agents are nucleoside reverse transcriptase inhibitors (NRTIs)
  - Tenofovir, emtricitabine, abacavir, lamivudine, zidovudine, didanosine, stavudine

For the exam, know that antiretroviral therapy is now recommended for ALL HIV-infected patients (regardless of CD4 count). Increased urgency to initiate antiretroviral therapy in following patient populations:

- AIDS-defining condition (including HIV-associated dementia and AIDS-associated malignancies)
- Acute opportunistic infection
- CD4 count <200 cells/mm^3
- HIV-associated nephropathy
- Hepatitis B or hepatitis C co-infection
- Pregnancy
- Acute HIV infection

For the exam, know the signature side effects for the major drug classes (NNRTIs, NRTIs, and PIs) and know the five antiviral regimens that are recommended for starting therapy in treatment-naïve patients:

- Darunavir + ritonavir + tenofovir (disoproxil fumarate or alafenamide) + emtricitabine
- Dolutegravir + abacavir + lamivudine (only for patients who are HLA-B*5701 negative)
- Dolutegravir + tenofovir (disoproxil fumarate or alafenamide) + emtricitabine
- Elvitegravir + cobicistat + tenofovir (disoproxil fumarate or alafenamide) + emtricitabine
- Raltegravir + tenofovir (disoproxil fumarate or alafenamide) + emtricitabine

A summary of acceptable initial combination regimens for antiretroviral naïve patients follows:

- PI-based regimen: PI (boosted with ritonavir or cobicistat) + 2 NRTIs

- Integrase inhibitor-based regimen: Integrase inhibitor + 2 NRTIs

Drugs of Choice

Prophylaxis of First-Episode Opportunistic Infections in Patients with HIV

Opportunistic Infection	Indication	First-Line Therapy
PJP	CD4 count <200 cells/mm^3 **OR** Oropharyngeal candidiasis **OR** History of AIDS-defining illness	TMP/SMX 1 DS tablet PO daily **OR** TMP/SMX 80/400 mg (single-strength [SS]) PO daily
Toxoplasma gondii encephalitis	Toxoplasma IgG (+) with CD4 count <100 cells/mm^3	TMP/SMX 1 DS tablet PO daily
Mycobacterium avium complex (MAC) disease	CD4 count <50 cells/mm^3	Azithromycin 1200 mg PO 1 × weekly **OR** Clarithromycin 500 mg PO BID **OR** Azithromycin 600 mg PO 2 × weekly

Treatment and Secondary Prophylaxis of AIDS-Associated Opportunistic Infections

Opportunistic Infection	First-Line Therapy/Duration
PJP	*Treatment:* TMP/SMX (IV/PO) ± corticosteroids* × 21 days *Secondary Prophylaxis:* TMP/SMX 1 DS tablet PO daily **OR** TMP/SMX 1 SS tablet PO daily
Toxoplasma gondii encephalitis	*Treatment:* Pyrimethamine (PO) + sulfadiazine (PO) + leucovorin[†] (PO) × ≥6 wk *Secondary Prophylaxis:* Pyrimethamine + sulfadiazine + leucovorin[†]
MAC disease	*Treatment:* Clarithromycin (or azithromycin) (PO) + ethambutol (PO) × ≥12 mo *Secondary Prophylaxis:* Clarithromycin (or azithromycin) + ethambutol
Mucocutaneous candidiasis	*Treatment:* Oropharyngeal: Fluconazole (PO) **OR** clotrimazole (troche) **OR** miconazole (buccal) **OR** itraconazole (PO) **OR** posaconazole (PO) **OR** nystatin × 7–14 days Esophageal: Fluconazole (IV/PO) **OR** itraconazole (PO) × 14–21 days *Secondary Prophylaxis:* Usually not recommended unless patients have frequent or severe recurrences
Cryptococcal meningitis	*Treatment:* Induction: Liposomal amphotericin B (IV) + Flucytosine (PO) × ≥2 wk Consolidation: Fluconazole (IV/PO) × ≥8 wk *Secondary Prophylaxis:* Fluconazole (PO)
Cytomegalovirus retinitis	*Treatment:* Ganciclovir (or foscarnet) (via intravitreal injection) × 1–4 doses over 7–10 days + valganciclovir (PO) × 14–21 days *Secondary Prophylaxis:* Valganciclovir (PO)

* Indications for adjunctive corticosteroid therapy for PJP include PaO_2 <70 mmHg (room air) **OR** alveolar-arterial O_2 gradient >35 mmHg.
†Leucovorin reduces the risk of bone marrow suppression associated with pyrimethamine.

Non-Nucleoside Reverse Transcriptase Inhibitors (NNRTIs)

Generic • Brand • Dose/Dosage Forms	Contraindications	Primary Side Effects	Key Monitoring	Pertinent Drug Interactions	Med Pearl
Mechanism of action – bind to an allosteric site on reverse transcriptase that results in a conformational change to the enzyme's active site					
Efavirenz • Sustiva • 600 mg PO QHS • Caps, tabs	None	• Rash • ↑ LFTs • Hyperlipidemia • Drowsiness • Dizziness • Insomnia • Abnormal vivid dreaming • Agitation • Depression • Suicidal thoughts • Hallucinations • Fat redistribution • QT interval prolongation	LFTs	• CYP2B6 and CYP3A4 substrate • CYP2C9 and CYP2C19 inhibitor • CYP2B6 and CYP3A4 inducer • ↑ risk of TDP with other drugs that prolong QT interval	• Can cause a false positive cannabinoid or benzodiazepine screening test • Take on an empty stomach
Etravirine • Intelence • 200 mg PO BID • Tabs	None	• Rash • Nausea • Hypersensitivity reaction • ↑ LFTs • Fat redistribution		• CYP3A4, CYP2C9, and CYP2C19 substrate • CYP2C9 and CYP2C19 inhibitor • CYP3A4 inducer	• May disperse tabs in water • Take with food
Nevirapine • Viramune, Viramune XR • IR: 200 mg PO daily × 2 wk, then 200 mg PO BID • ER: 200 mg PO daily (of IR) × 2 wk, then 400 mg PO daily (of ER) • Suspension, tabs (IR and ER)	Moderate or severe hepatic impairment	• Rash • ↑ LFTs • Fat redistibution		CYP2B6 and CYP3A4 substrate and inducer	• Risk of hepatotoxicity in men and women with CD4 count >400 and >250 cells/mm^3, respectively • Hepatotoxicity often associated with a rash • 2-wk lead-in period with IR helps to ↓ rash
Rilpivirine • Edurant • 25 mg PO daily • Tabs	Concurrent use with carbamazepine, oxcarbazepine, phenobarbital, phenytoin, rifampin, rifapentine, PPIs, dexamethasone, and St. John's wort	• Rash • ↑ LFTs • Depression • Insomnia • Headache • Fat redistribution		• CYP3A4 substrate • Does not inhibit or induce CYP450 enzymes • H$_2$-antagonists, PPIs, and antacids may ↓ absorption (avoid concomitant use of PPIs; may use H$_2$-antagonists or antacids [need to space administration])	• Requires ≥500-calorie meal • ↑ virologic failure with high baseline HIV RNA (>100,000 copies/mL)

Nucleoside Reverse Transcriptase Inhibitors (NRTIs)

Generic • Brand • Dose/Dosage Forms	Contraindications	Primary Side Effects	Key Monitoring	Pertinent Drug Interactions	Med Pearl
Mechanism of action – triphosphate moiety competes with natural substrates for incorporation into proviral DNA that is developed by reverse transcriptase					
Abacavir • Ziagen • 300 mg PO BID or 600 mg PO daily • Solution, tabs	• Discontinue drug promptly and do not rechallenge in patients with hypersensitivity • HLA-B*5701 positive • Moderate or severe hepatic impairment	• Hypersensitivity reaction • Lactic acidosis • Hepatomegaly with steatosis • Fat redistribution	Hypersensitivity symptoms (fever, rash, N/V/D, abdominal pain, malaise, fatigue, dyspnea, cough)	None	Perform HLA-B*5701 test prior to initiating therapy: only use if negative
Didanosine • Videx, Videx EC • ER: ≥60 kg: 400 mg PO daily (250 mg PO daily when used with tenofovir disoproxil fumarate); 25 to <60 kg: 250 mg PO daily (200 mg PO daily when used with tenofovir disoproxil fumarate) • Solution: ≥60 kg: 200 mg PO BID (250 mg PO daily when used with tenofovir disoproxil fumarate); <60 kg: 125 mg PO BID (200 mg PO daily when used with tenofovir disoproxil fumarate) • ER caps, solution	Concurrent use with allopurinol or ribavirin	• Peripheral neuropathy • Pancreatitis • Lactic acidosis • Hepatomegaly with steatosis • Hepatotoxicity • Fat redistribution • N/V/D • Optic neuritis	LFTs	• Tenofovir ↑ levels (↓ didanosine dose) • Ganciclovir ↑ levels • Methadone ↓ levels (use ER didanosine) • ↓ FQ, ketoconazole, and itraconazole levels (space administration)	• Do not crush or open ER caps • Reconstitute powder for oral solution with water or antacid • Adjust dose in renal impairment • Take on an empty stomach (0.5 hr before or 2 hr after meal)
Emtricitabine • Emtriva • Caps: 200 mg PO daily • Solution: 240 mg PO daily • Caps, solution	None	• N/V/D • Hyperpigmentation of palms/soles • Lactic acidosis • Hepatomegaly with steatosis	None	None	Adjust dose in renal impairment

Nucleoside Reverse Transcriptase Inhibitors (NRTIs) *(cont'd)*

Generic • Brand • Dose/Dosage Forms	Contraindications	Primary Side Effects	Key Monitoring	Pertinent Drug Interactions	Med Pearl
Lamivudine • Epivir • 150 mg PO BID or 300 mg PO daily • Solution, tabs	None	• N/V/D • Pancreatitis • Lactic acidosis • Hepatomegaly with steatosis • Fat redistribution	Monitor viral load more frequently with oral solution	None	• Also active against hepatitis B (Epivir HBV) • Adjust dose in renal impairment
Stavudine • Zerit • ≥60 kg: 40 mg PO BID • <60 kg: 30 mg PO BID • Caps, solution	None	• Peripheral neuropathy • Pancreatitis • Lactic acidosis • Hepatomegaly with steatosis • Hepatotoxicity • Fat redistribution • Hyperlipidemia	LFTs	Additive risk of pancreatitis with concurrent didanosine	Adjust dose in renal impairment
Tenofovir Viread (disoproxil fumarate) • 300 mg PO daily • Powder, tabs Vemlidy (alafenamide) • 25 mg PO daily (only indicated for hepatitis B; only available in combination products for HIV) • Tabs	CrCl <30 mL/min (alafenamide)	• Renal impairment (> with disoproxil fumarate) • Fanconi syndrome • ↓ bone mineral density (> with disoproxil fumarate) • Lactic acidosis • Hepatomegaly with steatosis • Headache • N/V/D	• SCr • Bone mineral density	• ↓ atazanavir levels • ↑ didanosine levels (↓ didanosine dose) • Lopinavir/ritonavir, atazanavir/ritonavir, darunavir/ritonavir, acyclovir, valacyclovir, ganciclovir, valganciclovir, aminoglycosides, and NSAIDs ↑ levels	• Also active against hepatitis B • Oral powder can be used if patient unable to swallow tabs • Oral powder should be mixed in soft food (NOT liquids) • Adjust dose of disoproxil fumarate in renal impairment • Alafenamide associated with ↓ risk of renal impairment and reduced bone density
Zidovudine • Retrovir • 300 mg PO BID • 1 mg/kg IV q4h until PO can be taken • Caps, injection, solution, tabs	Concurrent ribavirin due to additive toxicity	• Anemia • Neutropenia • Headache • N/V • Myopathy • Lactic acidosis • Hepatomegaly with steatosis • Fat redistribution • Hyperlipidemia • Nail pigmentation	CBC with differential	None	• Can be used to prevent maternal-fetal HIV transmission • Adjust dose in renal impairment

Protease Inhibitors (PIs)

Generic • Brand • Dose/Dosage Forms	Contraindications	Primary Side Effects	Key Monitoring	Pertinent Drug Interactions	Med Pearl
Mechanism of action – inhibit HIV protease enzyme from processing the gag-pol polyprotein precursor, thereby preventing development and maturation of new HIV particles					
Atazanavir • Reyataz • Therapy naïve: 300 mg PO daily (400 mg PO daily when used with efavirenz) + ritonavir 100 mg PO daily (or cobicistat 150 mg PO daily) **OR** 400 mg PO daily (if unable to tolerate ritonavir) • Therapy experienced: 300 mg PO daily + ritonavir 100 mg PO daily (or cobicistat 150 mg PO daily) • Caps, powder	Concurrent use with alfuzosin, rifampin, irinotecan, triazolam, ergot derivatives, St. John's wort, lovastatin, simvastatin, pimozide, lurasidone sildenafil (for pulmonary hypertension), indinavir, and nevirapine	• Indirect hyper-bilirubinemia • PR interval prolongation • Hyperlipidemia • Hepatotoxicity • N/V • Hyperglycemia • Fat redistribu-tion • Cholelithiasis • Nephrolithiasis • Renal impair-ment • Rash	• LFTs • Bilirubin • Lipids • Blood glucose • Electro-cardio-gram (ECG)	• CYP3A4 inhibitor and substrate • H_2-antagonists, PPIs, and antacids may ↓ absorption (follow guide-lines for using in combination)	• Oral powder used in children ≥3 mo and 10 to <25 kg • Oral powder can be used in adults if patient unable to swallow tabs • Take with food • Adjust dose in hepatic impairment
Darunavir • Prezista • Therapy naïve or therapy experienced (with no da-runavir mutations): 800 mg PO daily + ritonavir 100 mg PO daily (or cobicistat 150 mg PO daily) • Therapy experienced (with ≥1 darunavir resistance associated substitution): 600 mg PO BID + ritonavir 100 mg PO BID • Suspension, tabs	Concurrent use with alfuzosin, dronedarone, colchicine, ranolazine, rifampin, triazolam, ergot derivatives, St. John's wort, lovastatin, simvastatin, pimozide, lurasidone, and silde-nafil (for pulmonary hypertension)	• Hyperlipidemia • Rash • Hepatotoxicity • N/V/D • Headache • Hyperglycemia • Fat redistribu-tion	• LFTs • Lipids • Blood glucose	• CYP3A4 inhibitor and substrate • CYP2C9 inducer	• Perform genotypic and/or phenotypic testing prior to initi-ating therapy • Use with caution in patients with sulfa allergy • Take with food
Fosamprenavir • Lexiva • Therapy naïve: 1,400 mg PO BID **OR** 1,400 mg PO daily + ritonavir 100–200 mg PO daily **OR** 700 mg PO BID + ritonavir 100 mg PO BID • Therapy experienced: 700 mg PO BID + ritonavir 100 mg PO BID • Suspension, tabs	Concurrent use with alfuzo-sin, flecainide, propafe-none, rifampin, triazolam, ergot derivatives, St. John's wort, lovastatin, simvastatin, pimo-zide, lurasidone, and sildenafil (for pulmonary hypertension)	• Hyperlipidemia • Rash • Headache • Hepatotoxicity • N/V/D • Hyperglycemia • Fat redistribution • Nephrolithiasis	• LFTs • Lipids • Blood glucose	• CYP3A4 inhibitor and substrate • H_2-antagonists ↓ levels	• Use with caution in patients with sulfa allergy • Adjust dose in hepatic impairment • Adults should take suspension without food; children should take suspension with food • Take tabs with meals if taking with ritonavir

Protease Inhibitors (PIs) *(cont'd)*

Generic • Brand • Dose/Dosage Forms	Contraindications	Primary Side Effects	Key Monitoring	Pertinent Drug Interactions	Med Pearl
Indinavir • Crixivan • 800 mg PO q8h **OR** 800 mg PO BID + ritonavir 100–200 mg PO BID • Caps	Concurrent use with alfuzosin, amiodarone, triazolam, alprazolam, ergot derivatives, lovastatin, simvastatin, pimozide, lurasidone, and sildenafil (for pulmonary hypertension)	• Hyperlipidemia • Hepatotoxicity • N/V/D • Nephrolithiasis • Indirect hyper-bilirubinemia • Hyperglycemia • Fat redistribution	• LFTs • Lipids • Bilirubin • Blood glucose	CYP3A4 inhibitor and substrate	• Patients are advised to drink six 8 oz glasses of water per day • Adjust dose in hepatic impairment • If taking *without* ritonavir, take with water 1 hr before or 2 hr after meals
Lopinavir/ritonavir • Kaletra • Lopinavir 400 mg/ritonavir 100 mg PO BID **OR** lopinavir 800 mg/ritonavir 200 mg PO daily • BID regimen must be used if patient has ≥3 lopinavir resistance associated substitutions • Solution, tabs	Concurrent use with alfuzosin, dronedarone, colchicine, rifampin, triazolam, ergot derivatives, elbasvir/grazoprevir, St. John's wort, lovastatin, simvastatin, ranolazine, pimozide, lurasidone, and sildenafil (for pulmonary hypertension)	• Hyperlipidemia • Pancreatitis • Hepatotoxicity • N/V/D • Hyperglycemia • Fat redistribution • PR interval prolongation • QT interval prolongation	• LFTs • Lipids • Blood glucose • ECG	CYP3A4 substrate and inhibitor	• Recommended PI for pregnant women (BID dosing only) • Oral solution contains alcohol and propylene glycol • Take oral solution with food
Nelfinavir • Viracept • 1,250 mg PO BID **OR** 750 mg PO TID • Tabs	Concurrent use with alfuzosin, amiodarone, quindine, rifampin, triazolam, ergot derivatives, St. John's wort, lovastatin, simvastatin, pimozide, lurasidone, and sildenafil (for pulmonary hypertension)	• N/D • Hyperlipidemia • Hyperglycemia • Fat redistribution • Hepatotoxicity	• LFTs • Lipids • Blood glucose	• CYP3A4 and CYP2C19 substrate • CYP3A4 inhibitor	• May disperse tabs in water • Take with food
Ritonavir • Norvir • 100–400 mg/day in 1–2 divided doses to boost other PIs • Caps, solution, tabs	Concurrent use with alfuzosin, amiodarone, dronedarone, colchicine, flecainide, propafenone, quindine, voriconazole (with ritonavir doses ≥800 mg/day), triazolam, ergot derivatives, St. John's wort, lovastatin, simvastatin, pimozide, lurasidone, and sildenafil (for pulmonary hypertension)	• Hyperlipidemia • Hepatotoxicity • N/V/D • Hyperglycemia • Fat redistribution • Paresthesia • Taste disturbance	• LFTs • Lipids • Blood glucose • ECG	• CYP3A4 and CYP2D6 substrate and inhibitor • CYP1A2, CYP2C9, and CYP2C19 inducer	• Only used for boosting • Oral solution contains alcohol • Take with food • Do NOT refrigerate oral solution

Protease Inhibitors (PIs) *(cont'd)*

Generic • Brand • Dose/Dosage Forms	Contraindications	Primary Side Effects	Key Monitoring	Pertinent Drug Interactions	Med Pearl
Saquinavir • Invirase • 1,000 mg PO BID + ritonavir 100 mg PO BID • Caps, tabs	• QT interval prolongation or concurrent use with other drugs that prolong QT interval • Complete atrioventricular block (in absence of pacemaker) • Severe hepatic impairment • Concurrent use with alfuzosin, amiodarone, cobicistat, dofetilide, lidocaine, flecainide, propafenone, quinidine, trazodone, rifampin, triazolam, ergot derivatives, St. John's wort, lovastatin, simvastatin, pimozide, lurasidone, and sildenafil (for pulmonary hypertension)	• PR interval prolongation • QT interval prolongation • Hyperlipidemia • Hepatotoxicity • N/V/D • Headache • Hyperglycemia • Fat redistribution	• LFTs • Lipids • Blood glucose • ECG	CYP3A4 substrate and inhibitor	Take with food
Tipranavir • Aptivus • Therapy experienced: 500 mg PO BID + ritonavir 200 mg PO BID • Caps, solution	• Moderate or severe hepatic impairment • Concurrent use with alfuzosin, amiodarone, flecainide, propafenone, quinidine, rifampin, triazolam, ergot derivatives, St. John's wort, lovastatin, simvastatin, pimozide, lurasidone, and sildenafil (for pulmonary hypertension)	• Hepatotoxicity • Intracranial hemorrhage • Rash • N/V/D • Hyperlipidemia • Hyperglycemia • Fat redistribution	• LFTs • Lipids • Blood glucose	• CYP3A4 substrate • CYP2D6 inhibitor • CYP1A2, CYP2C19, and CYP3A4 inducer • Antiplatelets, anticoagulants, and vitamin E ↑ risk of bleeding	• Not for therapy naïve patients • Use with caution in patients with sulfa allergy • Take with food if used with ritonavir tabs • Oral solution contains propylene glycol • Do NOT refrigerate oral solution

Integrase Inhibitors

Generic • Brand • Dose/Dosage Forms	Contraindications	Primary Side Effects	Key Monitoring	Pertinent Drug Interactions	Med Pearl
Mechanism of action – inhibit integration of proviral DNA into host CD4 T-cell genome					
Dolutegravir • Tivicay • Therapy naïve or therapy experienced, integrase inhibitor naïve: 50 mg PO daily • Integrase inhibitor experienced with certain integrase inhibitor associated resistance substitutions: 50 mg PO BID • Tabs	Concurrent use with dofetilide	• Hypersensitivity reaction • Insomnia • Headache • Depression or suicidal thoughts (primarily in patients with pre-existing psychiatric conditions)	None	• ↑ dofetilide and metformin levels • Etravirine, efavirenz, nevirapine, fosamprenavir/ritonavir, and tipranavir/ritonavir ↓ levels • Carbamazepine, oxcarbazepine, phenytoin, phenobarbital, St. John's wort, and rifampin ↓ levels • Absorption ↓ with antacids and products containing iron, magnesium, aluminum, calcium, or zinc (give dolutegravir 2 hr before or 6 hr after these medications)	↑ dose to 50 mg PO BID when used with carbamazepine, efavirenz, fosamprenavir/ritonavir, tipranavir/ritonavir, or rifampin
Elvitegravir • Only available in combination products	None	• N/D • Depression or suicidal thoughts (primarily in patients with pre-existing psychiatric conditions)	None	• CYP3A4 substrate • Atazanavir, lopinavir/ritonavir, ketoconazole ↑ levels • Carbamazepine, efavirenz, didanosine, bosentan, oxcarbazepine, phenytoin, phenobarbital, rifampin, rifabutin, dexamethasone, and St. John's wort ↓ levels • Absorption ↓ with antacids and products containing iron, magnesium, aluminum, calcium, or zinc (space administration by ≥2 hr) • May ↑ ketoconazole, rifabutin, bosentan, and buprenorphine levels • May ↓ naloxone and methadone levels	Take with food

Integrase Inhibitors *(cont'd)*

Generic • Brand • Dose/Dosage Forms	Contraindications	Primary Side Effects	Key Monitoring	Pertinent Drug Interactions	Med Pearl
Raltegravir • Isentress • Therapy naïve or patients who are virologically suppressed on initial regimen of 400 mg PO BID: 1,200 mg PO daily • Therapy experienced: 400 mg PO BID • Chewable tabs, powder for suspension, tabs	None	• N/D • Headache • Rash • ↑ creatinine kinase • Muscle weakness • Insomnia • Depression or suicidal thoughts (primarily in patients with pre-existing psychiatric conditions)	None	• Rifampin ↓ levels • Absorption ↓ with antacids containing aluminum or magnesium (space administration)	• ↑ dose to 800 mg PO BID when used with rifampin • Chewable tabs and suspension for children

Cytochrome P450 Inhibitor

Generic • Brand • Dose/Dosage Forms	Contraindications	Primary Side Effects	Key Monitoring	Pertinent Drug Interactions	Med Pearl
Mechanism of action – CYP3A inhibitor used to ↑ systemic exposure to the CYP3A substrates, atazanavir and darunavir					
Cobicistat • Tybost • Therapy naïve or experienced: 150 mg PO daily + atazanavir 300 mg PO daily **OR** 150 mg PO daily + darunavir 800 mg PO daily • Tabs	Concurrent use with alfuzosin, dronedarone, irinotecan, rifampin, triazolam, ergot derivatives, St. John's wort, lovastatin, simvastatin, pimozide, lurasidone, sildenafil (for pulmonary hypertension), nevirapine, indinavir, carbamazepine, phenytoin, phenobarbital, ranolazine, colchicine	• ↑ SCr/↓ CrCl (monitor closely if SCr ↑ by >0.4 mg/dL) • Jaundice • Nausea	SCr/CrCl	• CYP2D6 and CYP3A substrate and inhibitor • ↑ risk of renal impairment when used with tenofovir (do not use combination if CrCl <70 mL/min)	• ↑ SCr by inhibiting renal tubular secretion • Take with food

CCR5 Inhibitor

Generic • Brand • Dose/Dosage Forms	Contraindications	Primary Side Effects	Key Monitoring	Pertinent Drug Interactions	Med Pearl
Mechanism of action – acts as an antagonist for the CCR5 receptor, a chemokine coreceptor that can facilitate HIV entry into CD4 T-cells					
Maraviroc • Selzentry • Use with strong CYP3A4 inhibitors (including PIs [except tipranavir/ritonavir] and elvitegravir/ritonavir): 150 mg PO BID • Use with strong CYP3A4 inducers (including efavirenz, etravirine, rifampin, phenytoin, phenobarbital, and carbamazepine): 600 mg PO BID • Use with other medications (including tipranavir/ritonavir, nevirapine, raltegravir, NRTIs and enfuvirtide): 300 mg PO BID • Solution, tabs	CrCl <30 mL/min with concurrent use of strong CYP3A4 inhibitors or inducers	• Abdominal pain • Cough • Dizziness • Joint/muscle pain • Rash • Hepatotoxicity • Orthostatic hypotension	• Tropism testing • LFTs • Blood pressure	CYP3A4 substrate	• Only for patients with CCR5-tropic HIV • Hepatotoxicity may be preceded by systemic hypersensitivity reaction (rash, eosinophilia) • Adjust dose in renal impairment

Fusion Inhibitor

Generic • Brand • Dose	Contraindications	Primary Side Effects	Key Monitoring	Pertinent Drug Interactions	Med Pearl
Mechanism of action – blocks conformational changes in gp41 on the surface of HIV that are required for HIV fusion with CD4 cell membranes					
Enfuvirtide • Fuzeon • 90 mg subcut BID • Injection	None	• Local injection site reactions (pain, erythema, induration, nodules and cysts, pruritus, ecchymosis) • Pneumonia • Hypersensitivity reactions	Injection sites	None	Only HIV medication available as subcut injection

Combination Products: See individual drug components for important points		
Brand	Components	Dosing
Atripla	Efavirenz, tenofovir disoproxil fumarate, emtricitabine	1 tablet PO daily
Combivir	Lamivudine, zidovudine	1 tablet PO BID
Complera	Rilpivirine, tenofovir disoproxil fumarate, emtricitabine	1 tablet PO daily
Descovy	Emtricitabine, tenofovir alafenamide	1 table PO daily
Epzicom	Abacavir, lamivudine	1 tablet PO daily
Evotaz	Atazanavir, cobicistat	1 tablet PO daily
Genvoya	Elvitegravir, cobicistat, emtricitabine, tenofovir alafenamide	1 tablet PO daily
Odefsey	Emtricitabine, rilpivirine, tenofovir alafenamide	1 tablet PO daily
Prezcobix	Darunavir, cobicistat	1 tablet PO daily
Stribild	Elvitegravir, cobicistat, emtricitabine, tenofovir disproxil fumarate	1 tablet PO daily
Triumeq	Dolutegravir, abacavir, lamivudine	1 tablet PO daily
Trizivir	Abacavir, lamivudine, zidovudine	1 tablet PO BID
Truvada	Emtricitabine, tenofovir disoproxil fumarate	1 tablet PO daily

TUBERCULOSIS

Guidelines Summary

The overall goals for treatment of TB are: (1) To cure the individual patient, and (2) to minimize the transmission of *Mycobacterium tuberculosis* to other persons.

- Risk factors
  - Location of birth (New York, New Jersey, California, Florida, and Texas account for 92% of cases)
  - Close contact (>40 hours per week) with TB patients
  - Increase in age
  - Race and ethnicity: Hispanics, African Americans, and Asian Pacific Islanders

- Successful treatment of TB has benefits for both the individual patient and the community in which the patient resides.

- Prescribing physician responsibility for treatment completion is a fundamental principle in TB control.

- Treatment of patients with TB is most successful within a comprehensive framework that addresses both clinical and social issues of relevance to the patient.

- It is strongly recommended that patient-centered care be the initial management strategy, regardless of the source of supervision. This strategy should always include an adherence plan that emphasizes directly observed therapy (DOT).

- Patients with TB caused by drug-susceptible organisms usually are treated initially with a four-drug regimen (rifampin, isoniazid, pyrazinamide, and ethambutol [RIPE]) followed by a two-drug continuation phase (rifampin and isoniazid).

Antitubercular Drugs

Generic • Brand • Dose/Dosage Forms	Contraindications	Primary Side Effects	Key Monitoring	Pertinent Drug Interactions	Med Pearl
Mechanism of action – inhibits mycolic acid synthesis resulting in disruption of the bacterial cell wall					
Isoniazid • Only available generically • Latent: 5 mg/day (max = 300 mg) PO daily × 6–9 mo **OR** 15 mg/kg (max = 900 mg) PO weekly × 6–9 mo • Active: multiple scenarios • Injection, syrup, tabs	• Hepatic impairment • Previous severe reactions (drug fever, chills, arthritis)	• Depression • Flushing • Jaundice	• LFTs • Sputum cultures	CYP2C19 and CYP2D6 inhibitor	• Severe and sometimes fatal hepatitis may occur within 3 mo of treatment • Drinking alcohol not recommended during treatment • Pyridoxine should be administered to prevent peripheral neuropathy
Mechanism of action – inhibits bacterial RNA synthesis by binding to the beta subunit of DNA-dependent RNA polymerase, blocking RNA transcription					
Rifampin • Rifadin • 10 mg/kg/day PO/IV (max = 600 mg/day) • Caps, injection	Concurrent use with PIs	• Numbness • Flu-like syndrome • Rash • Red discoloration of bodily fluids • Neutropenia/leukopenia	• LFTs • CBC • Sputum cultures • Chest x-ray	CYP1A2, CYP2C9, CYP2C19 and CYP3A4 inducer	None
Mechanism of action – kills mycobacteria replicating in macrophages; exact mechanism is not known					
Pyrazinamide • Only available generically • 40–55 kg: 1,000 mg/day PO • 56–75 kg: 1,500 mg/day PO • 76–90 kg: 2,000 mg/day PO (max dose) • Tabs	• Acute gout • Hepatic impairment	• Malaise • Anorexia • Hepatotoxicity	• LFTs • Uric acid levels • Sputum cultures • Chest x-ray	None	Typically used for the first 2 mo of therapy
Mechanism of action – suppresses mycobacteria multiplication by interfering with RNA synthesis					
Ethambutol • Myambutol • 15–25 mg/kg/day (max = 1,600 mg/day) • Tabs	Optic neuritis	• Myocarditis • Headache • Gout • Hepatotoxicity	• Baseline and periodic (monthly) visual testing • LFTs	Aluminum hydroxide ↓ absorption (separate by 4 hr)	Optic neuritis manifests as ↓ red-green color perception, ↓ visual field

PRACTICE QUESTIONS

1. Which of the following medications should NOT be given to a 1-year-old child?

    (A) Amoxicillin
    (B) Cefuroxime
    (C) Clindamycin
    (D) Penicillin
    (E) Tetracycline

2. Which of the following medications would be appropriate for the treatment of *Pseudomonas aeruginosa*?

    (A) Ampicillin
    (B) Cefepime
    (C) Ceftriaxone
    (D) Erythromycin
    (E) Clindamycin

3. A patient admitted to the hospital is diagnosed with aspergillosis. Which of the following antimicrobial agents would be MOST appropriate to initiate in this patient?

    (A) Acyclovir
    (B) Caspofungin
    (C) Chloramphenicol
    (D) Nystatin
    (E) Tigecycline

4. Patients taking which of the following antimicrobial agents should be counseled to wear sunscreen because of the risk of photosensitivity? (Select ALL that apply.)

    (A) Bactrim
    (B) Biaxin
    (C) Cleocin
    (D) Factive
    (E) Vibramycin

5. Which of the following drugs used in the treatment of tuberculosis can cause orange-red discoloration of a patient's urine?

    (A) Isoniazid
    (B) Ethambutol
    (C) Pyrazinamide
    (D) Rifampin
    (E) Streptomycin

6. A woman diagnosed with a sexually transmitted disease picks up her antibiotic prescription at her local pharmacy. The pharmacist counsels her that she should not drink alcoholic beverages while taking this medication because it may lead to an unpleasant reaction. Which of the following antibiotics has MOST likely been prescribed for this patient?

   (A) Azithromycin
   (B) Cefixime
   (C) Doxycycline
   (D) Metronidazole
   (E) Penicillin VK

7. An 85-year-old female patient has been hospitalized with an infection. She has a creatinine clearance of 25 mL/min. Which of the following antibiotics does NOT need to be dose-adjusted in this patient?

   (A) Ceftriaxone
   (B) Gentamicin
   (C) Meropenem
   (D) Piperacillin-tazobactam
   (E) Vancomycin

8. Which of the following antibiotics is the first-line treatment for *Pneumocystis jiroveci* pneumonia?

   (A) Acyclovir
   (B) Azithromycin
   (C) Ciprofloxacin
   (D) Fluconazole
   (E) Trimethoprim-sulfamethoxazole

9. Which of the following is an acceptable antiviral regimen for a treatment-naïve patient with HIV?

   (A) Abacavir + didanosine + zidovudine
   (B) Efavirenz + nevirapine + emtricitabine
   (C) Darunavir + ritonavir + atazanavir
   (D) Tenofovir + emtricitabine + raltegravir
   (E) Dolutegravir + tipranavir + stavudine

10. Acyclovir is available in which of the following formulations?
    (Select ALL that apply.)

    (A) Capsule
    (B) Injection
    (C) Sublingual film
    (D) Topical ointment
    (E) Transdermal patch

ANSWERS AND EXPLANATIONS

1. **E**

Tetracycline should not be given to children younger than 9 years of age, as it can cause enamel hypoplasia or permanent tooth discoloration, therefore choice (E) is correct. The other medications can be administered safely to children.

2. **B**

Cefepime, a fourth-generation cephalosporin, is the only antibiotic listed that would treat an infection caused by *Pseudomonas aeruginosa*; therefore, choice (B) is correct.

3. **B**

Aspergillosis is a serious fungal infection. Both caspofungin (B) and nystatin (D) are considered antifungal agents; however, nystatin is used topically (as an oral suspension for thrush or as topical cream/ointment/powder) for local infections caused by *Candida* spp. Caspofungin is administered intravenously and can be used for the treatment of aspergillosis; thus, choice (B) is correct. Acyclovir (A) is an antiviral agent. Tigecycline (E) and chloramphenicol (C) are used for bacterial infections.

4. **A, D, E**

Fluoroquinolones, sulfonamides, and tetracyclines are associated with an increased risk of photosensitivity. Therefore, patients receiving Bactrim (trimethoprim/sulfamethoxazole) (A), Factive (gemifloxacin) (D), or Vibramycin (doxycycline) (E) should be counseled to wear sunscreen during the course of therapy. Neither Biaxin (clarithromycin) (B) nor Cleocin (clindamycin) (C) is associated with photosensitivity.

5. **D**

Rifampin (D) can cause an orange-red discoloration of all bodily fluids (e.g., tears, saliva, urine). Rifabutin can also cause this discoloration of bodily fluids. Isoniazid (A), ethambutol (B), pyrazinamide (C), and streptomycin (E) do not cause discoloration of the urine.

6. **D**

Metronidazole should not be taken with alcohol as this may lead to a disulfiram-like reaction, which can manifest as severe flushing, headache, nausea, vomiting, or chest and abdominal pain. Although patients generally should not take any of their medications with alcohol, the concomitant use with metronidazole can lead specifically to this very unpleasant reaction; therefore, answer (D) is correct.

7. **A**

Ceftriaxone (A) is eliminated via both biliary and renal excretion. Therefore, the dose of this antibiotic does not need to be adjusted in patients with renal impairment. The dose of gentamicin (B), meropenem (C), piperacillin-tazobactam (D), and vancomycin (E) would all need to be adjusted in this patient with a CrCl of 25 mL/min.

8. **E**

Trimethoprim/sulfamethoxazole (E) is the drug of choice for the treatment of *Pneumocystis jiroveci* pneumonia, provided that the patient does not have a sulfa allergy. Alternative medications, including dapsone, pentamidine, or atovaquone, can be used for the treatment of this opportunistic infection in patients with a sulfa allergy.

9. **D**

The regimen consisting of tenofovir + emtricitabine + raltegravir (D) is an acceptable approach for management of a treatment-naïve patient with HIV because it contains 2 nucleoside reverse transcriptase inhibitors (NRTIs) (tenofovir and emtricitabine) and an integrase inhibitor (raltegravir). Other acceptable antiviral regimens include those that contain a protease inhibitor (PI) (boosted with ritonavir or cobicistat) + 2 NRTIs. Choice (A) contains 3 NRTIs (abacavir + didanosine + zidovudine). Choice (B) contains 2 non-nucleoside reverse transcriptase inhibitors (NNRTIs) (efavirenz and nevirapine) + 1 NRTI (emtricitabine). Choice (C) contains 3 PIs (darunavir + ritonavir + atazanavir). Choice (E) contains an integrase inhibitor (dolutegravir), a PI (tipranavir), and a NRTI (stavudine). None of these four regimens is acceptable for the management of a treatment-naïve patient with HIV.

10. **A, B, D**

Acyclovir is available as a capsule (A), an intravenous injection (B), and a topical ointment (D). This drug is also available as a tablet, oral suspension, buccal tablet, and topical cream. Acyclovir is not available as a sublingual film (C) or a transdermal patch (E).

Pulmonary Disorders

This chapter covers the following diseases:

- **Asthma**
- **Chronic obstructive pulmonary disease**

ASTHMA

Assessment and Monitoring

Once asthma is diagnosed, accurate classification of severity (prior to treatment initiation) and control (for patients on treatment) is essential. Classification is based upon considerations of both impairment and risk, including frequency of symptoms, nighttime awakenings, interference with normal activity, use of a short-acting β_2 agonist (for those on treatment), lung function (spirometry or peak flow), and exacerbations. Assessment varies based upon age (0–4 years, 5–11 years, and 12 years and older). Tables follow for classification of asthma severity and asthma control in patients age 12 years and older.

Classification of Asthma Severity (12 Years and Older)

	Intermittent	Persistent		
		Mild	**Moderate**	**Severe**
Symptoms	≤2 days/week	>2 days /week but not daily	Daily	Throughout the day
Nighttime awakenings	≤2 × /month	3–4 × /month	>1 × /week but not nightly	Often 7 × /week
Short-acting β2-agonist use for symptom control	≤2 days/week	>2 days/week but not daily	Daily	Several times per day
Interference with normal activity	None	Minor limitation	Some limitation	Extreme limitation

Classification of Asthma Severity (12 Years and Older)   *(cont'd)*

	Intermittent	Persistent		
		Mild	**Moderate**	**Severe**
Lung function	• Normal FEV1 between exacerbations • FEV1 >80% predicted • FEV1/FVC normal	• FEV1 ≥80% predicted **OR** • FEV1/FVC normal	• FEV1 60–79% predicted **OR** • FEV1/FVC reduced 5%	• FEV1 <60% predicted **OR** • FEV1/FVC reduced >5%
Exacerbations (requiring oral corticosteroids)	0–1/year (see note)	≥2/year (see note)		
	Consider severity and interval since last exacerbation. Frequency and severity may fluctuate over time for patients in any severity category.			
	Relative annual risk of exacerbations may be related to FEV1.			

Adapted from National Heart, Lung and Blood Institute, National Asthma Education and Prevention Program, Expert Panel Report 3: Guidelines for the Diagnosis and Management of Asthma—Full Report, 2007. www.nhlbi.nih.gov/files/docs/guidelines/asthgdln.pdf.

Classification of Asthma Control (12 Years and Older)

	Well Controlled	**Not Well Controlled**	**Very Poorly Controlled**
Symptoms	≤2 days/week	>2 days/week	Throughout the day
Nighttime awakenings	≤2 × /month	1–3 × /week	≥4 × /week
Interference with normal activity	None	Some limitation	Extreme limitation
Short-acting β$_2$-agonist use for symptom control	≤2 days/ week	>2 days/week	Several times per day
FEV1 or peak flow	>80% predicted/ personal best	60–80% predicted/ personal best	<60% predicted/ personal best
Validated questionnaires ATQ ACQ ACT	0 ≤0.75 ≥20	1–2 ≥1.5 16–19	3–4 N/A ≤15
Exacerbations	0–1/year	≥2/year	
	Consider severity and interval since last exacerbation.		
Progressive loss of lung function	Evaluation requires long-term follow-up care.		
Treatment-related adverse effects	Medication side effects can vary in intensity from none to very troublesome and worrisome. The level of intensity does not correlate to specific levels of control but should be considered in the overall assessment of risk.		

Adapted from National Heart, Lung and Blood Institute, National Asthma Education and Prevention Program, Expert Panel Report 3: Guidelines for the Diagnosis and Management of Asthma—Full Report, 2007. www.nhlbi.nih.gov/files/docs/guidelines/asthgdln.pdf.

Guidelines Summary

General Principles of Asthma Management

Long-term goals:

- Minimize exacerbations
- Maintain good control of daily symptoms
- Limit fixed airflow limitation
- Minimize side effects of treatment
- Patient's own self-identified goals

Medication categories:

- Controller therapy: Used for maintenance treatment. Decreases airway inflammation, controls symptoms, and decreases risk of exacerbation and declining lung function.
- Rescue therapy: Used as needed for relief of breakthrough symptoms.
- Add-on therapy: Used in severe asthma to address persistent symptoms despite high-dose inhaled corticosteroids (ICS) and long-acting beta agonist (LABA) therapy.

Control-based management:

- Continuous cycle of assessment, treatment, monitoring.
- Stepwise therapy based upon severity and level of control.
- Inhaled corticosteroids are the mainstay of therapy for all persistent asthma.

Asthma Treatment Summary

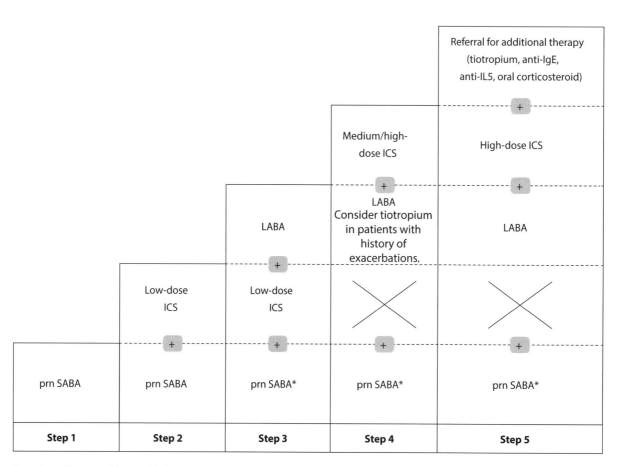

Step 6 per NAEPP is addition of daily oral corticosteroids.

Abbreviations: ICS = inhaled corticosteroid; LABA = long-acting β-2 agonist; prn = as needed;
SABA = short-acting β-2 agonist
* Low-dose ICS/formoterol is reliever therapy for those taking low-dose ICS/formoterol or low-dose beclametasone/formoterol controller therapies.
Adapted from GINA 2017 guidelines

Inhaled Corticosteroids

Generic • Brand • Dose/Dosage Forms	Contraindications	Primary Side Effects	Key Monitoring	Pertinent Drug Interactions	Med Pearl
Mechanism of action – glucocorticoid receptor agonist with an affinity for the receptor resulting in anti-inflammatory and immunosuppressive properties, and antiproliferative actions					
Fluticasone • Flovent Diskus, Flovent HFA • 88–440 mcg BID	Primary treatment of acute bronchospasm	• Throat irritation • Cough • Oral candidiasis • Upper respiratory tract infection • Sinusitis	• FEV1 • Peak flow • Other PFTs • Hypothalamic-pituitary-adrenal axis suppression	• CYP3A4 substrate • Cobicistat (component of Stribild) and ritonavir may ↑ levels	• HFA formulation for Flovent • Most potent corticosteroid
Fluticasone furoate ☆ • Arnuity Ellipta • 100–200 mcg daily					
Fluticasone propionate • Armonair RespiClick • 55–232 mcg BID					
Budesonide ☆ • Pulmicort Flexhaler, Pulmicort Respules • Flexhaler: 180–720 mcg BID • Respules: 0.25–1 mg/day					Respules are the only nebulized corticosteroid
Mometasone • Asmanex HFA, Asmanex Twisthaler • HFA: 100–200 mcg BID • Twisthaler: 110–880 mcg/day					Twisthaler is true once daily
Beclomethasone ☆ • QVAR • 40–320 mcg BID					HFA formulation
Flunisolide • Aerospan • 160–320 mcg BID					HFA formulation
Ciclesonide • Alvesco • 80 mcg BID (max = 640 mcg/day)					Drug is a solution aerosol so no shaking is required

Short-Acting β₂ Agonists

Generic • Brand • Dose/Dosage Forms	Contraindications	Primary Side Effects	Key Monitoring	Pertinent Drug Interactions	Med Pearl
Mechanism of action – relaxes bronchial smooth muscle by acting on β₂ receptors in the lungs					
Albuterol☆ • Ventolin HFA, Proventil HFA, ProAir HFA, ProAir Respiclick • Metered-dose inhaler (MDI): 2 inhalations every 4–6 hr prn (90 mcg/inhalation) • Neb: 2.5 mg 3–4 × / day prn	Hypersensitivity	• Dose-dependent • Angina • Arrhythmias • Chest discomfort • Cough • Tremor	• FEV1 • Peak flow • Blood pressure • HR	Nonselective β-blockers ↓ effects	• Excessive use can ↑ risk of death • Nebulizer is compatible with budesonide, cromolyn, ipratropium
Levalbuterol☆ • Xopenex, Xopenex HFA • MDI: 2 inhalations every 4–6 hr prn (45 mcg/inhalation) • Neb: 0.63 mg TID	Hypersensitivity	• Tremor • Rhinitis • Tachycardia			Fewer cardiac side effects than albuterol

Long-Acting β₂ Agonists

Generic • Brand • Dose/Dosage Forms	Contraindications	Primary Side Effects	Key Monitoring	Pertinent Drug Interactions	Med Pearl
Mechanism of action – relaxes bronchial smooth muscle					
Salmeterol • Serevent Diskus • 50 mcg/inhalation • 1 inhalation BID (max = 2 puffs/day)	• Primary treatment of acute bronchospasm • Presence of tachyarrhythmias • Monotherapy	• Headache • Hypertension • Dizziness • Chest pain • Throat irritation	• FEV1 • Peak flow	• CYP3A4 substrate • Cobicistat (component of Stribild) and ritonavir may ↑ levels	• LABAs may ↑ the risk of asthma-related deaths; should be used only in adjunct therapy with inhaled corticosteroids
Formoterol • Only available in combination products in US (for asthma)	• Hypersensitivity • Monotherapy	• Headache • Hypertension • Dizziness • Chest pain • Throat irritation	• FEV1 • Peak flow	Nonselective β-blockers ↓ effects	

Immunomodulators

Generic • Brand • Dose/Dosage Forms	Contraindications	Primary Side Effects	Key Monitoring	Pertinent Drug Interactions	Med Pearl
Mechanism of action – IgG monoclonal antibody which inhibits IgE receptor on mast cells and basophils					
• Omalizumab • Xolair • 150–375 mg subcut every 2–4 wk, based on weight and serum IgE	Primary treatment of acute bronchospasm	• Pain and bruising of injection sites • Anaphylaxis • Neuromuscular pain	Be prepared for anaphylaxis	None	Do not administer >150 mg per injection site
Mechanism of action – interleukin-5 antagonist which ↓ production and survival of eosinophils; however, the mechanism of action in asthma has not been definitively established					
Mepolizumab • Nucala • 100 mg subcut every 4 wk	Hypersensitivity	• Anaphylaxis • Injection site reaction • Antibody development • Herpes zoster activation	• FEV1 • Peak flow • Other PFTs	None	• Add-on therapy for severe asthma with eosinophilic phenotype • Zoster vaccination recommended prior to use
Reslizumab • Cinqair • 3 mg/kg IV every 4 wk	Hypersensitivity	• Anaphylaxis • ↑ creatine kinase • Antibody development	• FEV1 • Peak flow • Other PFTs	None	Add-on therapy for severe asthma with eosinophilic phenotype

Leukotriene Receptor Antagonists

Generic • Brand • Dose/Dosage Forms	Contraindications	Primary Side Effects	Key Monitoring	Pertinent Drug Interactions	Med Pearl
Mechanism of action – selective leukotriene receptor antagonist of leukotrienes D4 and E4					
Montelukast☆ • Singulair • 4–10 mg PO HS • Tabs, chewable tabs, and granules	Hypersensitivity	• Behavioral changes (agitation, hostility, anxiety, depression, hallucinations, insomnia, irritability, suicidal thoughts) • Headache • Churg-Strauss syndrome (rare)	Behavioral changes	None	Approved for adults and children ≥1 yr
Zafirlukast • Accolate • 10–20 mg PO BID		• ↑ liver function tests (LFTs) • Headache • Insomnia • Depression	LFTs	• CYP2C9 substrate • CYP2C9 and CYP3A4 inhibitor • May ↑ effects of warfarin • CYP2C9 inhibitors may ↑ effects • CYP2C9 inducers may ↓ effects	Must be taken on empty stomach

Other Asthma Medications

Generic • Brand • Dose/Dosage Forms	Contraindications	Primary Side Effects	Key Monitoring	Pertinent Drug Interactions	Med Pearl
Mechanism of action – prevents the mast cells from releasing histamine and leukotrienes					
Cromolyn • Only available generically • 60–80 mg/day • Nebulization solution	Primary treatment of acute bronchospasm	• Cough and irritation • Unpleasant taste • ↑ sneezing	PFTs	None	• Safety is the primary advantage of this drug • May take 4–6 wk for full benefit • Approved for adults and children > 2 yr
Mechanism of action – 5-lipoxygenase inhibitor limits neutrophil and monocyte aggregation					
Zileuton • Zyflo, Zyflo CR • IR: 600 mg PO 4 × /day • CR: 1,200 mg PO BID	Acute liver disease	• ↑ LFTs • Headache	• LFTs at baseline, then every 4 wk × 3 mo, then every 2–3 mo for the rest of the yr, then periodically • Peak flow	• CYP1A2, CYP2C9, and CYP3A4 substrate • CYP1A2 inhibitor • May ↑ effects/toxicity of theophylline and warfarin	• 4 × /day dose is disadvantage for IR • CR should be taken with food
Mechanism of action – methylxanthine causes bronchodilation by ↑ tissue concentrations of cyclic adenine monophosphate					
Theophylline ☆ • Theo-24, Theocron, Elixophyllin • 10 mg/kg/day PO up to 600 mg/day • Liquid, sustained-release tabs, and caps	Allergy to corn-derived dextrose	• Tachycardia • Nausea/vomiting • Central nervous system (CNS) stimulation • Theophylline toxicity (persistent, repetitive vomiting)	• Theophylline concentrations (10–20 mcg/mL) • Heart rate • CNS effects	• CYP1A2 substrate • CYP1A2 inhibitors may ↑ effects/toxicity • CYP1A2 inducers may ↓ effects	Dosage adjustments should be in small increments (maximum: 25%); ↓ dose by 25% in older adult patients
Aminophylline • Only available generically • Dose is diagnosis- and age-dependent • Injection	Hypersensitivity to theophylline				Theophylline dose is 80% of aminophylline dose

Combination Products: See individual drug components for important points		
Brand	**Components**	**Dosing**
Advair Diskus, Advair HFA, Airduo Respiclick	Fluticasone + Salmeterol	Diskus: 1 inhalation BID HFA: 2 inhalations BID Respiclick: 1 inhalation BID
Breo Ellipta	Fluticasone + Vilanterol	1 inhalation daily
Dulera	Mometasone + Formoterol	2 inhalations BID
Symbicort	Formoterol + Budesonide	2 inhalations BID

CHRONIC OBSTRUCTIVE PULMONARY DISEASE

Classification of Airflow Severity

- GOLD I: mild COPD: FEV1 ≥80% predicted
- GOLD II: moderate COPD: 50% ≤FEV1 <80% predicted
- GOLD III: severe COPD: 30% ≤FEV1 <50% predicted
- GOLD IV: very severe COPD: FEV1 <30% predicted

Classification of COPD Exacerbation Risk

- Group A: mild to moderate airflow limitation, low risk of exacerbation
- Group B: mild to moderate airflow limitation, low risk of exacerbation with more symptoms than group A
- Group C: severe to very severe airflow limitation, high risk of exacerbation
- Group D: severe to very severe airflow limitation, high risk of exacerbation with more symptoms than group C

Guidelines Summary

Treatment is based on the **G**lobal Initiative for Chronic **O**bstructive **L**ung **D**isease (GOLD).

- Goals of therapy:
  - Reduce symptoms
  - Reduce frequency and severity of exacerbations
  - Improve health status and exercise tolerance
- Treatment approach to stable COPD:
  - Influenza and pneumococcal (PPSV 23) vaccination should be offered for all patients who smoke and all patients with diagnosed COPD.
  - Smoking cessation should be encouraged for all patients who smoke.
  - Short-acting inhaled bronchodilators, including β_2 agonists and anticholinergics, can be used as needed in patients in Group A.
  - Long-acting inhaled bronchodilators, including LABAs and long-acting anticholinergics, are first-line pharmacological therapy for patients in Groups B, C, and D.
  - Long-acting inhaled bronchodilators may be combined for enhanced efficacy if monotherapy is insufficient.
  - ICS are recommended as an addition to long-acting bronchodilator therapy for Groups C and D.

- Roflumilast may reduce exacerbations for patients with severe or very severe COPD and frequent exacerbations not adequately controlled with long-acting bronchodilator therapy.
- Theophylline should be reserved for patients unable to access or afford long-acting inhaled bronchodilators.

■ Treatment approach to exacerbations:

- Exacerbation diagnosis is based on clinical presentation of significant change in daily symptoms and sputum production.
- Goal of therapy is to minimize impact of the current exacerbation and prevent future exacerbations.
- Use of short-acting bronchodilators and systemic corticosteroids (prednisone 40 mg daily for 5 days) can shorten recovery time.
- Oral antibiotics may be considered in patients with ↑ sputum purulence. Use is most clearly indicated in patients with mechanical ventilation or all three cardinal symptoms (↑ dyspnea, ↑ sputum production, and ↑ sputum purulence).
- Choice of antibiotic is based upon local bacterial resistance patterns.

COPD Treatment Summary

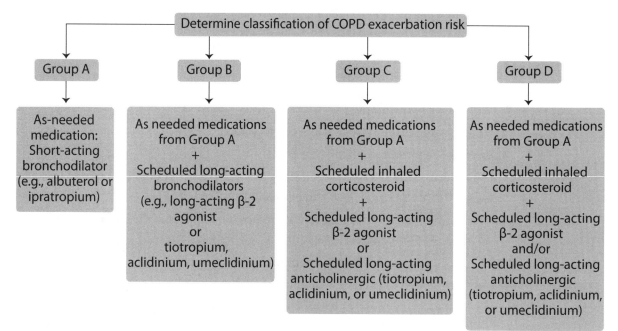

Medications for COPD

(See Asthma section for additional drug tables including ICS, short-acting bronchodilators, and methylxanthines.)

Long-Acting Bronchodilators

Generic • Brand • Dose	Contraindications	Primary Side Effects	Key Monitoring	Pertinent Drug Interactions	Med Pearl
Mechanism of action – long-acting β_2-adrenergic agonist; relaxes bronchial smooth muscle					
Indacaterol • Arcapta Neohaler • 75 mcg daily Arformoterol • Brovana • 15 mcg BID Formoterol • Perforomist • 20 mcg BID Salmeterol • Serevent Diskus • 50 mcg/ inhalation • 1 inhalation BID Olodaterol • Striverdi Respimat • 2 inhalations daily	Monotherapy in the treatment of asthma	• Cough • Chest pain • Headache • Nasopharyn- gitis	• PFTs • HR	Nonselective β-blockers	• Indacaterol, arformoterol, formoterol, and olodaterol not approved for the treatment of asthma • Arformoterol and formoterol available as nebulizer solution
Mechanism of action – blocks acetylcholine at the parasympathetic sites in bronchial smooth muscle, causing bronchodilation					
Ipratropium☆ • Atrovent HFA • MDI: 2 inhalations 4 × /day (max = 12 puffs/24 hrs) • Nebulizer: 500 mcg every 6–8 hr	• Hypersensitivity • Peanut allergy (due to soya lecithin) • Does not apply to Atrovent HFA	• Upper respiratory tract infection • Palpitation • Xerostomia • Pharyngeal irritation	• FEV1 • Peak flow • Other PFTs	Avoid use with other anticholinergic inhalers	• Not recommended for initial treatment of acute episode of bronchospasm • Anticholinergic side effects are possible. Be careful in BPH, narrow-angle glaucoma, and myasthenia gravis
Tiotropium☆ • Spiriva Han- dihaler, Spiriva Respimat • Handihaler: 1 cap (18 mcg) via inhalation daily • Respimat: 2 inhalations daily	Contains lactose				

Long-Acting Bronchodilators *(cont'd)*

Generic • Brand • Dose	Contraindications	Primary Side Effects	Key Monitoring	Pertinent Drug Interactions	Med Pearl
Aclidinium • Tudorza Pressair • 1 inhalation BID	Hypersensitivity to milk protein	[Same as above]	[Same as above]	[Same as above]	[Same as above]
Umeclidinium • Incruse Ellipta • 1 inhalation daily	Hypersensitivity to milk protein				
Glycopyrrolate • Seebri Neohaler • 1 cap (15.6 mcg) by inhalation BID	Hypersensitivity	• Upper respiratory tract infection • Nasopharyngitis			

Phosphodiesterase-4 Inhibitor

Generic • Brand • Dose	Contraindications	Primary Side Effects	Key Monitoring	Pertinent Drug Interactions	Med Pearl
Mechanism of action – inhibits phosphodiesterase-4 leading to an accumulation of cyclic AMP					
Roflumilast • Daliresp • 500 mcg daily	Hepatic impairment (Child-Pugh class B or C)	• Diarrhea • Weight loss • Nausea • Gynecomastia	• Weight • LFTs	• CYP1A2 and CYP3A4 substrate • CYP1A2 and CYP3A4 inhibitors may ↑ effects • CYP1A2 and CYP3A4 inducers may ↓ effects	Not indicated for relieving acute bronchospasms or for use as monotherapy of COPD

Combination Products: See individual drug components for important points		
Brand	**Components**	**Dosing**
Advair Diskus	Fluticasone + Salmeterol	1 inhalation BID
Anoro Ellipta	Umeclidinium + Vilanterol	1 inhalation daily
Bevespi Aerosphere	Glycopyrrolate + Formoterol	2 inhalations BID
Breo Ellipta	Fluticasone + Vilanterol	1 inhalation daily
Combivent Respimat	Ipratropium + Albuterol	1 inhalation 4×/day
Stiolto Respimat	Tiotropium + Olodaterol	2 inhalations daily
Symbicort	Budesonide + Formoterol	2 inhalations BID
Utibron Neohaler	Glycopyrrolate + Indacaterol	1 cap inhaled BID

PRACTICE QUESTIONS

1. What is Zyflo's mechanism of action?

    (A) Selective leukotriene-receptor antagonist of leukotrienes D4 and E4
    (B) 5-lipoxygenase inhibitor limits neutrophil and monocyte aggregation
    (C) Methylxanthine causes bronchodilation by increasing tissue concentrations of cyclic adenine monophosphate
    (D) Relaxes bronchial smooth muscle by stimulating beta-2 receptors

2. The device used to measure forced vital capacity is called a

    (A) tonometer.
    (B) optomyometer.
    (C) sphygmomanometer.
    (D) spirometer.
    (E) gonioscope.

3. QVAR is indicated for which of the following scenarios? (Select ALL that apply.)

    (A) Asthma
    (B) Emphysema
    (C) Chronic brochitis
    (D) Smoking cessation

4. Which of the following include fluticasone as an active ingredient? (Select ALL that apply.)

    (A) Flonase
    (B) Flovent
    (C) Spiriva
    (D) Pulmicort

5. Patient counseling that includes the need for the patient to rinse his or her mouth and spit after use is applicable to which medication?

    (A) Breo Ellipta
    (B) Arcapta Neohaler
    (C) Xopenex HFA
    (D) Servent Diskus

6. Which of the following should ALWAYS be used in combination with an inhaled corticosteroid in the treatment of asthma?

(A) Budesonide
(B) Cromolyn
(C) Formoterol
(D) Levalbuterol

7. A patient with GOLD 2 risk Group B presents with persistent dyspnea and cough despite smoking cessation and intermittent use of short acting bronchodilator therapy. Which therapy option would be most appropriate to initiate?

(A) Spiriva Respimat
(B) Pulmicort Flexhaler
(C) Theophylline
(D) Roflumilast

ANSWERS AND EXPLANATIONS

1. **B**

The challenging aspect of this question is that Zyflo is classified as a leukotriene modifier (A), like Accolate or Singulair, but the two have different mechanisms of action. Zyflo's mechanism is an inhibitor of 5-lipoxygenase versus an antagonist at the receptor. Choice (C) is the mechanism of theophylline and choice (D) is the mechanism of albuterol.

2. **D**

A spirometer is a gasometer used for measuring respiratory gases, so (D) is correct. A tonometer (A) determines pressure or tension within the eye. An optomyometer (B) is an instrument for determining the relative power of the extrinsic muscles of the eye. A sphygmomanometer (C) measures arterial blood pressure. A gonioscope (E) measures the lens angle in relationship to the eye.

3. **A**

QVAR is an inhaled corticosteroid that is indicated only for the maintenance and prophylactic treatment of asthma, so (A) is the only correct answer.

4. **A, B**

Flonase and Flovent contain fluticasone. Spiriva (C) contains tiotropium. Pulmicort (D) contains budesonide.

5. **A**

Breo Ellipta contains fluticasone, which is an inhaled corticosteroid. Counseling for inhaled corticosteroids should include having the patient rinse his or her mouth with water and spit it out to reduce the risk of thrush or hoarseness. The other medications listed do not contain an inhaled corticosteroid and therefore do not require the patient to rinse his or her mouth after use.

6. **C**

Formoterol is a long-acting beta-2 agonist that needs to be administered in conjunction with an inhaled corticosteroid. Use of long-acting beta-2 agonists without the use of an inhaled corticosteroid has been associated with increased risk of asthma-related deaths. Budesonide is an inhaled corticosteroid and should not be used with another inhaled corticosteroid. Cromolyn and levalbuterol do not need to be administered with an inhaled corticosteroid, although they often are.

7. **A**

Long-acting bronchodilators (long-acting beta-2 agonists or long-acting anticholinergics) such as tiotropium are the mainstay of therapy in COPD. This would be the most appropriate therapy for this patient in risk group B with persistent symptoms. Pulmicort Flexhaler (B) is an inhaled corticosteroid and would be appropriate add-on therapy should the patient need additional therapy after long-acting bronchodilator therapy is optimized. Theophylline (C) is a xanthine oxidase inhibitor. Use of this class is reserved for patients who are unable to access or afford long-acting inhaled bronchodilator therapy. Roflumilast (D) is reserved for severe cases with frequent exacerbations.

Endocrine Disorders

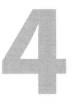

This chapter covers the following diseases:

- **Diabetes mellitus**
- **Hypothyroidism**
- **Hyperthyroidism**
- **Polycystic ovarian syndrome**

DIABETES MELLITUS

Guidelines Summary

- American Diabetes Association (ADA) Guideline Goals
  - Preprandial glucose 80–130 mg/dL
  - Postprandial glucose <180 mg/dL
  - A1c <7%
  - Blood pressure <140/90 mmHg
  - Goals should be individualized

Patient education is integral to successful management of diabetes. Diabetes education should be conducted through an interdisciplinary approach.

Dietary education should focus on medical nutrition therapy provided by a registered dietitian.

Exercise should include 150 min/week of moderate intensity aerobic activity or 75 min/week of vigorous aerobic activity.

- Insulin replacement is necessary in type 1 DM and is generally initiated at 0.5–1 units/kg/day.
  - Analog-based basal bolus regimen (50% basal, 50% bolus [divided into 3 meals]); **OR**
  - Human insulin–based split-mixed regimen (70% A.M.; 30% P.M. [each dose $\frac{2}{3}$ NPH to $\frac{1}{3}$ Regular])
- Insulin regimens are adjusted based upon patient response (self-monitored blood glucose [SMBG]).
- Metformin is first-line therapy for patients with type 2 DM unless contraindicated.
- Second-line options include insulin, sulfonylureas, dipeptidyl-peptidase 4 (DPP-4) inhibitors, glucagon-like peptide-1 (GLP-1) agonists, sodium-glucose cotransporter 2 (SGLT-2) inhibitors, and thiazolidinediones (TZD).
- Second-line selection is made based upon patient-specific considerations of efficacy needed, risk of hypoglycemia/weight gain, other side effects, and cost.
- New data is emerging indicating potential cardiovascular risk reduction with the use of empagliflozin and liraglutide.

Treatment Algorithm

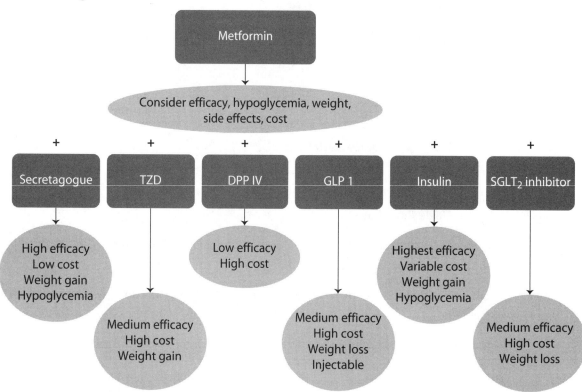

Insulin

Generic • Brand	Onset	Peak	Duration	Comments
Rapid-acting				• Hypoglycemia is the most common side effect. It is defined as blood sugar <70 mg/dL and must be treated as soon as recognized. • Insulin dosage is individually based due to sensitivity; 0.5–1.0 units/kg/day for the average nonobese patient. • Duration of action is prolonged in renal failure.
Aspart☆ • NovoLog	5–15 min	30–90 min	<5 hr	
Lispro U-100☆ Lispro U-200 • Humalog	5–15 min	30–90 min	<5 hr	
Glulisine • Apidra	5–15 min	30–90 min	<5 hr	
Short-acting				
Regular☆ • Humulin R (OTC)	30–60 min	2–3 hr	5–8 hr	
Inhaled, regular • Afrezza	30–60 min	2–3 hr	5–8 hr	
Intermediate, basal				
NPH (Neutral Protamine Hagedorn)☆ • Humulin N (OTC)	2–4 hr	4–10 hr	10–16 hr	
Long-acting, basal				
Glargine U-100☆ • Basaglar, Lantus	2–4 hr	No peak	20–24 hr	
Detemir☆ • Levemir	3–8 hr	No peak	6–24 hr	
Glargine U-300 • Toujeo	2–4 hr	No peak	22–24 hr	
Degludec • Tresiba	1–3 hr	No peak	42 hr	

Insulin   *(cont'd)*

Generic • Brand	Onset	Peak	Duration	Comments
Premixed				[Same as above]
75% Lispro protamine/ 25% lispro • Humalog Mix 75/25	5–15 min	Dual	10–16 hr	
50% Lispro protamine / 50% lispro • Humalog Mix 50/50	5–15 min	Dual	10–16 hr	
50% Aspart protamine / 50% aspart • NovoLog Mix 50/50	5–15 min	Dual	10–16 hr	
70% Aspart protamine / 30% aspart • NovoLog Mix 70/30	5–15 min	Dual	10–16 hr	
70% Degludec/30% aspart • Ryzodeg	5–15 min	Dual	<5 hr (aspart); 42 hr (degludec)	
70% NPH / 30% regular • 70/30 (OTC)	30–60 min	Dual	10–16 hr	
• OTC insulin is available without a prescription. • Rapid-acting insulin should be given at time of meal ingestion, no more than 15 minutes from eating. • Regular insulin should be given 30 minutes prior to meal due to delayed onset of action.				

Sulfonylureas

Generic • Brand • Dose & Max	Contraindications	Primary Side Effects	Key Monitoring	Pertinent Drug Interactions	Med Pearl
Sulfonylureas, first generation – stimulate insulin release from the pancreatic beta cells					
Tolbutamide • Only available generically • 250 mg–3 g daily Tolazamide • Only available generically • 100 mg–1 g daily Chlorpropamide • Diabinese • 100–500 mg daily	• Type 1 DM • Sulfa allergy • Creatinine clearance (CrCl) <50 mL/min (chlorpropamide)	• Hypoglycemia • Weight gain	• Fasting plasma glucose (FPG) • A1c every 3 mo • S/S hypoglycemia	• Tolbutamide = CYP2C9 substrate and inhibitor • Chlorpropamide = CYP2C9 substrate • Chronic ethanol ingestion may ↓ hypoglycemic effect	Response plateaus after half maximum dose

Sulfonylureas *(cont'd)*

Generic • Brand • Dose & Max	Contraindications	Primary Side Effects	Key Monitoring	Pertinent Drug Interactions	Med Pearl
Sulfonylureas, second generation – stimulate insulin release from the pancreatic beta cells					
Glyburide☆ • DiaBeta, Glynase • 1.25–20 mg/day (given daily BID) • Micronized: 0.75–12 mg/day (given daily BID) Glipizide☆ • Glucotrol, Glucotrol XL • 2.5–40 mg/day Glimepiride☆ • Amaryl • 1–8 mg daily	• Type 1 DM • Sulfa allergy	• Hypoglycemia • Weight gain	• FPG • A1c every 3 mo • S/S hypoglycemia	• CYP2C9 substrates • CYP2C9 inhibitors may ↑ effects • CYP2C9 inducers may ↓ effects • Chronic ethanol ingestion may ↓ hypoglycemic effect	• Response plateaus after half maximum dose • Administer with meals

Meglitinides

Generic • Brand • Dose & Max	Contraindications	Primary Side Effects	Key Monitoring	Pertinent Drug Interactions	Med Pearl
Mechanism of action – in presence of glucose, stimulate insulin release from the pancreatic beta cells					
Repaglinide • Prandin • 0.5–16 mg/day (taken BID–4 × /day)	• Type 1 DM • Concurrent use of gemfibrozil	• Hypoglycemia • Weight gain	• Postprandial plasma glucose • A1c every 3 mo • S/S hypoglycemia	• CYP2C8 and CYP3A4 substrate • CYP2C8 and CYP3A4 inhibitors may ↑ effects • CYP2C8 and CYP3A4 inducers may ↓ effects	• Faster acting and shorter duration than sulfonylureas • Recommended for postprandial hyperglycemia • Administer each dose 15–30 min before meals
Nateglinide • Starlix • 60–120 mg TID	Type 1 DM			• CYP2C9 and CYP3A4 substrate • CYP2C9 and CYP3A4 inhibitors may ↑ effects • CYP2C9 and CYP3A4 inducers may ↓ effects	

Biguanide

Generic • Brand • Dose & Max	Contraindications	Primary Side Effects	Key Monitoring	Pertinent Drug Interactions	Med Pearl
Mechanism of action – ↓ hepatic glucose production, ↓ intestinal absorption of glucose, and improves insulin sensitivity					
Metformin☆ • Glucophage, Glucophage XR • IR: 500–2,550 mg/day (in 2–3 divided doses) • XR: 500–2,000 mg daily	• CrCl < 30 mL/min • Lactic acidosis • Severe heart failure • Radiocontrast dyes (discontinue 48 hr before and after procedure)	• Diarrhea • Flatulence • Lactic acidosis • Vitamin B_{12} deficiency	• Serum creatinine (SCr) • Hemoglobin/ hematocrit • Vitamin B12 concentrations • FPG • A1c every 3 mo	Cimetidine may ↑ effects	• Black box warning: lactic acidosis • Maximum daily dose for IR is 2,550 mg

Alpha-Glucosidase Inhibitors

Generic • Brand • Dose & Max	Contraindications	Primary Side Effects	Key Monitoring	Pertinent Drug Interactions	Med Pearl
Mechanism of action – inhibit pancreatic alpha-amylase and alpha-glucosidases, block carbohydrate hydrolysis to glucose; $\downarrow$ postprandial blood glucose					
Acarbose • Precose • 25–100 mg TID	• Cirrhosis • Inflammatory bowel disease • Intestinal obstruction	• Abdominal pain • Diarrhea • Flatulence	• Liver function tests (LFTs) every 3 mo × 1 yr • Postprandial plasma glucose • A1c every 3 mo	• Sulfonylureas and insulin $\uparrow$ risk of hypoglycemia	• Must treat hypoglycemia with simple carbohydrate such as glucose • Administer with food
Miglitol • Glyset • 25–100 mg TID			• Postprandial plasma glucose • A1c every 3 mo		

Thiazolidinediones

Generic • Brand • Dose & Max	Contraindications	Primary Side Effects	Key Monitoring	Pertinent Drug Interactions	Med Pearl
Mechanism of action – PPAR-gamma activator, which improves insulin sensitivity					
Rosiglitazone • Avandia • 2–8 mg daily	• Liver disease • Unstable heart failure • Previous myocardial infarction • Osteopenia or osteoporosis • History of bladder cancer	• Edema • Hepatotoxicity	• LFTs at baseline and periodically • FPG • A1c every 3 mo	• CYP2C8 substrates • CYP2C8 inhibitors may $\uparrow$ effects • CYP2C8 inducers may $\downarrow$ effects	• Potential link to $\uparrow$ risk of cardiovascular events; controversial
Pioglitazone ☆ • Actos • 15–45 mg daily					• Thought to have better lipid profile than rosiglitazone

Amylinomimetic

Generic • Brand • Dose & Max	Contraindications	Primary Side Effects	Key Monitoring	Pertinent Drug Interactions	Med Pearl
Mechanism of action – amylin cosecreted with insulin $\downarrow$ postprandial blood sugars, prolonging gastric emptying, $\downarrow$ postprandial glucagon secretion, and caloric intake through centrally mediated appetite suppression					
Pramlintide • Symlin • 15–120 mcg subcut daily	• Gastroparesis • Hypoglycemia unawareness	• Nausea • Severe hypoglycemia	• Blood sugars (before and after meals and HS) • A1c every 3 mo • S/S hypoglycemia	• May delay absorption of other drugs due to $\uparrow$ gastric emptying time (administer other medications 1 hr prior to pramlintide) • Sulfonylureas and insulin $\uparrow$ risk of hypoglycemia ($\downarrow$ dose of mealtime insulin by 50% when starting pramlintide)	Adjunctive treatment *with* mealtime insulin

GLP-1 Receptor Agonists

Generic • Brand • Dose & Max	Contraindications	Primary Side Effects	Key Monitoring	Pertinent Drug Interactions	Med Pearl
Mechanism of action – analogs of GLP-1, which ↑ insulin secretion, ↑ B-cell growth/replication, slow gastric emptying, and ↓ food intake					
Exenatide ☆ • Byetta (IR) • 5–10 mcg subcut BID • Bydureon (ER) • 2 mg subcut once weekly	• CrCl <30 mL/min • Family history of medullary thyroid carcinoma (ER) • Multiple endocrine neoplasia syndrome type 2 (ER)	• Nausea • Hypoglycemia • ↓ appetite • Weight loss • Pancreatitis • Thyroid tumors	• FPG • A1c every 3 mo • S/S pancreatitis • S/S hypoglycemia • Thyroid tumors	• May delay absorption of other drugs due to ↑ gastric emptying time (administer other medications 1 hour prior) • Sulfonylureas and insulin ↑ risk of hypoglycemia	• IR: Administer within 60 min before main meals of day • ER: Reconstitute prior to injection, must be injected immediately after reconstitution; administer without regard to meals; administer missed dose within 3 days
Liraglutide • Victoza • 0.6–1.8 mg subcut daily	• Family history of medullary thyroid carcinoma • Multiple endocrine neoplasia syndrome type 2				• Administer without regard to meals • Saxenda used for chronic weight management
Albiglutide • Tanzeum • 30–50 mg subcut once weekly					• Reconstitute prior to injection, must be injected within 8 hours of reconstitution • Administer without regard to meals • Administer missed dose within 3 days
Lixisenatide • Adlyxin • 10 mcg subcut daily × 14 days then 20 mcg subcut daily					Administer within 1 hr of 1st meal of day
Dulaglutide • Trulicity • 0.75–1.5 mg subcut once weekly		• Nausea • Hypoglycemia • ↓ appetite • Weight loss • Pancreatitis • Thyroid tumors • Tachycardia • PR interval prolongation • Atrioventricular block	• FPG • A1c every 3 mo • S/S pancreatitis • S/S hypoglycemia • Thyroid tumors • Heart rate • Electrocardiogram		• Administer without regard to meals • Administer missed dose within 3 days

DPP-4 Inhibitors

Generic • Brand • Dose & Max	Contraindications	Primary Side Effects	Key Monitoring	Pertinent Drug Interactions	Med Pearl
Mechanism of action – prolong the active incretin levels of GLP-1 and glucose-dependent insulinotropic polypeptide (GIP)					
Sitagliptin ☆ • Januvia • 25–100 mg daily	None	• Hypoglycemia • Arthralgias • Pancreatitis	• Blood urea nitrogen (BUN)/SCr • FPG • A1c every 3 mo • S/S pancreatitis • S/S hypoglycemia	• Sulfonylureas and insulin ↑ risk of hypoglycemia • May ↑ digoxin concentrations	• 100-mg dose is preferred unless patient has renal impairment • Adjust dose in renal impairment
Saxagliptin • Onglyza • 2.5–5 mg daily		• Hypoglycemia • Arthralgias • Pancreatitis • Heart failure	• BUN/SCr • FPG • A1c every 3 mo • S/S pancreatitis • S/S hypoglycemia • S/S heart failure	• CYP3A4 substrate • CYP3A4 inhibitors may ↑ effects; ↓ dose to 2.5 mg daily when used with strong CYP3A4 inhibitors • CYP3A4 inducers may ↓ effects • Sulfonylureas and insulin ↑ risk of hypoglycemia	Adjust dose in renal impairment
Linagliptin • Tradjenta • 5 mg daily		• Hypoglycemia • Arthralgias • Pancreatitis	• FPG • A1c every 3 mo • S/S pancreatitis • S/S hypoglycemia	• CYP3A4 and P-glycoprotein (P-gp) substrate • CYP3A4 or P-gp inhibitors may ↑ effects • CYP3A4 or P-gp inducers may ↓ effects • Sulfonylureas and insulin ↑ risk of hypoglycemia	No renal dose adjustment
Alogliptin • Nesina • 25 mg daily		• Hypoglycemia • Arthralgias • Pancreatitis • Heart failure	• BUN/SCr • FPG • A1c every 3 mo • S/S pancreatitis • S/S hypoglycemia • S/S heart failure • LFTs (at baseline)	• Sulfonylureas and insulin ↑ risk of hypoglycemia	Adjust dose in renal and hepatic impairment

SGLT2 Inhibitors

Generic • Brand • Dose & Max	Contraindications	Primary Side Effects	Key Monitoring	Pertinent Drug Interactions	Med Pearl
Mechanism of action – ↓ reabsorption of filtered glucose from tubular lumen, ↑ glucosuria					
Canagliflozin • Invokana • 100–300 mg daily	• Hypersensitivity • CrCl <30 mL/min	• Genitourinary infections (especially in females) • Dehydration • Hyperkalemia • Hypotension • DKA • Fractures • Acute kidney injury • Urosepsis/ pyelonephritis • Hypoglycemia • ↑ low-density lipoprotein cholesterol (LDL-C)	• BUN/SCr • FPG • A1c every 3 mo • S/S hypoglycemia • Blood pressure • Serum potassium (K+) • LDL-C • S/S heart failure • LFTs (at baseline) • S/S genital fungal infections or urinary tract infections	• Rifampin, phenytoin, phenobarbital, and ritonavir may ↓ effects • May ↑ digoxin concentrations • Diuretics may ↑ risk of volume depletion and hypotension • Sulfonylureas and insulin ↑ risk of hypoglycemia	Administer before first meal of the day
Dapagliflozin • Farxiga • 5–10 mg daily				• Diuretics may ↑ risk of volume depletion and hypotension • Sulfonylureas and insulin ↑ risk of hypoglycemia	
Empagliflozin • Jardiance • 10–25 mg daily	• Hypersensitivity • CrCl < 45 mL/min				• Administer in A.M. • Administer without regard to meals

Combination Products

See individual drug components for important points		
Brand	**Components**	**Maximum Daily Dose**
Actoplus Met, Actoplus Met XR	Actoplus Met = Pioglitazone + Metformin Actoplus Met XR = Pioglitazone + Metformin ER	Actoplus Met: Pioglitazone 45 mg/metformin 2,550 mg Actoplus Met XR: Pioglitazone 45 mg/metformin ER 2,000 mg
Avandamet	Rosiglitazone + Metformin	Rosiglitazone 8 mg/metformin 2,000 mg
Avandaryl (only available generically)	Rosiglitazone + Glimepiride	Rosiglitazone 8 mg/glimepiride 4 mg
Duetact	Pioglitazone + Glimepiride	Pioglitazone 45 mg/glimepiride 8 mg
Glucovance	Glyburide + Metformin	Glyburide 20 mg/metformin 2,000 mg
Glyxambi	Empagliflozin + Linagliptin	Empagliflozin 25 mg/linagliptin 5 mg
Invokamet	Canagliflozin + Metformin	Cangliflozin 300 mg/metformin 2,000 mg
Janumet, Janumet XR	Janumet = Sitagliptin + Metformin Janumet XR = Sitagliptin + Metformin ER	Janumet: Sitagliptin 100 mg/metformin 2,000 mg Janumet XR: Sitagliptin 100 mg/metformin ER 2,000 mg
Jentadueto, Jentadueto XR	Jentadueto = Linagliptin + Metformin Jentadueto XR = Linagliptin + Metformin ER	Jentadueto: Linagliptin 5 mg/metformin 2,000 mg Jentadueto XR: Linagliptin 5 mg/metformin ER 2,000 mg
Kazano	Alogliptin + Metformin	Alogliptin 25 mg/metformin 2,000 mg

Combination Products *(cont'd)*

Brand	Components	Maximum Daily Dose
Kombiglyze XR	Saxagliptin + Metformin ER	Saxagliptin 5 mg/metformin ER 2,000 mg
Metaglip (only available generically)	Glipizide + Metformin	Glipizide 20 mg/metformin 2,000 mg
Oseni	Alogliptin + Pioglitazone	Alogliptin 25 mg/pioglitazone 45 mg
Qtern	Dapagliflozin + Saxagliptin	Dapagliflozin 10 mg/saxagliptin 5 mg
Prandimet	Repaglinide + Metformin	Repaglinide 10 mg/metformin 2,500 mg
Soliqua	Insulin Glargine + Lixisenatide	Insulin glargine 60 units/lixisenatide 20 mcg
Synjardy and Synjardy XR	Synjardy = Empagliflozin + Metformin Synjardy XR = Empagliflozin + Metformin ER	Synjardy: Empagliflozin 25 mg/metformin 2,000 mg Synjardy XR: Empagliflozin 25 mg/metformin ER 2,000 mg
Xigduo XR	Dapagliflozin + Metformin ER	Dapagliflozin 10 mg/metformin ER 2,000 mg
Xultophy	Insulin Degludec + Lixisenatide	Insulin degludec 50 units/lixisenatide 1.8 mg

HYPOTHYROIDISM

Guidelines Summary

The treatment and management of chronic thyroiditis and clinical hypothyroidism must be tailored to the individual patient. Many clinical endocrinologists treat the goiter of chronic thyroiditis with levothyroxine, even in patients with normal levels of TSH, and all physicians will treat clinical hypothyroidism with levothyroxine replacement therapy.

- TSH is the primary marker for medication monitoring. Because thyroid hormone functions on a negative feedback loop, elevated levels indicate hypothyroid state and low levels indicate hyperthyroid state.

- Initial dose of levothyroxine is 1.7 mcg/kg/day. Adjust doses in 10–25 mcg/day increments based upon clinical response. Half-life of levothyroxine is approximately 1 week. TSH monitoring and dose adjustments occur at 4–8 week intervals.

Medications for Hypothyroidism

Generic • Brand • Dose	Contraindications	Primary Side Effects	Key Monitoring	Pertinent Drug Interactions	Med Pearl
Mechanism of action – T4 is c onverted to T3 and exerts many metabolic effects through control of DNA transcription and protein synthesis					
Levothyroxine☆ (T4) • Synthroid, Levoxyl, Unithroid • Tab: 25–300 mcg daily • Also available as injection Liothyronine (T3) • Cytomel, Triostat • 5–100 mcg daily • Injection, tabs	• Recent myocardial infarction or thyrotoxicosis • Uncorrected adrenal insufficiency	• Angina • Anxiety • Alopecia • ↑ LFTs • Tachycardia	• TSH • T3 • T4 • Free T4 • Heart rate • Blood pressure • Weight	Absorption may be ↓ by: cholestyramine, aluminum-containing medications, sucralfate, sodium polystyrene sulfonate, phenytoin, carbamazepine, rifampin	• T4: not the active compound; must be converted to T3 to become active • Thyroid treatment may also be used to augment depression treatment • Narrow therapeutic index drug • Often involved in medication errors
Desiccated thyroid☆ T4 (80%) T3 (20%) • Armour, Thyroid • 15–120 mg daily • Tab	• Hypersensitivity to beef or pork • Recent myocardial infarction or thyrotoxicosis • Uncorrected adrenal insufficiency				• Same as above • Origin: hog, cow, sheep • 80% T4 and 20% T3 is to mimic natural physiologic production
Liotrix • Thyrolar • Levothyroxine 12.5–100 mcg/liothyronine 3.1–25 mcg daily • Tabs	• Uncorrected adrenal cortical insufficiency • Untreated thyrotoxicosis				Liotrix is LT4/LT3 which is T4:T3 ratio; this ratio is 4:1

HYPERTHYROIDISM

Guidelines Summary

Symptomatic Management

Therapy targeting symptoms of hyperthyroidism (primarily tachycardia) is recommended in elderly patients, those with resting heart rate >90 beats per minute, and patients with preexisting cardiovascular disease. Oral β-blockers are the mainstay of therapy; see Cardiovascular Disorders chapter for details on this drug class.

Antithyroid Therapy

Three treatment modalities are available for Graves' disease: surgical intervention, antithyroid drugs, and radioactive iodine.

- In the United States, radioactive iodine is currently the treatment of choice for Graves' disease. Many clinical endocrinologists prefer an ablative dose of radioactive iodine, but some prefer use of a smaller dose in an attempt to render the patient euthyroid. Ablative therapy with radioactive iodine yields quicker resolution of the hyperthyroidism than does small-dose therapy, and thereby minimizes potential hyperthyroid-related morbidity.

- Although thyroidectomy for Graves' disease was frequently used in the past, it is now uncommonly performed in the United States unless coexistent thyroid cancer is suspected.

- Antithyroid medications, methimazole and propylthiouracil, have been used since the 1940s and are prescribed in an attempt to achieve a remission. The remission rates are variable, and relapses are frequent. Patients in whom remission is most likely to be achieved are those with mild hyperthyroidism and small goiters. Antithyroid drug treatment is not without the risk of adverse reactions, including minor rashes, and, in rare instances, agranulocytosis and hepatitis.

Medications for Hyperthyroidism

Generic • Brand • Dose	Contraindications	Primary Side Effects	Key Monitoring	Pertinent Drug Interactions	Med Pearl
Mechanism of action – inhibits synthesis of thyroid hormones by blocking the oxidation of iodine in the thyroid gland					
Propylthiouracil • Only available generically • Initial: 300–600 mg/day in 3–4 divided doses • Maintenance: 50–300 mg/day in 2–3 divided doses	Hypersensitivity	• Benign transient leukopenia (white blood cell [WBC] count <4,000/mm^3) • Pruritic maculo-papular rash • Arthralgias • Fever • Hepatotoxicity • Lupus-like syndrome	• WBC with differential • LFTs • TSH • T3 • T4	May ↑ effects of warfarin	• Clinical improvement approx. 4–8 weeks • Side effects with propylthiouracil more common with higher doses and in children • Rash may be treated with antihistamine • Severe side effects may require discontinuation of therapy • "PTU" is an error-prone abbreviation; avoid use • Tapering doses may start once clinical improvement seen • Correction of hyperthyroidism may alter disposition of • β-blockers, digoxin, and theophylline • Propylthiouracil preferred in pregnancy
Methimazole • Tapazole • Initial: 15–60 mg/day in 3 divided doses • Maintenance: 5–30 mg/day	Hypersensitivity				

POLYCYSTIC OVARY SYNDROME

Guidelines Summary

Treatment is based on a symptoms approach for anovulation, amenorrhea, ovulation induction, and hirsutism.

Anovulation and Amenorrhea

- Hormonal contraceptives (oral, patch, or vaginal ring) are first-line therapy to regulate or restore irregular or absent menses. The agents also improve symptoms of hirsutism and acne.
- Weight-reduction through a combination of calorie restriction and exercise are important; they affect and improve insulin resistance.
- Progestin, including medroxyprogesterone acetate, is often used to induce menses.
- Insulin-sensitizing agents, including metformin, pioglitazone, and rosiglitazone, are used to ↓ insulin resistance primarily in patients with type 2 DM or in those with IFG.

Ovulation Induction

- Lifestyle modifications, especially weight loss, will assist with ovulation induction.
- Clomiphene citrate is used to induce ovulation for up to 6 months.
- Ovarian drilling with laser or diathermy can be considered but is not recommended.
- Insulin-sensitizing agents, such as metformin and thiazolidinediones, can induce ovulation.

Hirsutism

- Oral contraceptives can reduce hair growth.
- Antiandrogens, including spironolactone, flutamide, insulin-sensitizing agents, and eflornithine can be used to ↓ hair growth.
- Mechanical hair removal, such as shaving, plucking, waxing, depilatory creams, electrolysis, and laser vaporization, can also be used.

Medications for Polycystic Ovary Syndrome

Generic • Brand • Dose	Contraindications	Primary Side Effects	Key Monitoring	Pertinent Drug Interactions	Med Pearl
Mechanism of action – inhibits secretion of pituitary gonadotropins, which prevents follicular maturation and ovulation; causes endometrial thinning					
Medroxyprogesterone☆ • Provera • Amenorrhea: 5–10 mg daily × 10 days	• History of deep venous thrombosis or pulmonary embolism • Pregnancy	• Headache • Weight changes • Edema • Menstrual irregularities	• Pregnancy should be ruled out • Symptoms of migraine	CPY3A4 substrate	Long-term use can lead to ↓ bone mineral density
Mechanism of action – Enclomiphene is less potent in inducing ovulation; however, it is rapidly absorbed and metabolized, allowing for the more potent zuclomiphene to act. Zuclomiphene inhibits normal estrogen negative feedback, which results in release of luteinizing hormone and follicle stimulating hormone; more potent than enclomiphene					
Clomiphene citrate (38% zuclomiphene; 62% enclomiphene) • Clomid • 50–100 mg daily × 5 days	• Liver disease • Abnormal uterine bleeding • Ovarian cysts • Uncontrolled thyroid or adrenal dysfunction • Pregnancy	• Ovarian enlargement • Hot flashes • Breast discomfort • Nausea • Bloating	• Pregnancy test • Menstrual cycle	May ↑ effects of ospemifene	Dosages ≥150 mg do not improve symptoms for PCOS
Mechanism of action – competes with aldosterone receptor sites in the distal tubules					
Spironolactone☆ • Aldactone • 50–200 mg daily	• Acute renal failure • Hyperkalemia • Pregnancy	• Gynecomastia • Hyperkalemia • Nausea • Cramping	• Blood pressure • Renal function • K$^+$	Use with angiotensin-converting enzyme inhibitors, angiotensin receptor blockers, K$^+$ supplements, or nonsteroidal anti-inflammatory drugs may ↑ risk of hyperkalemia	Adjust dose in renal impairment
Mechanism of action – nonsteroidal antiandrogen that inhibits androgen uptake or inhibits binding to androgen in target tissue					
Flutamide • Only available generically • 125–250 mg BID-TID	• Severe hepatic impairment • Pregnancy	• Gynecomastia • Hot flashes • Breast tenderness • Galactorrhea • ↓ libido	LFTs monthly for 4 mo, then periodically	CYP1A2 substrate	Most cases of liver failure occur within first 3 months of therapy

Medications for Polycystic Ovary Syndrome *(cont'd)*

Generic • Brand • Dose	Contraindications	Primary Side Effects	Key Monitoring	Pertinent Drug Interactions	Med Pearl
Mechanism of action – inhibitor of 5-alpha reductase, which results in the inhibition of conversion of testosterone to dihydrotestosterone					
Finasteride ☆ • Proscar, Propecia • 2.5–5 mg daily	Pregnancy	• Impotence • Ejaculation disturbances • ↓ libido • Orthostatic hypotension	Absolute need for dual forms of birth control	None	Women should avoid contact with crushed or broken tablets and the semen from a male partner exposed to finasteride (teratogen)
Mechanism of action – inhibits ornithine decarboxylase, the rate-limiting enzyme in biosynthesis of putrescine, spermin, and spermidine (rapid dividing cell most susceptible)					
Eflornithine • Vaniqa • Apply BID	Hypersensitivity	• Acne • Pruritus • Alopecia • Stinging	None	None	• Used to ↓ unwanted facial hair • Do not wash affected area for 8 hr following application • Onset of action 4–8 wk

PRACTICE QUESTIONS

1. Patients with overactive thyroid may present with which of the following symptoms?

   (A) Weight loss
   (B) Heat intolerance
   (C) Heart palpitations
   (D) Goiter
   (E) All of the above

2. A patient comes to the pharmacy and tells you that her blood sugars were 126 and 127 mg/dL fasting on two occasions. She wants some advice because her doctor didn't have time to talk with her. What is the main point you will be addressing with this woman?

   (A) This patient does not have diabetes because the doctor did the same test.
   (B) This patient has diabetes but does not need formal education; she should just watch what she eats and exercise more.
   (C) This patient doesn't have diabetes but might develop it soon.
   (D) This patient has diabetes, needs a formal diabetes education class, and is likely a candidate for metformin.

3. How many days can Humalog stay out of the refrigerator and be considered safe to administer?

   (A) 1 day
   (B) 28 days
   (C) 56 days
   (D) 90 days
   (E) 180 days

4. A 62-year-old woman (5'2″, 180 lb) with type 2 diabetes, history of medullary thyroid carcinoma, osteopenia, and stage 3 chronic kidney disease (CrCl = 45 mL/min) presents for routine follow-up. Current medications include metformin 1 g BID, lisinopril 10 mg PO daily, calcium carbonate/vitamin D 600/400 BID, and aspirin 81 mg PO daily. Labs today include A1c 7.6%, AST 20 IU/L, ALT 22 IU/L and K 4.2 mEq/L. Which of the following is the most appropriate recommendation?

   (A) Initiate Bydureon 2 mg SC once each week.
   (B) Initiate pioglitazone 30 mg PO once daily.
   (C) Initiate insulin glargine 40 units once daily.
   (D) Initiate sitagliptin 50 mg PO daily.

5. Which of the following medications is contraindicated in a patient with heart failure?

   (A) Exenatide
   (B) Sitagliptin
   (C) Glimepiride
   (D) Pioglitazone

6. Which of the following medications is MOST likely to cause hypoglycemia?

   (A) Metformin
   (B) Glipizide
   (C) Sitagliptin
   (D) Exenatide

7. Which of the following mechanisms MOST accurately describes the action of exenatide?

   (A) Mimics glucagon-like peptide-1
   (B) Inhibits gluconeogenesis in the liver
   (C) Inhibits the dipeptidyl peptidase IV enzyme
   (D) Increases insulin sensitivity in the periphery

8. A 65-year-old woman (5′2″, 182 lb) with hypertension, heart failure (NHYA Class I), and history of pancreatitis is newly diagnosed with type 2 diabetes. Medications include lisinopril 20 mg PO daily, carvedilol 6.25 mg PO BID, and aspirin 81 mg PO daily. Serum laboratory results today include A1c 8.3%, creatinine 1.6 mg/dL, ALT 35 IU/L, and BNP 20 pg/mL. A prescription is written for metformin. Which of the following statements is the BEST evaluation of this therapy?

   (A) Appropriate drug; no contraindications present
   (B) Inappropriate drug; contraindicated due to pancreatitis
   (C) Inappropriate drug; contraindicated due to heart failure
   (D) Inappropriate drug; contraindicated due to renal function

9. A 72-year-old man with hypothyroidism is treated with levothyroxine 88 mcg PO daily for 6 weeks. His TSH returns at 18 mIU/L (normal range 0.4–4 mIU/L). Which of the following is the most appropriate recommendation?

   (A) Increase levothyroxine dose to 100 mcg PO daily, recheck TSH in 2 weeks.
   (B) Increase levothyroxine dose to 100 mcg PO daily, recheck TSH in 6 weeks.
   (C) Decrease levothyroxine dose to 75 mcg PO daily, recheck TSH in 2 weeks.
   (D) Decrease levothyroxine dose to 75 mcg PO daily, recheck TSH in 6 weeks.

10. Which of the following is an appropriate patient education to provide for a patient on oral levothyroxine?

    (A) Take medication after a high-fat meal.
    (B) Take medication on an empty stomach.
    (C) Take medication without regard to meals.
    (D) Take medication with a glass of milk.

ANSWERS AND EXPLANATIONS

1. E

Weight loss, heat intolerance, heart palpitations, and goiter are all commonly seen symptoms with hyperthyroid disorders. Other common symptoms include nervousness, emotional lability, bowel frequency, irregular menses, and increased appetite.

2. D

This patient has diabetes and needs a formal diabetes education class. Metformin is first line therapy. Choice (A) is not correct because this woman does have diabetes—her fasting blood sugar was verified and was ≥126 mg/dL. Although the doctor caught the disease early, the patient still needs to seek formal education as this will lead to the best management.

3. B

Most unopened insulin preparations are stable at normal temperatures for 28 days. They should not be used if frozen or exposed to temperature greater than 98.6°F. Once opened (in use), vials may be stored in the refrigerator or for up to 28 days at room temperature.

4. D

Sitagliptin 50 mg PO daily is an appropriate agent to lower the A1c as needed and at an appropriate dose for renal function (30–50 mL/min = 50 mg daily). Bydureon (A) would be inappropriate for this patient due to the history of medullary thyroid carcinoma. Pioglitazone (B) would not be a good choice due to its potential to decrease bone mineral density; this patient has osteopenia. Although insulin glargine (C) would be an appropriate option, the dose of 40 units daily is too high for a starting dose.

5. D

Pioglitazone is contraindicated in a patient with heart failure. Thiazolidinediones have a side effect profile that includes fluid retention/edema and have demonstrated increases in heart failure exacerbations. The class should be avoided in patients with heart failure, especially NYHA classes III and IV.

6. B

Sulfonylureas such as glipizide have the greatest risk of hypoglycemia among the listed agents. Metformin (A) does not cause hypoglycemia as monotherapy. Although sitagliptin (C) and exenatide (D) can cause hypoglycemia, the risk is significantly lower than with secretagogues.

7. **A**

Exenatide is a glucagon-like peptide agonist that, by mimicking this incretin hormone, results in glucose-dependent insulin secretion, slowed gastric emptying, and diminished glucagon secretion postprandially.

8. **D**

Metformin is contraindicated in female patients with serum creatinine ≥1.4 mg/dL and males with serum creatinine ≥1.5 mg/dL. Pancreatitis (B) is not a contraindication to the use of metformin. Decompensated heart failure (C) is a contraindication to the medication, but this patient's heart failure is currently compensated (NYHA class I).

9. **B**

The TSH elevation indicates that the patient remains hypothyroid and requires a higher dose of levothyroxine. The half-life of levothyroxine is ~1 week; therefore, TSH levels are checked at 4–8 weeks to allow medication to reach steady state.

10. **B**

Levothyroxine is best and most consistently absorbed when taken on an empty stomach. Taking it with a high-fat meal (A), other food (C), or milk (D) would decrease absorption.

Neurological Disorders

This chapter covers the following disease states:

- **Multiple sclerosis**
- **Epilepsy**
- **Parkinson's disease**
- **Migraine headache**
- **Alzheimer's disease**

MULTIPLE SCLEROSIS

Guidelines Summary

The clinical management of MS should include consideration of treatment for acute exacerbations, altering the disease process, and alleviating ongoing symptoms related to the disease.

Disease-modifying drugs (DMDs) are used to alter the disease process. Treatment with interferon beta or glatiramer should be initiated as soon as possible after diagnosis in patients with relapsing disease. Therapies should be continued indefinitely except in the case of intolerable side effects, clear lack of benefit, or new therapy considerations.

Acute exacerbations—The cornerstone of therapy for acute exacerbations is IV corticosteroids. Methylprednisolone is most commonly used at 50–100 mg/day for 3–10 days. Oral prednisone may also be considered, but there is not strong evidence for using oral corticosteroids. Although corticosteroids have been shown to be very effective in the treatment of acute exacerbations, they do not alter the disease process.

Altering disease process—DMDs are the therapy of choice in altering the MS disease process. The currently approved DMDs include: interferon-β1a (Avonex and Rebif), interferon-β1b (Betaseron and Extavia), peginterferon β1a (Plegridy), glatiramer acetate (Copaxone), natalizumab (Tysabri), mitoxantrone (Novantrone), dimethyl fumarate (Tecfidera), teriflunomide (Aubagio), fingolimod (Gilenya), alemtuzumab (Lemtrada), and daclizumab (Zinbryta).

- The interferon agents and glatiramer acetate are considered first-line DMDs.
- Natalizumab may be considered if a patient cannot tolerate or has a poor response to another MS medication.
- Dimethyl fumarate, teriflunomide, fingolimod, alemtuzumab, and daclizumab are approved for relapsing MS.
- Mitoxantrone is approved to treat worsening relapsing-remitting MS and secondary progressive MS.
- Patients are generally treated with one DMD at a time, but worsening disease can be treated with combination DMD + mitoxantrone pulse therapy.

Symptom management—Dalfampridine (Ampyra) is used to improve walking in patients with MS.

Medications for Multiple Sclerosis

Generic • Brand • Dose & Max	Contraindications	Primary Side Effects	Key Monitoring Parameters	Pertinent Drug Interactions	Med Pearls
Disease-Modifying Drugs					
Mechanism of action – anti-inflammatory and immunomodulatory effects are exerted through binding of interferon to human cell-surface receptors and subsequent ↓ T-cell production of pro-inflammatory cytokines, ↓ production of pro-inflammatory lymphocytes, and ↑ production of anti-inflammatory lymphocytes					
Interferon-β1a • Avonex, Rebif • Avonex: 30 mcg IM weekly • Rebif: 4.4–8.8 mcg subcut 3 times weekly × 2 wk, then 11–22 mcg subcut 3 times weekly × 2 wk, then 22–44 mcg 3 times weekly Interferon-β1b • Betaseron, Extavia • 0.0625 mg subcut every other day; ↑ dose by 0.0625 mg every 2 wk to target dose of 0.25 mg subcut every other day Peginterferon-β1a • Plegridy • 63 mcg subcut on day 1, then 94 mcg subcut on day 15, then 125 mcg subcut every 2 wk starting on day 29	• Hypersensitivity to interferon-β or human albumin • Allergy to other interferons	• Flu-like symptoms (fever, chills, fatigue, muscle aches) • Injection site reactions • Anemia • Thrombocytopenia • Hepatotoxicity • Depression	• Liver function tests (LFTs) • Complete blood count (CBC)	None	• Acetaminophen or nonsteroidal anti-inflammatory drugs (NSAIDs) can ↓ flu-like symptoms • Neutralizing antibodies may develop, rendering the drug less efficacious

Medications for Multiple Sclerosis   *(cont'd)*

Generic • Brand • Dose & Max	Contraindications	Primary Side Effects	Key Monitoring Parameters	Pertinent Drug Interactions	Med Pearls
Mechanism of action – influences immature CD4 cells to become less inflammatory, thereby suppressing demyelination and preventing nerve fiber damage					
Glatiramer acetate • Copaxone, Glatopa • 20 mg subcut daily or 40 mg subcut 3 times/week	Hypersensitivity to the drug or to mannitol	• Injection site reactions • Postinjection reactions (chest pain, palpitations)	Injection reactions	• Avoid use of live vaccines	Does not produce neutralizing antibodies
Mechanism of action – ↓ central inflammation by binding to sphingosine 1-phosphate receptors					
Fingolimod • Gilenya • 0.5 mg PO daily	• Myocardial infarction • Unstable angina • Transient ischemic attack/cerebrovascular accident • New York Heart Association class III/IV or decompensated heart failure (HF) • Atrioventricular (AV) block/sick sinus syndrome • QTc interval ≥500 msec • Concurrent use with class Ia or III antiarrhythmic	• Bradycardia • AV block • Hypertension • Infection • Macular edema • Dyspnea • ↑ LFTs • Diarrhea • Headache • Flu-like syndrome • HF • QT interval prolongation • Hypersensitivity reactions • Posterior reversible encephalopathy syndrome (PRES) • Progressive multifocal leukoencephalopathy (PML)	• Heart rate (HR) • Blood pressure (BP) • CBC • Electrocardiogram (ECG) • Ophthalmologic exam • LFTs • S/S of HF • S/S of PRES or PML • S/S of infection	• Class Ia and class III anti-arrhythmics may ↑ risk of bradycardia and AV block • Avoid use of live vaccines • Use with QT-interval prolonging agents may ↑ risk of torsades de pointes (TdP)	Give zoster vaccination prior to administration, if needed
Mechanism of action – monoclonal antibody inhibits pro-inflammatory interactions within vascular endothelial cells and parenchymal brain cells					
Natalizumab • Tysabri • 300 mg IV infusion every 4 wk	• Hypersensitivity • Current or history of PML	• Infusion reactions (rash, drowsiness, fever, chills, hypotension, nausea, shortness of breath) • ↑ LFTs • Infection • Headache • Fatigue • Arthralgia • PML	• MRI (baseline, and repeated if PML suspected) • LFTs • Infusion reactions • S/S of infection	Other DMDs ↑ risk of PML	• Reserved for patients who have not responded to other DMDs • Should be used as monotherapy only • Available only through a restrictive prescribing program (MS-TOUCH) • Also indicated for Crohn's disease

Medications for Multiple Sclerosis *(cont'd)*

Generic • Brand • Dose & Max	Contraindications	Primary Side Effects	Key Monitoring Parameters	Pertinent Drug Interactions	Med Pearls
Mechanism of action – ↓ migration of T cells into the CNS by arresting the cell cycle and interfering with DNA repair and RNA synthesis					
Mitoxantrone • Only available generically • 12 mg/m² IV infusion every 3 mo; max cumulative dose = 140 mg/m²	Hypersensitivity	• HF • Nausea • Neutropenia • Alopecia • Menstrual irregularities • Infection	• Echocardiogram (left ventricular ejection fraction [LVEF] at baseline and prior to each IV infusion) • CBC with differential • LFTs • S/S of infection	Avoid use of live vaccines	Discontinue therapy if LVEF <50% or clinically significant decline in LVEF
Mechanism of action – activates nuclear factor–like 2 pathway, ↓ inflammatory response to oxidative stress					
Dimethyl fumarate • Tecfidera • 120 mg PO BID × 7 days, then 240 mg PO BID	Hypersensitivity	• Dermatitis • Flushing • ↑ LFTs • Lymphopenia • Nausea/vomiting/diarrhea (N/V/D) • Hypersensitivity reaction • PML • Infection	• CBC with differential (baseline, 6 mo, then every 6–12 mo) • S/S of PML • S/S of infection • LFTs	May ↓ effectiveness and ↑ toxicity of live vaccines	May give with food or give aspirin 325 mg 30 min before to ↓ flushing
Mechanism of action – inhibits pyrimidine synthesis, ↓ proliferation and inflammation					
Teriflunomide • Aubagio • 7–14 mg PO daily	• Hypersensitivity • Severe hepatic impairment • Pregnancy • Women of reproductive potential without adequate contraception	• Hepatotoxicity • Rash • Hypersensitivity reaction • Hypertension • Infection • Interstitial lung disease • Peripheral neuropathy • Neutropenia • Headache • Alopecia • N/D	• CBC with differential • LFTs (monthly for first 6 mo) • BP • Renal function • PPD (prior to initiation) • Pregnancy test (prior to initiation) • S/S of infection	• CYP2C8 inhibitor • CYP1A2 inducer • May ↓ effects of warfarin • Avoid use of live vaccines	• Counsel males and females on appropriate use of contraception during therapy (teratogenic) • Screen for tuberculosis (TB) prior to initiating therapy

Medications for Multiple Sclerosis   *(cont'd)*

Generic • Brand • Dose & Max	Contraindications	Primary Side Effects	Key Monitoring Parameters	Pertinent Drug Interactions	Med Pearls
Mechanism of action – monocolonal antibody to CD52 receptors which causes the depletion of lymphocytes to CD52 receptors which causes the depletion of lymphocytes					
Alemtuzumab • Lemtrada • 12 mg IV daily × 5 days, then 12 mg daily × 3 days 12 months later	HIV infection	• Autoimmune conditions • Bone marrow suppression • Infection • Infusion reactions • Pulmonary fibrosis • PML • Thyroid disease • Malignancy (melanoma)	• CBC with differential • S/S of infection • Thyroid stimulating hormone • S/S of infusion reactions • S/S of PML • Malignancy • S/S of pulmo-nary fibrosis • Renal function • Urinalysis • Skin exam	Avoid use of live vaccines	• REMS program • Premedicate with cortico-steroids for first 3 days of each treatment course • Initiate antiviral therapy (to prevent herpes infection) on 1st day of therapy and continue for 2 mo or until CD4+ cell count >200/m^3
Mechanism of action – monoclonal antibody inhibitor of IL-2					
Daclizumab • Zinbryta • 150 mg subcut monthly	• Hypersensitivity • Hepatic impairment • Autoimmune hepatitis	• Hepatotoxicity • Autoimmune disorders • Photosensitivity • N/D • Hypersensitivity reaction • Infection • Depression • Suicidal thoughts	• LFTs • S/S of infection	Avoid use of live vaccines	• REMS program • Screen for TB and hepatitis B/C prior to initiating therapy
Symptom Management					
Mechanism of action – potassium channel blocker; ↑ action potential in demyelinated axon					
Dalfampridine • Ampyra • 10 mg PO every 12 hr	• History of seizures • Moderate–severe renal impairment (creatinine clearance ≤50 mL/min) • Hypersensitivity	• Seizures • Anaphylaxis • Urinary tract infection • Dizziness • Insomnia • Headache • Nausea • Balance disturbance	• Renal function • Walking ability	None	• Indicated to improve walking in patients with MS • Seizure risk is dose-dependent

EPILEPSY

Guidelines Summary

- Goals of treatment include a lack of seizure activity, minimal medication side effects of treatment, and improved quality of life.

- Treatment with antiepileptic drugs (AEDs) is warranted for patients that experience multiple seizures or have significantly affected quality of life. AED choice is based on the specific seizure type, the patient's age, comorbidities, ability to adhere to the regimen, and insurance coverage.

- AED monotherapy is preferred, but some patients may require combination therapy.

- First-line AEDs for partial seizures include carbamazepine, phenytoin, lamotrigine, valproic acid, and oxcarbazepine.

- First-line AEDs for generalized absence seizures include valproic acid and ethosuximide.

- First-line AEDs for tonic-clonic seizures include phenytoin, carbamazepine, and valproic acid.

- Alternative AEDs include gabapentin, topiramate, levetiracetam, zonisamide, tiagabine, primidone, felbamate, lamotrigine, phenobarbital, lacosamide, vigabatrin, and perampanel.

- The Food and Drug Administration (FDA) issued an alert regarding the relationship between the use of AEDs and suicidality (including suicidal behavior or ideation). Pooled analyses completed by the FDA indicated a significant ↑ of suicidality for patients treated with AEDs when compared to those given placebo. All AEDs appear to ↑ the risk similarly. Manufacturers of all AEDs are now required to include a boxed warning in their prescribing information and to include a medication guide for patients in their product labeling regarding the risk of suicide.

Antiepileptic Drugs

Generic • Brand • Dose/Dosage Forms	Contraindications	Primary Side Effects	Key Monitoring Parameters	Med Pearls
Mechanism of action –inhibits voltage-gated sodium channels, thereby depressing electrical transmission in the nucleus ventralis anterior of the thalamus				
Carbamazepine ☆ • Carbatrol, Epitol, Equetro, Tegretol, Tegretol XR, Carnexiv • 200–1,600 mg/day in 2–4 divided doses • ER caps/tabs, injection suspension, tabs	• Bone marrow suppression • Concomitant use with monoamine oxidase inhibitors (MAOIs) or non-nucleoside transcriptase inhibitors	• Dizziness • Drowsiness • Unsteadiness • N/V • Blurred vision • Aplastic anemia • Agranulocytosis • Rash (Stevens-Johnson syndrome possible) • Hyponatremia	• CBC with differential • Suicidal ideation • Serum drug concentrations (4–12 mcg/mL) • Serum sodium (Na+) concentrations • Seizure occurrence	• First-line for partial seizures and generalized tonic-clonic seizures • ↑ risk of Stevens-Johnson syndrome in patients with HLA-B*1502 allele (Asian descent)
Mechanism of action – thought to ↑ gamma amino butyric acid (GABA) concentrations in the brain				
Valproic acid (divalproex sodium) ☆ • Depakote, Depakote ER, Depakene, Depacon • 10–60 mg/kg/day • Caps, delayed-release caps/tabs, ER tabs, injection, solution, sprinkle caps	• Hypersensitivity • Hepatic impairment • Urea cycle disorders • Known porphyria • Use in pregnant women for migraine prevention	• Hepatotoxicity • Thrombocytopenia • Hyperammonemia • Weight gain • Pancreatitis • Headache • Somnolence • Dizziness • Alopecia	• Serum drug concentrations (50–100 mcg/mL) • LFTs • CBC • Serum ammonia concentrations • Suicidal ideation • Seizure occurrence	• First-line for partial, generalized, tonic-clonic, and absence seizures • Highly teratogenic • Also indicated for treatment of mania and migraine prophylaxis
Mechanism of action – promotes neuronal sodium efflux, thereby stabilizing the threshold against hyperexcitability				
Phenytoin ☆ • Dilantin • 100–200 mg TID • Caps, chewable tabs, injection, suspension	Hypersensitivity	• Nystagmus • Ataxia • Slurred speech • Dizziness • Insomnia • Headache • Tremor • Gingival hyperplasia • Rash (Stevens-Johnson syndrome possible)	• Serum drug concentrations (10–20 mcg/mL) • Suicidal ideation • Seizure occurrence	• First-line option for partial and generalized tonic-clonic seizures • Abrupt discontinuation should be avoided (may precipitate status epilepticus) • Takes 7–10 days to reach steady state • Therapeutic concentration must be corrected for hypoalbuminemia (serum albumin <4 g/dL): corrected phenytoin concentration = measured total concentration/([0.2*albumin] + 0.1) • ↑ risk of Stevens-Johnson syndrome in patients with HLA-B*1502 allele (Asian descent)

Antiepileptic Drugs   (cont'd)

Generic • Brand • Dose/Dosage Forms	Contraindications	Primary Side Effects	Key Monitoring Parameters	Med Pearls
Mechanism of action – depresses motor cortex and elevates the threshold of the CNS to convulsive stimuli				
Ethosuximide • Zarontin • 250–1,500 mg/day in divided doses • Caps, solution	Hypersensitivity	• Ataxia • Drowsiness • N/V/D • Blood dyscrasias • Rash (Stevens-Johnson syndrome possible)	• CBC • Suicidal ideation • Serum drug concentrations (40–100 mcg/mL) • Seizure occurrence	Used ONLY for absence seizures
Mechanism of action – blocks voltage-sensitive sodium channels, resulting in stabilization of hyperexcitable neuronal membranes				
Oxcarbazepine ☆ • Oxtellar XR, Trileptal • IR: 300–600 mg BID • ER: 600–1,200 mg daily • ER tabs, suspension, tabs	Hypersensitivity	• Sedation • Dizziness • Ataxia • Nausea • Rash (Stevens-Johnson syndrome possible) • Hyponatremia • Angioedema	• Suicidal ideation • Serum Na$^+$ concentrations • Seizure occurrence	• Adjust dose in renal impairment • 25–30% risk of cross-sensitivity in patients allergic to carbamazepine • ↑ risk of Stevens-Johnson syndrome in patients with HLA-B*1502 allele (Asian descent)
Felbamate • Felbatol • 1,200–3,600 mg/day in 3–4 divided doses • Suspension, tabs	• Hypersensitivity • Blood dyscrasias • Hepatic impairment	• Aplastic anemia • Acute liver failure • Anorexia • N/V • Insomnia • Headache	• CBC • LFTs • Suicidal ideation • Seizure occurrence	• AST or ALT ≥2 × upper limit of normal requires discontinuation • Not a first-line agent; reserved for refractory cases
Lamotrigine ☆ • Lamictal, Lamictal XR • IR: 25–700 mg/day in 1–2 divided doses • ER: 25–600 mg daily • Chewable tabs, ER tabs, ODTs, tabs	Hypersensitivity	• Rash (Stevens-Johnson syndrome possible) • Blood dyscrasias • Aseptic meningitis • Diplopia • Dizziness • Headache	• Rash • Suicidal ideation • S/S of aseptic meningitis • CBC • Seizure occurrence	• Risk of rash ↑ when combined with valproate • First-line option for partial seizures • Slow dose titration necessary (to minimize risk for rash) • May cause false-positive for phencyclidine (PCP) • Adjust dose in hepatic impairment
Lacosamide • Vimpat • 50–200 mg BID • Injection, solution, tabs	None	• N/V • Ataxia • Dizziness • PR interval prolongation • AV block • Headache • Fatigue • Diplopia • Tremor	• Suicidal ideation • ECG (in patients with conduction abnormalities, on negative chronotropic drugs or with cardiovascular disease) at baseline and at steady state or when receiving IV • Seizure occurrence	• Schedule V controlled substance • Adjust dose in renal or hepatic impairment

Antiepileptic Drugs *(cont'd)*

Generic • Brand • Dose/Dosage Forms	Contraindications	Primary Side Effects	Key Monitoring Parameters	Med Pearls
Mechanism of action – although structurally similar to GABA, pharmacological effects in epilepsy are not fully understood				
Gabapentin ☆ • Neurontin • 300–1,200 mg TID • Caps, solution, tabs	Hypersensitivity	• Dizziness • Fatigue • Somnolence • Ataxia • Weight gain • Angioedema • Behavioral disturbances (aggression, agitation, anger, anxiety, depression, hostility, nervousness) • Difficulty concentrating • Restlessness	• Suicidal ideation • Seizure occurrence	• No significant CYP450 drug interactions • Adjust dose in renal impairment • Also used for various neuropathies
Mechanism of action – blocks voltage-dependent sodium channels, augments GABA activity, antagonizes glutamate receptors				
Topiramate ☆ • Qudexy XR, Topamax, Trokendi XR • IR: 25–200 mg BID • ER: 50–400 mg daily • ER caps, sprinkle caps, tabs	Hypersensitivity	• Difficulty concentrating • Confusion • Memory issues • Speech problems • Depression • Somnolence • Fatigue • Dizziness • Headache • Weight loss • Kidney stones • Angle closure glaucoma • Visual field defects • ↓ sweating • Hyperthermia • Metabolic acidosis • Hyperammonemia • Encephalopathy • Paresthesia	• Suicidal ideation • Serum bicarbonate concentrations • Serum ammonia concentration (if unexplained lethargy, vomiting, or mental status changes) • Intraocular pressure • Seizure occurrence	• Adjust dose in renal impairment • Slow titration necessary to minimize side effects • Teratogenic • Also indicated for migraines

Antiepileptic Drugs (cont'd)

Generic • Brand • Dose/Dosage Forms	Contraindications	Primary Side Effects	Key Monitoring Parameters	Med Pearls
Mechanism of action – not well understood, thought to inhibit calcium channels and facilitate GABA transmission				
Levetiracetam ☆ • Keppra, Keppra XR, Spritam, Roweepra • IR: 500–1500 mg BID • ER: 1,000–3,000 mg daily • ER tabs, injection, ODTs, solution, tabs	None	• Dizziness • Behavioral disturbances (aggression, agitation, anger, anxiety, depression, hostility, nervousness) • Psychotic symptoms • Somnolence • Fatigue • Rash (Stevens-Johnson syndrome possible) • Ataxia • Anemia • Neutropenia • Hypertension	• Renal function • Suicidal ideation • CNS disturbances • BP (in children) • CBC with differential • Seizure occurrence	• Adjust dose in renal impairment • No significant drug interactions • Do not chew or crush IR tabs
Mechanism of action – elevates seizure threshold by ↓ postsynaptic excitability through stimulation of postsynaptic GABA inhibitory responses				
Phenobarbital ☆ • Only available generically • 60–200 mg/day in 2–3 divided doses • Elixir, injection, solution, tabs	• Severe liver impairment • Hypersensitivity • Porphyria • Dyspnea or airway obstruction	• Sedation • Nystagmus • Ataxia • Agitation • Hyperactivity • Headache • Nausea • Agranulocytosis • Rash (Stevens-Johnson syndrome possible) • Behavior changes • Intellectual blunting • Mood change • Respiratory depression (IV)	• Serum concentrations 20–40 mcg/mL • CBC with differential • LFTs • Suicidal ideation • Seizure occurrence	• Schedule IV controlled substance • Drug of choice for neonatal seizures • Frequency of side effects limits use • Titrate dose slowly to minimize side effects • Takes 3–4 wk to reach steady-state
Primidone • Mysoline • 750–2,000 mg/day in 3–4 divided doses • Tabs			• Serum concentrations 5–12 mcg/mL • CBC with differential • LFTs • Suicidal ideation • Seizure occurrence	Metabolized to phenobarbital
Mechanism of action – potent and specific inhibitor of GABA uptake into neuronal elements, thereby enhances GABA activity by ↓ its removal from the neuronal space				
Tiagabine • Gabitril • 32–56 mg/day in 2–4 divided doses • Tabs	Hypersensitivity	• Dizziness • Fatigue • Difficulty concentrating • Speech problems • Confusion • Somnolence • Rash (Stevens-Johnson syndrome possible) • Nervousness • Tremor • Blurred vision • Depression • Weakness	• Suicidal ideation • Seizure occurrence	Take with food

Antiepileptic Drugs *(cont'd)*

Generic • Brand • Dose/Dosage Forms	Contraindications	Primary Side Effects	Key Monitoring Parameters	Med Pearls
Mechanism of action – irreversible inhibition of gamma-aminobutyric acid transaminase (GABA-T), thereby ↑ the levels of GABA within the brain				
Vigabatrin • Sabril • 500 mg BID, then ↑ daily dose by 500 mg at weekly intervals (max dose = 1,500 mg BID) • Packet for oral solution, tabs	None	• Permanent vision loss • Anemia • Fatigue • Somnolence • Peripheral neuropathy • Edema • Tremor • Memory impairment • Weight gain • Confusion	• Ophthalmologic exam (every 3 mo) • Suicidal ideation • CBC • Seizure occurrence	• Adjust dose in renal impairment • Black box warning due to ophthalmologic effects • Available only through special REMS program
Mechanism of action – blocks voltage-dependent sodium and calcium channels, thereby ↓ repetitive neuronal firing				
Zonisamide ☆ • Zonegran • 100–600 mg/day in 1–2 divided doses • Caps	Hypersensitivity to zonisamide or sulfonamides	• Depression • Psychotic symptoms • Difficulty concentrating • Speech problems • Somnolence • Fatigue • Dizziness • Nausea • Rash (Stevens-Johnson syndrome possible) • Aplastic anemia • Agranulocytosis • ↓ sweating • Hyperthermia • Metabolic acidosis • Kidney stones • ↑ blood urea nitrogen/ serum creatinine	• Suicidal ideation • Renal function • Serum bicarbonate concentrations • Seizure occurrence	• Takes up to 2 wk to achieve steady-state • Teratogenic
Mechanism of action – modulates calcium influx at the nerve terminals, thereby inhibiting excitatory neurotransmitter release				
Pregabalin ☆ • Lyrica • 150–600 mg/day in 2–3 divided doses • Caps, solution	Hypersensitivity	• Angioedema • Somnolence • Dizziness • Peripheral edema	• Suicidal ideation • Presence of edema • Seizure occurrence	• Schedule V controlled substance • Adjust dose in renal impairment • Also indicated for neuropathic pain and fibromyalgia

Antiepileptic Drugs *(cont'd)*

Generic • Brand • Dose/Dosage Forms	Contraindications	Primary Side Effects	Key Monitoring Parameters	Med Pearls
Mechanism of action – antagonistic effects of ionotropic alpha-amino-3-hydroxy-5-methyl-4-isoxazolepropionic acid (AMPA) glutamate receptor				
Perampanel • Fycompa • 2–12 mg at bedtime • Suspension, tabs	None	• Dizziness • Gait disturbance • Headache • Somnolence • Fatigue • Behavioral disturbances (aggression, agitation, anger, anxiety, depression, hostility, nervousness) • Depression • Weight gain	• Suicidal ideation • Weight • Seizure occurrence	• Schedule III controlled substance • Adjust dose in renal impairment
Mechanism of action – mechanism is not well understood, but may be attributed to selective affinity for synaptic vesicle protein 2A (SV2A)				
Brivaracetam • Briviact • 25–100 mg BID • Injection, solution, tabs	Hypersensitivity	• Somnolence • Dizziness • Fatigue • Gait disturbance • Behavioral disturbances (aggression, agitation, anger, anxiety, depression, hostility, nervousness) • Psychotic symptoms • Angioedema • N/V	• Suicidal ideation • Seizure occurrence	• Schedule V controlled substance • Adjust dose in hepatic impairment

Selected AED Drug Interactions

AED	Interacting Medication	Effect
Carbamazepine • 3A4 substrate • Strong CYP1A2, CYP2C19, CYP2C8, CYP2C9, and CYP3A4 inducer	Abiraterone	↓ Abiraterone
	Apixaban	↓ Apixaban
	Bortezomib	↓ Bortezomib
	Cimetidine	↑ Carbamazepine
	Clozapine	↓ Clozapine
	Dabigatran	↓ Dabigatran
	Dolutegravir	↓ Dolutegravir
	Doxycycline	↓ Doxycycline
	Dronedarone	↓ Dronedarone
	Erythromycin	↑ Carbamazepine
	Everolimus	↓ Everolimus
	Fluoxetine	↑ Carbamazepine
	Ibrutinib	↓ Ibrutinib
	Isoniazid	↑ Carbamazepine
	Itraconazole	↓ Itraconazole
	Oral contraceptives	↓ Contraceptives
	Perampanel	↓ Perampanel
	Phenobarbital	↓ Carbamazepine, ↓ phenobarbital
	Phenytoin	↓ Carbamazepine, ↓ phenytoin
	Rivaroxaban	↓ Rivaroxaban
	Theophylline	↓ Theophylline
	Warfarin	↓ Warfarin
Valproic acid	Carbamazepine	↓ Valproic acid, ↑ carbamazepine
	Lamotrigine	↑ Lamotrigine
	Phenobarbital	↓ Valproic acid, ↑ phenobarbital
	Phenytoin	↓ Valproic acid, ↓ phenytoin
	Primidone	↓ Valproic acid, ↑ phenobarbital
Phenytoin • CYP2C19 and CYP2C9 substrate • Strong CYP2C19, CYP2C8, CYP2C9, and CYP3A4 inducer	Abiraterone	↓ Abiraterone
	Antacids	↓ Phenytoin
	Apixaban	↓ Apixaban
	Carbamazepine	↓ Phenytoin
	Cimetidine	↑ Phenytoin
	Clozapine	↓ Clozapine
	Dabigatran	↓ Dabigatran
	Dolutegravir	↓ Dolutegravir
	Dronederone	↓ Dronederone
	Fluconazole	↑ Phenytoin
	Isoniazid	↑ Phenytoin
	Oral contraceptives	↓ Contraceptives
	Perampanel	↓ Perampanel
	Phenobarbital	↑ or ↓ Phenytoin
	Rivaroxaban	↓ Rivaroxaban
	Ticagrelor	↓ Ticagrelor
	Warfarin	↑ Phenytoin, ↑ anticoagulant effect

Selected AED Drug Interactions   *(cont'd)*

AED	Interacting Medication	Effect
Ethosuximide • CYP3A4 substrate	Phenytoin Valproic acid	↑ Phenytoin ↑ or ↓ Ethosuximide
Oxcarbazepine • CYP3A4 inducer	Cobicistat Dolutegravir Elvitegravir Ledipasvir Oral contraceptives Perampanel Phenobarbital Phenytoin Sofosbuvir	↓ Cobicistat ↓ Dolutegravir ↓ Elvitegravir ↓ Ledipasvir ↓ Contraceptives ↓ Perampanel, ↑ oxcarbazepine ↓ Oxcarbazepine ↓ Oxcarbazepine ↓ Sofosbuvir
Felbamate • CYP3A4 substrate	Carbamazepine Phenobarbital Phenytoin Valproic acid	↓ Carbamazepine, ↓ felbamate ↑ Phenobarbital, ↓ felbamate ↑ Phenytoin, ↓ felbamate ↑ Valproic acid
Perampanel • CYP3A4 substrate	Buprenorphine Carbamazepine Oxcarbazepine Phenytoin Progestins	↑ CNS depressant effect ↓ Perampanel ↓ Perampanel ↓ Perampanel ↓ Progestins
Lacosamide • CYP2C19, CYP2C9, and CYP3A4 substrate	Carbamazepine Phenobarbital Phenytoin	↓ Lacosamide ↓ Lacosamide ↓ Lacosamide
Lamotrigine	Carbamazepine Phenobarbital Phenytoin Primidone Valproic acid	↓ Lamotrigine ↓ Lamotrigine ↓ Lamotrigine ↓ Lamotrigine ↑ Lamotrigine
Topiramate	Carbamazepine Oral contraceptives Phenytoin Simeprevir Valproic acid	↓ Topiramate ↓ Contraceptives ↓ Topiramate ↓ Simeprevir ↓ Valproic acid
Phenobarbital • CYP2C19 substrate • Strong CYP1A2, CYP2C8, CYP2C9, and CYP3A4 inducer	Apixaban Dronederone Felbamate Oral contraceptives Phenytoin Rivaroxaban Simeprevir Valproic acid	↓ Apixaban ↓ Dronederone ↑ Phenobarbital ↓ Contraceptives ↑ Phenobarbital ↓ Rivaroxaban ↓ Simeprevir ↑ Phenobarbital

Selected AED Drug Interactions   *(cont'd)*

AED	Interacting Medication	Effect
Primidone • Strong CYP1A2, CYP2C8, CYP2C9, and CYP3A4 inducer	Carbamazepine Corticosteroids Phenytoin Valproic acid	↓ Primidone, ↑ phenobarbital ↓ Corticosteroids ↓ Primidone, ↑ phenobarbital ↑ Primidone, ↓ phenobarbital
Tiagabine • CYP3A4 substrate	Carbamazepine Phenytoin	↓ Tiagabine ↓ Tiagabine
Vigabatrin	Clonazepam Phenytoin	↑ Clonazepam ↓ Phenytoin
Zonisamide • CYP3A4 substrate	Carbamazepine Phenobarbital Phenytoin	↓ Zonisamide ↓ Zonisamide ↓ Zonisamide
Brivaracetam • CYP2C19 substrate	Phenytoin	↓ Brivaracetam

PARKINSON'S DISEASE

Summary of Treatment Recommendations

- Initial therapy generally consists of either a dopamine agonist or carbidopa/levodopa.
  - Patients ≥65 years of age or those with significant disability due to their PD should receive carbidopa/levodopa as initial therapy.
  - Patients <65 years of age may receive a dopamine agonist as initial therapy.
  - Inadequate response to maximum tolerable doses of initial therapy with a dopamine agonist or carbidopa/levodopa should result in the addition of the alternate medication.
  - Subsequently, COMT inhibitors may be added to ongoing carbidopa/levodopa therapy, and adjunctive therapies such as amantadine or anticholinergics may also be utilized.
  - Anticholinergic agents are primarily useful for the treatment of tremor-predominant PD but should be used with caution in elderly patients and avoided in patients with pre-existing cognitive impairment.
  - Because dopamine agonists and carbidopa/levodopa are aimed at increasing the available dopamine in the CNS, side effects such as hallucinations and delusions are possible. Psychiatric side effects which occur at the lowest effective doses of these drugs may be treated with the antipsychotic medication, quetiapine.

Medications for Parkinson's Disease

Generic • Brand • Dose/Dosage Forms	Contraindications	Primary Side Effects	Key Monitoring Parameters	Pertinent Drug Interactions	Med Pearls
Mechanism of action – unknown, thought to enhance dopamine release and inhibit dopamine reuptake, also acts as an NMDA receptor antagonist					
Amantadine • Only available generically • 100–200 mg BID • Caps, solution, tabs	Hypersensitivity	• Confusion • Nightmares • Hallucinations • Insomnia • Nervousness • Irritability	• Renal function • Response to therapy • Mental status • BP	None	Adjust dose in renal impairment
Mechanism of action – monoamine-oxidase (MAO) B inhibitors: inhibit the catabolism of dopamine by selectively inhibiting the monoamine oxidase B enzyme					
Selegiline • Eldepryl, Zelapar • Cap/tab: 5 mg BID • ODT: 1.25–2.5 mg daily • Caps, ODTs, tabs	• Hypersensitivity • Concurrent use with meperidine, methadone, dextromethorphan, tramadol, or MAOIs	• Nausea • Hallucinations • Insomnia • Depression • Orthostasis • Impulse control disorders • Hypertensive crisis (if high-tyramine foods are ingested)	• BP • Response to therapy • Presence of anxiety or agitation • Suicidal ideation • S/S of serotonin syndrome	Use with meperidine, other opioid analgesics, dextromethorphan, tramadol, selective serotonin reuptake inhibitors (SSRIs), serotonin-norepinephrine reuptake inhibitors (SNRIs), tricyclic antidepressants (TCAs), cyclobenzaprine, triptans, or St. John's wort may ↑ risk of serotonin syndrome	• Avoid tyramine-containing foods • Should not be abruptly discontinued • Discontinue 14 days prior to surgery if possible; should not be taken with general anesthesia • Transdermal patch (Emsam) used for depression
Rasagiline • Azilect • 0.5–1 mg daily • Tabs	• Hypersensitivity • Concurrent use with meperidine, methadone, tramadol, MAOIs, cyclobenzaprine, dextromethorphan, or St. John's wort	• Hypertension • Nausea • Orthostasis • Somnolence • Hallucinations • Impulse control disorders • Hypertensive crisis (if high-tyramine foods are ingested)	• Response to therapy • BP • S/S of serotonin syndrome	• CYP1A2 substrate • CYP1A2 inhibitors may ↑ effects • CYP1A2 inducers may ↓ effects • Use with meperidine, other opioid analgesics, dextromethorphan, tramadol, SSRIs, SNRIs, TCAs, cyclobenzaprine, triptans, or St. John's wort may ↑ risk of serotonin syndrome	• Avoid tyramine-containing foods >150 mg • Should not be abruptly discontinued • Adjust dose in hepatic impairment
Xadago • Safinamide • 50–100 mg daily • Tabs	• Hypersensitivity • Concurrent use with meperidine, methadone, tramadol, MAOIs, cyclobenzaprine, dextromethorphan, or St. John's wort	• Dyskinesia • Hypertension • Orthostatic hypotension • Falls • Nausea • ↑ LFTs	• Response to therapy • BP • S/S of serotonin syndrome	Use with meperidine, other opioid analgesics, dextromethorphan, tramadol, SSRIs, SNRIs, TCAs, cyclobenzaprine, triptans, or St. John's wort may ↑ risk of serotonin syndrome	• Avoid tyramine-containing foods >150 mg

Medications for Parkinson's Disease (cont'd)

Generic • Brand • Dose/Dosage Forms	Contraindications	Primary Side Effects	Key Monitoring Parameters	Pertinent Drug Interactions	Med Pearls
Mechanism of action – levodopa is a direct precursor to dopamine and is converted to dopamine once it crosses the blood-brain barrier; carbidopa is a dopa decarboxylase inhibitor; it is necessary to combine carbidopa with levodopa in order to prevent the peripheral degradation of levodopa prior to entry into the blood-brain barrier.					
Carbidopa/levodopa☆ • Duopa, Rytary, Sinemet, Sinemet CR • Carbidopa 75–300 mg/day in 3–4 divided doses (75 mg required, side effects if >300 mg/day) • Levodopa 100–2,000 mg/day in 3–4 divided doses • Enteral suspension, CR caps, ER tabs, ODTs, tabs	• Hypersensitivity • Narrow-angle glaucoma • Concurrent use with MAOIs	• N/V • Orthostasis • Confusion • Hallucinations • Wearing-off fluctuations • Dyskinesias • Somnolence • Impulse control disorders	• Response to therapy • Presence of side effects • BP	• Nonselective MAOIs may cause hypertensive crisis • Pyridoxine (vitamin B6) ↓ effectiveness of levodopa	• IR tabs and CR caps/tabs often used simultaneously • CR is less bioavailable (~30% less) than IR • Duopa is indicated for PEG-J tube administration
Mechanism of action – dopamine agonists: directly stimulate striatal dopamine receptors					
Bromocriptine (ergot derivative) • Parlodel • 1.25–50 mg BID • Caps, tabs	• Uncontrolled hypertension • Sensitivity to ergot alkaloids • Pregnancy • Postpartum with history of coronary artery disease	• Valvular fibrosis • Nausea • Hallucinations • Dizziness • Drowsiness • Orthostasis • Impulse control disorders	• Response to therapy • Presence of side effects • BP	• ↓ levodopa dose by 20–30% when initiating • Metoclopramide and antipsychotics ↓ effects	Cardiac side effects ↓ clinical use; nonergot derivatives used much more commonly
Pramipexole☆ (nonergot derivative) • Mirapex, Mirapex ER • IR: 0.125–1.5 mg TID • ER: 0.375–4.5 mg daily • ER tabs, tabs	None	• N/V • Constipation • Orthostasis • Hallucinations • Somnolence • Syncope • Impulse control disorders	• Response to therapy • Presence of side effects • BP	• ↓ levodopa dose by 20–30% when initiating • Metoclopramide and antipsychotics ↓ effects	• Adjust dose in renal impairment • Titrate dose slowly and taper upon discontinuation • Also indicated for restless leg syndrome
Ropinirole☆ (nonergot derivative) • Requip, Requip XL • IR: 0.25–8 mg TID • ER: 2–24 mg daily • ER tabs, tabs	Hypersensitivity				• Titrate dose slowly and taper upon discontinuation • Also indicated for restless leg syndrome

Medications for Parkinson's Disease *(cont'd)*

Generic • Brand • Dose/Dosage Forms	Contraindications	Primary Side Effects	Key Monitoring Parameters	Pertinent Drug Interactions	Med Pearls
Rotigotine • Neupro • 2–8 mg daily • Transdermal patch	Hypersensitivity	• Application site reactions • N/V • Orthostasis • Hallucinations • Somnolence • Syncope • Impulse control disorders • Hypertension • Tachycardia • Edema	• Response to therapy • Presence of side effects • BP • HR	Metoclopramide and anti-psychotics ↓ effects	• Apply daily • Titrate dose slowly and taper upon discontinuation • Also indicated for restless leg syndrome
Mechanism of action – COMT inhibitors: inhibit the degradation of dopamine through inhibition of the catechol-O-methyltransferase enzyme					
Tolcapone • Tasmar • 100–200 mg TID • Tabs	• Hypersensitivity • Hepatic impairment • History of nontraumatic rhabdomyolysis or hyperpyrexia and confusion due to medication	• Hepatic failure • Dyskinesias • N/V/D • Orthostasis • Hallucinations • Somnolence • Syncope • Impulse control disorders • Rhabdomyolysis	• LFTs • Response to therapy • Presence of side effects • BP	• May ↑ effects of MAOIs (avoid concurrent use of nonselective MAOIs) • ↑ activity of drugs known to be metabolized by COMT (dopamine, dobuta-mine, isoproterenol, methyldopa)	• Reserved for third-line therapy in patients that do not respond adequately to carbidopa/levodopa and do-pamine agonists • Administer with carbidopa/levodopa
Entacapone • Comtan • 200–1,600 mg daily (divided up to 8 × daily; administered with each dose of carbidopa/levodopa) • Tabs	Hypersensitivity	• Dyskinesias • N/V/D • Hallucinations • Urine discolor-ation (brown-orange) • Orthostasis • Hallucinations • Somnolence • Syncope • Impulse control disorder	• Response to therapy • Presence of side effects • BP	• May ↑ effects of MAOIs (avoid concurrent use of nonselective MAOIs) • ↑ activity of drugs known to be metabolized by COMT (dopamine, dobutamine, isoproterenol, methyldopa)	• Reserved for third-line therapy in patients that do not respond adequately to carbidopa/levodopa and dopamine agonists • Preferred over tolcapone, as no fatal liver injury has been reported with this agent • Administer with carbidopa/levodopa
Combination product: Levodopa/carbidopa/entacapone (Stalevo)					

Medications for Parkinson's Disease   (cont'd)

Generic • Brand • Dose/Dosage Forms	Contraindications	Primary Side Effects	Key Monitoring Parameters	Pertinent Drug Inter-actions	Med Pearls
Mechanism of action – anticholinergics: through diminished activity of acetylcholine, help to ↓ the relative ↑ in activity compared to dopamine, thereby ↓ tremor					
Benztropine ☆ • Cogentin • 0.5–6 mg/day in 2–4 divided doses • Injection, tabs	Hypersensitivity	• Dry mouth • Blurred vision • Constipation • Urinary retention • Confusion • Memory impairment • Hallucinations	• Response to therapy • Presence of side effects	Additive anticholinergic side effects when co-administered with other anticholinergic medications	• Use with caution in elderly patients who are at risk for mental status changes with anticholinergic medications • Primarily used for tremor and/or drooling
Trihexyphenidyl • Only available generically • 1–15 mg/day in 3–4 divided doses • Solution, tabs	None				
Mechanism of action – second-generation atypical antipsychotic; inverse agonist and antagonist activity at 5-HT2A and 5-HT2C receptors					
Pimavanserin • Nuplazid • 17–34 mg daily • Tabs	None	• Edema • Confusion • Hallucination • Gait disturbance • QT interval prolongation	• ECG • Response to therapy	• CYP3A4 substrate • CYP3A4 inhibitors may ↑ toxicity/effect (↓ pimavanserin dose to 17 mg/day) • CYP3A4 inducers may ↓ effect • Use with QT-interval prolonging agents may ↑ risk of TdP	Indicated to treat hallucinations and delusions associated with PD psychosis

MIGRAINE HEADACHE

Summary of Treatment Recommendations

- Migraine treatment is divided into abortive treatment, rescue treatment, and prophylactic treatment. Most patients will respond to abortive treatment and can be controlled without the addition of rescue or prophylactic therapy.

- Abortive treatment options include analgesics (over-the-counter [OTC] and prescription), NSAIDs (detailed in bone and joint chapter), ergotamine and dihydroergotamine, serotonin agonists, and butorphanol. Over-the-counter analgesics, prescription non-opioid analgesics, and NSAIDs are reserved for patients with mild symptoms.

- The serotonin agonists are the mainstay of abortive therapy options for patients with moderate to severe symptoms. Various dosage forms are available and there is only slight variability between the efficacy and safety of available agents. Patients may respond to one agent in this class and not to another; therefore, trial and error is often the approach taken.

- For patients who have >2 headaches/week or >8 headaches/month, or who do not have an adequate response to abortive therapy, prophylactic therapy may be warranted.
- Available prophylactic agents include antihypertensive medications such as propranolol, atenolol, and metoprolol (detailed in cardiovascular chapter); antidepressant medications such as amitriptyline, paroxetine, fluoxetine, and sertraline (detailed in psychiatric disorders chapter); and anticonvulsant medications such valproic acid, gabapentin, tiagabine, and topiramate (detailed earlier in this chapter). In general, migraine prophylactic doses are low compared to normal doses of these medications.

Medications for Migraine

Generic • Brand • Dose/Dosage Forms	Contraindications	Primary Side Effects	Key Monitoring Parameters	Pertinent Drug Interactions	Med Pearls
Analgesics					
Acetaminophen, aspirin, caffeine • Excedrin Migraine, Anacin • 2 tabs at onset, then every 6 hr PRN • Tabs	• Hypersensitivity to any component • Pregnancy	Minimal	• Response to therapy • Presence of side effects	Other acetaminophen-containing meds (do not exceed 4 g/day)	Available OTC
Aspirin or acetaminophen with butalbital and caffeine☆ • Fiorinal, Fioricet • 1–2 tabs every 4–6 hrs PRN (max = 6 doses/day)	• Hypersensitivity to any component • Pregnancy	• Tachycardia • Dizziness • Drowsiness • Insomnia • Orthostatic hypotension	• Response to therapy • Presence of side effects	Alcohol ↑ CNS depression with butalbital	• Limit to 4 tabs/day and use max of 2 days/wk • Dependence may develop with continued use
Isometheptene/dichloralphenazone/APAP • Nodolor • 2 caps at onset, then 1 cap every hr PRN (max = 6 capsules/24 hr)	• Glaucoma • Severe renal disease • Hypertension • Cardiovascular disease • Cerebrovascular accident • MAOI use	• Dizziness • Skin rash	• Response to therapy • Presence of side effects	Use with MAOIs may ↑ risk for hypertensive crisis	Max 6 caps/day; 20 caps/mo

Medications for Migraine   *(cont'd)*

Generic • Brand • Dose/Dosage Forms	Contraindications	Primary Side Effects	Key Monitoring Parameters	Pertinent Drug Interactions	Med Pearls
Mechanism of action – exert serotonergic agonist activity, resulting in vasoconstriction					
Ergotamine tartrate • Ergomar • 1 tab at onset, then 1 tab every 30 min PRN • Not to exceed 3 tabs/day or 5 tabs/wk • SL tabs	• Hypersensitivity • Peripheral arterial disease • Coronary artery disease • Hypertension • Hepatic or renal impairment • Concurrent use of strong 3A4 inhibitors • Pregnancy	• Chest pain • Myocardial infarction • Hypertension • Tachycardia • Nausea • Valvular fibrosis	• Response to therapy • Presence of side effects • BP • HR	• CYP3A4 substrate • CYP3A4 inhibitors may ↑ effects/ toxicity • CYP3A4 inducers may ↓ effects	Potential for dependence with long-term use
Dihydroergotamine • DHE 45, Migranal • IV, IM, or subcut: 1 mg at onset, repeated at 1-hr intervals (max = 2 mg/day IV or 3 mg/day subcut or IM) • Nasal: 1 spray (0.5 mg) in each nostril; repeat in 15 min with spray in each nostril (max = 3 mg/day)	• Hypersensitivity • Peripheral arterial disease • Coronary artery disease • Hypertension • Hepatic or renal impairment • Concurrent use of strong 3A4 inhibitors • Pregnancy • Within 24 hr of triptan product • Within 2 wk of MAOI				

Medications for Migraine   *(cont'd)*

Mechanism of action – serotonin agonists (triptans): serotonin 5HT1 receptor agonists, resulting in vasoconstriction in the cerebral vasculature

Generic • Brand • Dose/Dosage Forms	Contraindications	Primary Side Effects	Key Monitoring Parameters	Pertinent Drug Interactions	Med Pearls
Sumatriptan☆ • Imitrex oral tablets • 25–100 mg at onset, may redose at >2 hr (max = 200 mg/day) • Imitrex or Alsuma subcut injection • 4–6 mg subcut; may repeat in 1 hr (max = 2 doses/day) • Imitrex nasal spray • 10–20-mg spray in 1 nostril at onset; may repeat after 2 hr (max = 40 mg/day) • Sumavel Dosepro, needle-free subcut injection • 6 mg subcut; may repeat in 1 hr (max = 12 mg/day) • Zembrace SymTouch subcut injection • 3 mg subcut; may repeat in 1 hr (max = 12 mg/day) • Onzetra Xsail powder for nasal inhalation • 22 mg, delivered by one nosepiece (11 mg in each nostril); may repeat in 2 hr (max = 44 mg/day)	• Coronary artery disease • Wolff-Parkinson-White syndrome • Stroke or transient ischemic attack • Peripheral arterial disease • Ischemic bowel disease • Uncontrolled hypertension • Within 24 hr of an ergot product • Within 2 wk of MAOI • Within 24 hr of strong 3A4 inhibitor (eletriptan) • Severe hepatic impairment (sumatriptan) • Severe renal or hepatic impairment (naratriptan)	• Fatigue • Dizziness • Flushing • Chest/neck/throat pressure • Unpleasant taste • Hypertension	• Response to therapy • Presence of side effects • BP	Use with meperidine, dextromethorphan, tramadol, SSRIs, SNRIs, TCAs, MAOIs, triptans, or St. John's wort may ↑ risk of serotonin syndrome	Onset: 30 min (PO); 15–30 min (intranasal); 10 min (subcut)
Zolmitriptan • Zomig, Zomig ZMT • Tabs: 1.25–2.5 at onset; may repeat in >2 hr if needed (max = 10 mg/day) • ODTs: 2.5 mg at onset; may repeat in >2 hr if needed (max = 10 mg/day) • Nasal spray: 2.5-mg spray in 1 nostril at onset; may repeat in >2 hr if needed (max = 10 mg/day)					Onset: 45 min

Medications for Migraine *(cont'd)*

Generic • Brand • Dose/Dosage Forms	Contraindications	Primary Side Effects	Key Monitoring Parameters	Pertinent Drug Interactions	Med Pearls
Naratriptan • Amerge • Tabs: 1–2.5 mg at onset; may repeat in >4 hr if needed (max = 5 mg/day)	[Same as above]	[Same as above]	[Same as above]	[Same as above]	Onset: 1–2 hr
Rizatriptan☆ • Maxalt, Maxalt MLT • Tabs, ODTs: 5–10 mg at onset; repeat in >2 hr if needed (max = 30 mg/day)					Onset: Within 2 hr
Almotriptan • Axert • Tabs: 6.25–12.5 mg at onset; repeat in >2 hr if needed (max = 2 doses/day)					Onset: 30 min
Eletriptan • Relpax • Tabs: 20–40 mg at onset; repeat in >2 hr if needed (max = 80 mg/day)					Onset: 30 min
Frovatriptan • Frova • Tabs: 2.5 mg at onset; repeat in > 2 hr if needed (max = 7.5 mg/day)					Onset: 3 hr
Combination product: Sumatriptan/naproxen (Treximet)					
Mechanism of action – butorphanol: mixed opioid agonist/antagonist with opioid analgesic properties					
Butorphanol • Only available generically • Nasal spray: 1 mg (1 spray) in 1 nostril at onset; may repeat in >1 hour; may then repeat in 3–4 hr after last dose if needed	• Hypersensitivity • Patients with a history of narcotic dependenc	• Somnolence • Dizziness • Nausea • Nasal congestion • Insomnia	• Response to therapy • Presence of adverse effects	Concurrent use of other CNS depressants will have additive adverse effects and should be avoided	• Schedule IV controlled substance • Not routinely used for migraines • High addiction potential

ALZHEIMER'S DISEASE

Guidelines Summary

- Goals of treatment include preservation of function and symptomatic slowing of cognitive decline. A commonly used benchmark is the change in MMSE within one year. Without therapy, MMSE would be expected to ↓ approximately 2–4 points per year. Therapeutic efficacy is often determined if MMSE ↓ by ≤2 points per year. None of the available therapies has an impact on halting disease progression or reversing pathophysiology.

- Cholinesterase inhibitors are the treatment of choice in mild to moderate AD. Although slight differences exist in the mechanism of action of these agents, there is no evidence to indicate greater efficacy with one agent over another. Agent selection is typically made based upon patient preference, cost, and potential for drug interactions. There is insufficient evidence to support a dose-response relationship within this class. It is currently recommended that patients be started on the lowest dose and titrated slowly to the typical maintenance dose.

- Memantine is the only currently available N-methyl-D-aspartate (NMDA) receptor antagonist and has been studied and approved in moderate to severe AD as either monotherapy or an adjunct to a cholinesterase inhibitor.

- The most widely accepted approach to treatment is to initiate a low dose of a cholinesterase inhibitor at the time of diagnosis with slow titration to a typical maintenance dose. After 6 months to 1 year, efficacy is assessed. If this therapy is not efficacious, the patient can be switched to an alternate cholinesterase inhibitor or memantine can be added (in moderate to severe disease).

Cholinesterase Inhibitors

Generic • Brand • Dose/Dosage Forms	Contraindications	Primary Side Effects	Key Monitoring Parameters	Pertinent Drug Interactions	Med Pearls
Mechanism of action – inhibit the activity of the cholinesterase enzyme, thereby allowing ↑ acetylcholine activity					
Donepezil ☆ • Aricept • 5 mg daily, then ↑ to 10 mg daily after 4–6 wk (max = 23 mg daily in moderate–severe AD) • ODTs, tabs Galantamine • Razadyne, Razadyne ER • IR: 4 mg BID × 4 wk, then 8 mg BID × ≥4 wk, then 12 mg BID • ER: 8 mg daily × 4 wk, then 16 mg daily × ≥4 wk, then 24 mg daily • ER caps, solution, tabs	Hypersensitivity	• N/V/D • Peptic ulcer disease • Weight loss • Urinary incontinence • Dizziness • Headache • Syncope • Salivation • Sweating • Bradycardia • AV block • Rash (Stevens-Johnson syndrome possible)	• Presence of side effects • ECG • HR • MMSE (at 6–12 mo intervals)	• May ↑ neuromuscular blockade with succinylcholine • Anticholinergic drugs ↓ efficacy • Cholinergic drugs ↑ toxicity	Slow titration can ↑ tolerability
Rivastigmine • Exelon • Caps: 1.5–6 mg BID • Patch: 4.6–13.3 mg daily • Caps, transdermal patch				• May ↑ neuromuscular blockade with succinylcholine • Anticholinergic drugs ↓ efficacy • Cholinergic drugs ↑ toxicity • Metoclopramide ↑ risk of extrapyramidal symptoms	• Capsules should be administered with meals • Also indicated for Parkinson-related dementia

NMDA Receptor Antagonist

Generic • Brand • Dose/Dosage Forms	Contraindications	Primary Side Effects	Key Monitoring Parameters	Pertinent Drug Interactions	Med Pearls
Mechanism of action – NMDA receptor antagonist, preventing detrimental effects of glutamate					
Memantine ☆ • Namenda, Namenda XR • IR: 5 mg daily × ≥1 wk, then 5 mg BID × ≥1 wk, then 5 mg A.M. and 10 mg P.M. × ≥1 wk, then 10 mg BID • ER: 7–28 mg daily • ER caps, solution, tabs	Hypersensitivity	• Confusion • Constipation • Dizziness • Headache • D/V • Hypertension	• Presence of side effects • BP • MMSE at 6–12 month intervals	• Carbonic anhydrase inhibitors and sodium bicarbonate may ↑ effects/toxicity	• Indicated for moderate–severe AD as monotherapy or in combination with cholinesterase inhibitor • Adjust dose in renal impairment
Combination product: Donepezil/memantine (Namzaric)					

PRACTICE QUESTIONS

1. What is recommended first-line for newly diagnosed multiple sclerosis?

   (A) Oral prednisone
   (B) Betaseron
   (C) Methylprednisolone
   (D) Natalizumab
   (E) Rebif + mitoxantrone

2. What patient counseling should be provided when dispensing an interferon injectable prescription for multiple sclerosis?

   (A) If the medication cannot be used within 1 month, freeze the syringe to allow beyond-date use.
   (B) Apply heat to the injection site before and after the injection.
   (C) Try to use the same injection site each time.
   (D) If the medication reaches room temperature, it is no longer usable and must be discarded.
   (E) NSAIDs may decrease the flu-like symptoms.

3. Which of the following is associated with the use of divalproex?

   (A) Hepatotoxicity
   (B) Hirsutism
   (C) Hypoglycemia
   (D) Renal dysfunction
   (E) Thrombocytosis

4. Which of the following medications is a contraindication to using sumatriptan?

   (A) Ibuprofen
   (B) Lisinopril
   (C) Phenelzine
   (D) Sertraline
   (E) Zolpidem

5. Which of the following is a contraindication to the use of rizatriptan? (Select ALL that apply.)

   (A) Uncontrolled hypertension
   (B) History of a stroke
   (C) Peripheral arterial disease (PAD)
   (D) Concomitant use of phenelzine
   (E) Concomitant use of naproxen

6. Which of the following medications should be AVOIDED with the use of donepezil? (Select ALL that apply.)

   (A) Diphenhydramine
   (B) Memantine
   (C) Amlodipine
   (D) Rivastigmine

7. Which of the following is a dopamine agonist?

   (A) Artane
   (B) Comtan
   (C) Mirapex
   (D) Sinemet

8. Which of the following medications, if added to a regimen containing apixaban, may cause a reduction in the efficacy of apixaban? (Select ALL that apply.)

   (A) Depakote
   (B) Dilantin
   (C) Keppra
   (D) Tegretol

9. Which of the following medications used to treat Parkinson's disease is formulated for PEG-J tube administration?

   (A) Duopa
   (B) Rytary
   (C) Sinemet CR

10. Which of the following disease states may memantine be used to treat?

    (A) Alzheimer's disease
    (B) Multiple sclerosis
    (C) Migraine
    (D) Parkinson's disease

ANSWERS AND EXPLANATIONS

1. **B**

Interferon agents (such as Betaseron, Avonex, and Rebif) and glatiramer acetate (Copaxone) are considered first-line disease-modifying drugs (DMDs) for the treatment of MS. Therefore, (B) is correct. Natalizumab (D) is reserved for patients who do not respond to traditional therapy. Treatment is usually initiated one agent at a time and, as the disease progresses, treatment with DMD + mitoxantrone pulse therapy (E) may be used. Corticosteroids (A and C) are the cornerstone of acute exacerbations but will play no role in treating the disease itself.

2. **E**

Acetaminophen or NSAIDs can reduce the flu-like symptoms associated with the interferon injections. The injectables for multiple sclerosis should never be frozen (A) and should always be protected from light. To ease the discomfort of the injections, ice—not heat (B)—can be applied to the injection site prior to the injection, and the injection site should be rotated each time (making choice C incorrect). It is perfectly fine and recommended to allow the injectable to reach room temperature prior to the injection (D), but it should otherwise be stored in the refrigerator.

3. **A**

Divalproex is associated with elevations in AST and ALT with potential hepatotoxicity. Hirsutism (B) is not correct as divalproex is associated with alopecia. Divalproex is not associated with hypoglycemia (C) and may be associated with hyperglycemia in rare instances. Divalproex does not cause renal dysfunction (D), and thrombocytosis (E) is not correct as divalproex is associated with thrombocytopenia.

4. **C**

The triptans are contraindicated if a patient has taken an MAOI within 2 weeks of using the triptan, as there is a risk of serotonin syndrome. NSAIDs may be taken with triptans; therefore, ibuprofen (A) is not a contraindication. Patients with uncontrolled HTN may not take triptans, but antihypertensive medications such as lisinopril (B) can be used. Sertraline (D) and zolpidem (E) may be used with triptans, but sertraline should be used with caution as there is a risk of serotonin syndrome with concomitant use.

5. **A, B, C, D**

Triptans cause vasoconstriction and cannot be used with ischemic heart or cerebrovascular disease. Patients with uncontrolled hypertension (A), history of a cerebrovascular accident or transient ischemic attack (B), PAD (C), or vasospastic condition should avoid the use of any triptan. Triptans also may cause serotonin syndrome if used within 2 weeks on an MAOI such as phenelzine (D), so the combination should be avoided. NSAIDs can be used with rizatriptan, so E is not correct.

6. **A, D**

Diphenhydramine is an anticholinergic agent that should not be used concomitantly with any acetylcholinesterase inhibitor, which may decrease the efficacy of the acetylcholinesterase inhibitor. Rivastigmine is also an acetylcholinesterase inhibitor; it should not be used together with any acetylcholinesterase inhibitor, as that would be a therapeutic duplication. Memantine (B) is an NMDA receptor antagonist and can be used in combination with acetylcholinesterase inhibitors. Amlodipine (C) may be used with acetylcholinesterase inhibitors.

7. **C**

Mirapex (pramipexole) is a dopamine agonist used for the treatment of Parkinson's disease. Artane (trihexphenidyl) (A) is an anticholinergic agent. Comtan (entacapone) (B) is a COMT inhibitor. Sinemet (carbidopa/levodopa) (D) is a decarboxylase inhibtor (carbidopa) combined with a dopamine precursor (levodopa). All agents can be used for the treatment of Parkinson's disease.

8. **B, D**

Dilantin (phenytoin) and Tegretol (carbamazepine) are both strong CYP3A4 inducers that will increase the metabolism of apixaban, possibly causing its therapeutic failure.

9. **A**

All 3 medications are formulations of carbidopa/levodopa. Duopa is an enteral suspension administered via continuous infusion through a PEG-J tube. Rytary (B) and Sinemet CR (C) are both long-acting formulations intended for oral administration.

10. **A**

Memantine (Namenda, Namenda XR) is an NMDA receptor antagonist that is used to treat moderate to severe Alzheimer's disease.

Gastrointestinal Disorders

This chapter covers the following diseases:

- **Gastroesophageal reflux disease/peptic ulcer disease**
- **Inflammatory bowel disease**

GASTROESOPHAGEAL REFLUX DISEASE/ PEPTIC ULCER DISEASE

Guidelines Summary

Gastroesophageal Reflux Disease

The goals of therapy are to relieve symptoms, promote healing of esophageal mucosa, prevent recurrence, and prevent complications.

- **Lifestyle modifications**
  - Unlikely to control symptoms, when used alone, in most patients
  - Dietary changes: Avoid foods that can worsen symptoms (alcohol, caffeine, chocolate, citrus juices, peppermint/spearmint, coffee, spicy foods, tomatoes, high-fatty meals, garlic, onions); avoid eating before bedtime; remain upright after meals
  - Weight loss
  - Smoking cessation
  - Head elevated off the bed by 6–8 inches
  - No tight-fitting clothes
  - No medications that can worsen symptoms

- **Pharmacological therapy**
  - Step 1: Antacids and over-the-counter (OTC) acid suppressants (H2RAs, omeprazole, lansoprazole, esomeprazole) can be used initially on an as-needed basis for intermittent or mild symptoms. If symptoms persist after 2 weeks, proceed to Step 2.
  - Step 2: PPI or H2RA (can be used at higher prescription doses).
    - » PPIs are considered more effective than H2RAs.
  - A promotility agent (e.g., metoclopramide) can be used as adjunctive therapy, if needed.

Peptic Ulcer Disease

The goals of therapy are to relieve symptoms, promote healing of the ulcer, eradicate *H. pylori* (if present), prevent recurrence, and prevent complications.

- **Lifestyle modifications:** Reduce stress, smoking cessation, discontinue NSAID use, avoid foods that can worsen symptoms
- **Pharmacological therapy**
  - *H. pylori*-associated ulcers: See treatment algorithm below (duration = 10–14 days, depending on regimen)

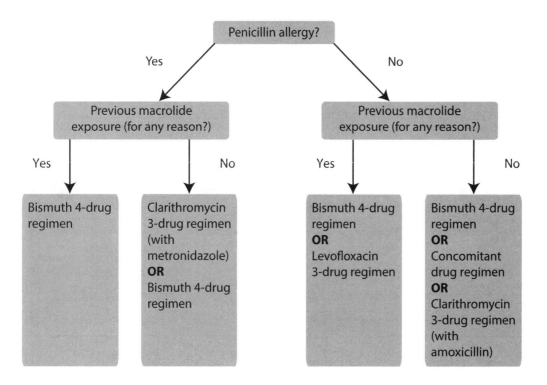

- NSAID-induced ulcers
  - » Treatment:
    - First-line therapy: PPI (duration of therapy = 6–8 weeks; may be longer if recurrent symptoms, heavy smoker, or continued NSAID use)
    - Second-line therapies: Misoprostol or H2RA
  - » Primary prevention:
    - Recommendations based on whether patient is at low, moderate, or high risk for NSAID GI toxicity (see Definitions) and the patient's risk for CV disease; high CV risk is defined by the patient's need for low-dose aspirin to prevent future CV events

	Low GI Risk	Moderate GI Risk	High GI Risk
Low CV Risk	NSAID alone	NSAID + PPI/misoprostol	Alternative therapy, if possible; or, cyclooxygenase-2 inhibitor + PPI/misoprostol
High CV Risk	Naproxen + PPI/ misoprostol	Naproxen + PPI/misoprostol	Avoid NSAIDs or cyclooxygenase-2 inhibitors; use alternative therapy

Antacids

Generic • Brand • Dose	Contraindications	Primary Side Effects	Key Monitoring	Pertinent Drug Interactions	Med Pearl
Mechanism of action – neutralize stomach acid and $\uparrow$ gastric pH					
Magnesium hydroxide/aluminum hydroxide • Mag-Al • 15 mL with meals and at bedtime Calcium carbonate • Tums, Maalox Chewables • 1–2 tabs q2h as needed	None	• Diarrhea (from magnesium [Mg^{2+}]) • Constipation (from aluminum [Al^{3+}] or calcium [Ca^{2+}])	S/S of GERD	• May bind to numerous drugs (separate from other drugs by at least 2 hr) • May $\downarrow$ absorption of drugs whose absorption is pH-dependent (e.g., itraconazole, ketoconazole, iron, atazanavir, nelfinavir, rilpivirine, mycophenolate mofetil, and erlotinib)	Use Mg^{2+}- and Al^{3+}- containing products with caution in patients with renal impairment

H$_2$ Receptor Antagonists

Generic • Brand • Dose	Dosage Forms	Primary Side Effects	Key Monitoring	Pertinent Drug Interactions	Med Pearl
Mechanism of action – reversibly inhibit histamine (H$_2$) receptors in the gastric parietal cells, which inhibits secretion of gastric acid					
Cimetidine • Tagamet HB • 200–1,600 mg/day	• Rx: Solution, tabs • OTC: Tabs	• Headache • Fatigue • Dizziness • Confusion • Gynecomastia (cimetidine)	S/S of GERD/PUD	• Cimetidine inhibits cytochrome P450 (CYP) enzymes to greater extent than the other drugs (inhibits CYP1A2, CYP2C19, CYP2D6, and CYP3A4) • May ↓ absorption of drugs whose absorption is pH-dependent (e.g., itraconazole, ketoconazole, iron, atazanavir, nelfinavir, rilpivirine, mycophenolate mofetil, and erlotinib)	Adjust dose of all H2RAs in renal impairment
Famotidine☆ • Pepcid • 20–80 mg/day	• Rx: Injection, suspension, tabs • OTC: Tabs				
Nizatidine • Only available generically • 150–300 mg/day	• Rx: Caps, solution				
Ranitidine☆ • Zantac • 75–300 mg/day	• Rx: Caps, injection, syrup, tabs • OTC: Tabs				
Combination product: Famotidine/calcium carbonate/magnesium hydroxide (Pepcid Complete)					

Proton Pump Inhibitors

Generic • Brand • Dose	Dosage Forms	Primary Side Effects	Key Monitoring	Pertinent Drug Interactions	Med Pearl
Mechanism of action – irreversibly inhibit H$^+$/K$^+$-ATPase in gastric parietal cells, which inhibits secretion of gastric acid					
Dexlansoprazole☆ • Dexilant • 30–60 mg/day	• Caps, orally disintegrating tabs (ODTs)	• Diarrhea • Headache	S/S of GERD/PUD	• May ↓ absorption of drugs whose absorption is pH-dependent (e.g., itraconazole, ketoconazole, iron, atazanavir, nelfinavir, rilpivirine, mycophenolate mofetil, and erlotinib) • May ↓ antiplatelet effects of clopidogrel • May ↑ effects/toxicity of methotrexate	May be associated with: • Osteoporosis-related fractures • ↓ Mg^{2+} • *Clostridium difficile* • Vitamin B$_{12}$ deficiency • Acute interstitial nephritis • Cutaneous/systemic lupus erythematosus
Esomeprazole☆ • Nexium, Nexium 24 hr • 20–40 mg/day	• Rx: Caps, granules for suspension, injection • OTC: Caps, tabs				
Lansoprazole☆ • Prevacid • 15–30 mg/day	• Rx: Caps, ODTs • OTC: Caps				
Omeprazole☆ • Prilosec • 20 mg/day	• Rx: Caps, granules for suspension • OTC: Tabs				
Pantoprazole☆ • Protonix • 20–40 mg/day	Granules for suspension, injection, tabs				
Rabeprazole☆ • Aciphex • 20 mg/day	Sprinkle capsules, tabs				
Combination products: Esomeprazole/naproxen (Vimovo) Omeprazole/sodium bicarbonate (Zegerid) Omeprazole/aspirin (Yosprala)					

Promotility Drug

Generic • Brand • Dose/Dosage Forms	Contraindications	Primary Side Effects	Key Monitoring	Pertinent Drug Interactions	Med Pearl
Mechanism of action – dopamine antagonist; ↑ LES pressure and accelerates gastric emptying					
Metoclopramide ☆ • Reglan, Metozolv ODT • 40–60 mg/day • Injection, ODTs, solution, tabs	Seizures	• Dizziness • Sedation • Diarrhea • Extrapyramidal symptoms (EPS)	• S/S of GERD • EPS	Use with antipsychotic agents may ↑ risk of EPS	• Can also be used for diabetic gastroparesis; erythromycin is an alternative • Adjust dose in renal impairment

Mucosal Protectant Drug

Generic • Brand • Dose/Dosage Forms	Contraindications	Primary Side Effects	Key Monitoring	Pertinent Drug Interactions	Med Pearl
Mechanism of action – nonabsorbable aluminum salt that forms bonds with damaged and normal GI tissue; complex forms protective cover over ulcerated area					
Sucralfate ☆ • Carafate • 4 g/day • Suspension, tabs	None	Constipation	S/S of PUD	May bind to numerous drugs (separate from other drugs by at least 2 hrs)	• Limited value in treatment of GERD; more useful in treatment of PUD • Use cautiously in patients with chronic kidney disease (↑ risk of Al^{3+} toxicity)

Prostaglandin Analog

Generic • Brand • Dose/Dosage Forms	Contraindications	Primary Side Effects	Key Monitoring	Pertinent Drug Interactions	Med Pearl
Mechanism of action – prostaglandin E1 analog; replaces protective prostaglandins inhibited by NSAID therapy					
Misoprostol • Cytotec • 400–800 mcg/day • Tabs	Pregnancy (abortifacient)	Diarrhea	S/S of PUD	None	• Women of childbearing age should have a pregnancy test before initiating therapy; educate regarding appropriate use of contraception • Can also be used for medical termination of pregnancy
Combination product: Misoprostol/diclofenac (Arthrotec)					

Helicobacter pylori First-Line Treatment Regimens (for PUD)

Proton Pump Inhibitor	Drug #2	Drug #3	Drug #4	Duration of Therapy	Comments
Three-Drug Regimen					
Esomeprazole 40 mg daily **OR** Lansoprazole 30 mg BID **OR** Omeprazole 20 mg BID **OR** Pantoprazole 40 mg BID **OR** Rabeprazole 20 mg BID	Amoxicillin 1,000 mg BID **OR** Metronidazole 500 mg TID (if penicillin allergy)	Clarithromycin 500 mg BID		14 days	• Clarithromycin 3-drug regimen • Prevpac is a compliance package that contains individual units of lansoprazole, amoxicillin, and clarithromycin • Omeclamox-Pak is a compliance package that contains individual units of omeprazole, amoxicillin, and clarithromycin
Esomeprazole 40 mg daily **OR** Lansoprazole 30 mg BID **OR** Omeprazole 20 mg BID **OR** Pantoprazole 40 mg BID **OR** Rabeprazole 20 mg BID	Amoxicillin 1,000 mg BID	Levofloxacin 500 mg daily		10–14 days	Levofloxacin 3-drug regimen
Four-Drug Regimen					
Esomeprazole 40 mg daily **OR** Lansoprazole 30 mg BID **OR** Omeprazole 20 mg BID **OR** Pantoprazole 40 mg BID **OR** Rabeprazole 20 mg BID	Bismuth subsalicylate 300 mg 4 × daily **OR** Bismuth subcitrate 120–300 mg 4 × daily	Metronidazole 250–500 mg 4 × daily **OR** Metronidazole 500 mg TID	Tetracycline 500 mg 4 × daily	10–14 days	• Bismuth 4-drug regimen • Pylera contains bismuth, metronidazole, and tetracycline in each capsule
Esomeprazole 40 mg daily **OR** Lansoprazole 30 mg BID **OR** Omeprazole 20 mg BID **OR** Pantoprazole 40 mg BID **OR** Rabeprazole 20 mg BID	Amoxicillin 1,000 mg BID	Clarithromycin 500 mg BID	Metronidazole 500 mg BID	10–14 days	Concomitant drug regimen

INFLAMMATORY BOWEL DISEASE

Severity of Disease: Ulcerative Colitis

- Mild: >4 stools/day (with or without blood), no systemic signs of toxicity, and normal erythrocyte sedimentation rate (ESR)
- Moderate: >4 stools/day and minimal signs of toxicity
- Severe: >6 stools/day (with blood) and evidence of toxicity (e.g., fever, tachycardia, anemia, or elevated ESR)

Severity of Disease: Crohn's Disease

- Mild-moderate: Ambulatory and able to tolerate oral intake without evidence of dehydration, systemic toxicity, abdominal tenderness, painful mass, intestinal obstruction, or >10% weight loss
- Moderate-severe: Fail to respond to treatment for mild-moderate disease or have fever, significant weight loss (>10%), abdominal mass/tenderness, intermittent nausea/vomiting (N/V) (without findings of obstruction), or significant anemia
- Severe/fulminant: Persistent symptoms despite the initiation of treatment with corticosteroids or biologic agents as outpatients or presenting with high fevers, persistent vomiting, evidence of intestinal obstruction, significant peritoneal signs (e.g., rebound tenderness, cachexia, or evidence of abscess)

Guidelines Summary

The goals of therapy are to induce and maintain remission, to prevent and resolve complications and systemic symptoms, and to maintain quality of life. There is no pharmacologic cure for these diseases; therefore, treatment focuses on management of symptoms.

- **Nonpharmacologic therapy**
  - Lifestyle changes/diet: Avoid foods that may worsen disease symptoms
  - Possible surgery when complications (e.g., fistulas, strictures, perforation) develop or to manage refractory disease

- **Pharmacologic therapy**
  - Adjunctive therapies: antidiarrheals (e.g., loperamide), antispasmodics (e.g., dicyclomine, propantheline, hyoscyamine)
  - Ulcerative colitis:
    » Treatment based upon whether inflammation is distal (below the splenic flexure; topical therapy appropriate) or extensive (proximal to the splenic flexure; requires systemic therapy)
    » Mild/moderate distal disease:
      - Active disease: Topical mesalamine (enema or suppository preferred), oral aminosalicylate, or topical corticosteroid
      - Maintenance of remission: Topical mesalamine or oral aminosalicylate
    » Mild/moderate extensive disease:
      - Active disease: Oral aminosalicylate (first-line), oral corticosteroids, azathioprine, 6-mercaptopurine, infliximab, adalimumab, golimumab, or vedolizumab
      - Maintenance of remission: Oral aminosalicylate (first-line), azathioprine, 6-mercaptopurine, infliximab, adalimumab, golimumab, or vedolizumab
    » Severe disease:
      - Infliximab (if urgent hospitalization not needed), intravenous (IV) corticosteroids (if urgent hospitalization needed), IV cyclosporine
  - Crohn's disease:
    » Mild/moderate active disease:
      - First-line: Oral aminosalicylate, budesonide (disease localized to ileum and/or right colon)
      - Second-line: Metronidazole, ciprofloxacin
    » Moderate/severe disease:
      - First-line: Prednisone
      - Second-line: Infliximab, adalimumab, certolizumab pegol, vedolizumab, natalizumab, methotrexate (IM or subcut)
    » Severe/fulminant disease:
      - First-line: IV corticosteroids
      - Second-line: IV cyclosporine or IV tacrolimus
    » Maintenance therapy:
      - First line: Azathioprine, 6-mercaptopurine, methotrexate, infliximab, adalimumab, certolizumab pegol, vedolizumab, or natalizumab

Aminosalicylates

Generic • Brand • Dose	Dosage Forms	Contraindications	Primary Side Effects	Key Monitoring	Med Pearl
Mechanism of action – ↓ inflammation in GI tract by inhibiting prostaglandin synthesis and subsequent production of various immune mediators; sulfasalazine is cleaved in colon to mesalamine (responsible for therapeutic effect) + sulfapyridine (causes side effects); olsalazine and balsalazide also contain mesalamine					
Sulfasalazine • Azulfidine, Azulfidine EN • Induction: 3–4 g/day • Maintenance: 2 g/day	Tabs, delayed-release (DR) (enteric-coated) tabs	• Aspirin allergy • Sulfa allergy • Glucose-6-phosphate dehydrogenase (G6PD) deficiency • Pregnancy (near term)	• Stevens-Johnson syndrome • Photosensitivity • N/V • Headache • Folate deficiency • Hemolytic anemia • Agranulocytosis • Hepatitis • Orange discoloration of bodily fluids	• S/S of IBD • Liver function tests (LFTs) (with sulfasalazine) • Complete blood count (CBC) (with sulfasalazine)	• Mesalamine, olsalazine, and balsalazide are not sulfa derivatives; are poorly absorbed from GI tract (better tolerated than sulfasalazine) • Folic acid should be given to patients on sulfasalazine • Sulfasalazine may ↑ effects of warfarin and oral hypoglycemics • All may ↓ absorption of digoxin
Mesalamine • Apriso, Asacol HD, Canasa, Delzicol, Lialda, Pentasa, Rowasa • Oral: *Induction* 2.4–4.8 g/day; *Maintenance*, 1.5–4 g/day • Rectal enema (Rowasa): 4 g at bedtime • Rectal suppository (Canasa): 1 g at bedtime	Extended-release (ER) caps, DR tabs, rectal enema, rectal suppository	• Aspirin allergy • G6PD deficiency	• Nausea • Diarrhea • Headache • Malaise		
Olsalazine • Dipentum • 1–3 g/day	Caps				
Balsalazide • Colazal, Giazo • 1.5–6.75 g/day	Caps, tabs				

Corticosteroids

Generic • Brand • Dose	Dosage Forms	Contraindications	Primary Side Effects	Key Monitoring	Med Pearl
Mechanism of action – quickly ↓ inflammation during acute exacerbations of IBD					
Budesonide • Entocort EC, Uceris • Entocort EC: *Initial*: 9 mg daily for up to 2 mo; *Maintenance*: 6 mg daily for up to 3 mo • Uceris (PO): 9 mg daily for up to 2 mo • Uceris (rectal foam): 1 metered dose (2 mg) BID for 2 wk, then 1 metered dose (2 mg) daily for 4 wk	DR caps, ER tabs, rectal foam	None	• Hyperglycemia • ↑ appetite • Insomnia • Hypertension • Edema • Adrenal suppression • Osteoporosis • Cataracts • Delayed wound healing	• S/S of IBD • Blood glucose • Blood pressure (BP) • Electrolytes	• Methylprednisolone and prednisone should only be used to treat acute exacerbation (4–8 wk) and then tapered • IV therapy given for severe exacerbations for 7–10 days, then switched to PO therapy • Budesonide has localized effect; has minimal systemic side effects • Entocort EC indicated for CD • Uceris indicated for UC
Methylprednisolone☆ • Solu-Medrol • 10–100 mg/day	Injection, tabs				
Prednisone☆ • Sterapred • 20–60 mg/day	Tabs				

Immunosuppressants

Generic • Brand • Dose	Contraindications	Primary Side Effects	Key Monitoring	Pertinent Drug Interactions	Med Pearl
Mechanism of action – ↓ production of inflammatory mediators (e.g., interleukins) through various mechanisms					
Azathioprine • Azasan, Imuran • 75–150 mg/day 6-Mercaptopurine • Purixan • 50–100 mg/day	• Pregnancy • Bone marrow suppression • Hepatic impairment	• Pancreatitis • Arthralgias • Nausea • Diarrhea • Rash • Bone marrow suppression • Hepatotoxicity	• Amylase/lipase (if symptoms) • CBC with differential • LFTs	• Allopurinol and febuxostat may ↑ risk of side effects (↓ azathioprine dose by 75% when used with allopurinol; avoid concomitant use with febuxostat) • Aminosalicylates may ↑ risk of side effects • May ↓ effects of warfarin	• 6-mercaptopurine is active metabolite of azathioprine • Adjust dose in renal impairment
Cyclosporine • Sandimmune • 4–8 mg/kg/day IV	Renal failure	• Hypertension • Nephrotoxicity • Hypomagnesemia • Infection • Anaphylaxis	• BP • Blood urea nitrogen (BUN)/ serum creatinine (SCr) • Electrolytes • S/S of infection • Cyclosporine levels	• CYP3A4 substrate and inhibitor • CYP3A4 inhibitors may ↑ levels/toxicity • CYP3A4 inducers may ↓ effects • May ↑ effects of other CYP3A4 substrates	• Used only for severe disease that has not responded to corticosteroids • Used only for 7–10 days
Methotrexate☆ • Rheumatrex • 15–25 mg/wk IM or subcut	• Pregnancy • Bone marrow suppression • Severe renal or hepatic impairment	• Hepatotoxicity • Bone marrow suppression • Pneumonitis • Rash • N/V • Diarrhea	• LFTs • CBC with differential • Chest x-ray (if symptoms)	• NSAIDs and salicylates ↑ risk of toxicity • Penicillins, sulfonamides, and tetracyclines may ↑ risk of toxicity	• Only effective for CD (useful for steroid-dependent and steroid-refractory CD) • Adjust dose in renal impairment

Biological Agents

Generic • Brand • Dose	Contraindications	Primary Side Effects	Key Monitoring	Pertinent Drug Interactions	Med Pearl
Mechanism of action – inhibit tumor necrosis factor (TNF)					
Adalimumab • Humira • 160 mg subcut on day 1 or over 2 days, then 80 mg 2 wk later (day 15), then 40 mg every other wk beginning day 29	None	• Headache • Rash • Injection site reactions • Anaphylaxis • Infection (especially tuberculosis [TB], fungal infections and hepatitis B virus [HBV] reactivation) • Lymphoma • Heart failure (HF) exacerbation • Bone marrow suppression • Lupus-like syndrome • Demyelinating disorders	• S/S of infection • S/S of HF • CBC with differential	Do not administer live vaccines	• PPD and HBV screening should be done before initiating treatment • Approved for moderately to severely active CD or UC in patients who have not responded despite adequate therapy with a corticosteroid or immunosuppressant
Certolizumab pegol • Cimzia • 400 mg subcut at 0, 2, and 4 wks; then 400 mg every 4 wk	None				• PPD and HBV screening should be done before initiating treatment • Only approved for moderately to severely active CD in patients who have not responded despite adequate therapy with a corticosteroid or immunosuppressant
Golimumab • Simponi • 200 mg subcut at wk 0, then 100 mg at wk 2, then 100 mg every 4 wk	None				• PPD and HBV screening should be done before initiating treatment • Only approved for moderately to severely active UC in patients who have not responded despite adequate therapy with a corticosteroid or immunosuppressant
Infliximab • Inflectra, Remicade • 5 mg/kg IV at 0, 2, and 6 wk; then every 8 wk	New York Heart Association class III or IV HF (for doses >5 mg/kg)	• Infusion reactions (hypotension, dyspnea, urticaria) • Delayed hypersensitivity reactions (fever, rash, myalgia, headache, sore throat, hand/facial edema, dysphagia, arthralgias) • Infection (especially TB, fungal infections, or HBV reactivation) • HF exacerbation • Bone marrow suppression • Lymphoma • Hepatotoxicity	• BP • LFTs • S/S of infection • S/S of HF • CBC with differential		• Delayed hypersensitivity reaction may occur as early as after 2nd dose • Premedicate with H_1 antagonist, H2RA, acetaminophen, and/or corticosteroid • PPD and HBV screening should be done before initiating treatment • Approved for moderately to severely active CD or UC in patients who have not responded despite adequate therapy with a corticosteroid or immunosuppressant

Biological Agents *(cont'd)*

Generic • Brand • Dose	Contraindications	Primary Side Effects	Key Monitoring	Pertinent Drug Interactions	Med Pearl
Mechanism of action – ↓ inflammation by binding to α4-subunit of integrins					
Natalizumab • Tysabri • 300 mg IV every 4 wk; discontinue if no response by wk 12	• Progressive multifocal leuko-encephalopathy (PML) • Concurrent use of TNF inhibitors or immunosuppres-sants	• PML (may be fatal) • Headache • Fatigue • Depression • Rash • Nausea • Arthralgia • Hypersensitivity reactions (hypotension, urticaria, fever, rash, rigors, nausea, flushing, dizziness, chest pain) • Anaphylaxis • Infection (especially opportunistic infections or herpes encephalitis meningitis) • Hepatotoxicity	• S/S of PML • Brain MRI (at baseline) • S/S of infection • LFTs	Do not administer live vaccines	• Patients need to be enrolled in CD-TOUCH program • Must be administered as monotherapy • Only approved for moderate to severely active CD in patients who are refractory to or unable to tolerate conventional therapies and TNF inhibitors
Mechanism of action – ↓ inflammation by binding to α4β7-subunit of integrins					
Vedolizumab • Entyvio • 300 mg IV at 0, 2, and 6 wk; then every 8 wk; discontinue if no response by wk 14	None	• Hypersensitivity reactions • Anaphylaxis • Infusion reactions • Infection (especially TB) • PML • Hepatotoxicity	• S/S of infection • S/S of PML • LFTs	Do not administer live vaccines	• Consider performing PPD before treatment • Approved for moderately to severely active CD or UC in patients who are refractory to or unable to tolerate TNF blocker or corticosteroid therapy

PRACTICE QUESTIONS

1. Remicade is the brand name for which of the following medications?

   (A) Azathioprine
   (B) Balsalazide
   (C) Budesonide
   (D) Cyclosporine
   (E) Infliximab

2. Which of the following is a contraindication for the use of metoclopramide?

   (A) Hyperkalemia
   (B) Myasthenia gravis
   (C) Porphyria
   (D) Seizure disorder
   (E) Sulfa allergy

3. A patient using NSAIDs for chronic pain develops a bleeding ulcer. Which of the following medications would be MOST appropriate to treat his condition?

   (A) Aluminum hydroxide
   (B) Bismuth subsalicylate
   (C) Calcium carbonate
   (D) Metoclopramide
   (E) Misoprostol

4. A patient who is taking warfarin for chronic atrial fibrillation develops GERD. Which of the following medications would MOST likely interact with the warfarin and increase this patient's risk for bleeding?

   (A) Cimetidine
   (B) Magnesium hydroxide
   (C) Misoprostol
   (D) Pantoprazole
   (E) Sucralfate

5. Which of the following reasons MOST likely explains why the plasma levels of ketoconazole are decreased in patients taking lansoprazole?

   (A) Lansoprazole induces the CYP450 enzymes that metabolize ketoconazole.
   (B) Ketoconazole requires an acidic environment for its oral absorption.
   (C) Lansoprazole binds acidic drugs in the GI tract.
   (D) Lansoprazole has prokinetic effects, which decrease GI transit time.
   (E) There is a competition for transport mechanisms in the GI tract.

6. Which of the following medications needs to be dose-adjusted in patients with renal impairment? (Select ALL that apply.)

    (A) Adalimumab
    (B) Budesonide
    (C) Esomeprazole
    (D) Metoclopramide
    (E) Ranitidine

7. A patient with UC has a history of anaphylaxis when taking trimethoprim/sulfamethoxazole. Which of the following medications would be safe to use for the treatment of UC in this patient? (Select ALL that apply.)

    (A) Asacol HD
    (B) Azulfidine
    (C) Dipentum
    (D) Simponi
    (E) Uceris

8. Which of the following characteristics is more likely to occur with UC than CD?

    (A) Confinement of the disease to the colon and rectum
    (B) Fistula formation
    (C) Cobblestone pattern of inflammation
    (D) Transmural lesion in the GI tract
    (E) Systemic complications

9. Which of the following supplements may be needed in a patient taking chronic sulfasalazine therapy for IBD?

    (A) Calcium carbonate
    (B) Folic acid
    (C) Iron
    (D) Vitamin B_{12}
    (E) Vitamin C

10. Which of the following baseline tests should be performed before a patient begins certolizumab pegol therapy for CD?

    (A) Brain MRI
    (B) LFTs
    (C) PPD
    (D) Serum creatinine
    (E) Uric acid

ANSWERS AND EXPLANATIONS

1. **E**

Remicade is the brand name for infliximab. Imuran is the brand name for azathioprine (A). Colazal is the brand name for balsalazide (B). Entocort EC or Uceris are brand names for oral budesonide (C). Sandimmune, Gengraf, and Neoral are brand names for cyclosporine (D).

2. **D**

Seizure disorder is a contraindication for the use of metoclopramide; therefore, choice (D) is correct.

3. **E**

The first-line therapy for an NSAID-induced ulcer is a PPI. However, no PPIs are listed as answer choices. Appropriate second-line therapies for an NSAID-induced ulcer are either misoprostol or an H_2RA. Misoprostol is a prostaglandin E1 analog that acts to replace protective prostaglandins that have been inhibited by NSAID therapy. Aluminum hydroxide (A), bismuth subsalicylate (B), calcium carbonate (C), and metoclopramide (D) would not be appropriate treatments for a NSAID-induced ulcer.

4. **A**

Cimetidine is a strong inhibitor of CYP3A4 and a moderate inhibitor of CYP1A2. It is also a weak inhibitor of CYP2C9. (R)-warfarin is a substrate of CYP3A4 and CYP1A2, while (S)-warfarin is a substrate of CYP2C9. Therefore, cimetidine has the potential to inhibit the metabolism of both the (S)- and (R)-enantiomers of warfarin, which could lead to an increased risk of bleeding. Magnesium hydroxide (B), misoprostol (C), pantoprazole (D), and sucralfate (E) do not inhibit the CYP450 system and therefore should not increase the risk of bleeding with warfarin.

5. **B**

The absorption of ketoconazole is pH-dependent; this antifungal drug requires an acidic environment to be adequately absorbed; therefore, the bioavailability of this drug decreases as gastric pH increases. By increasing gastric pH, lansoprazole may reduce the absorption of ketoconazole, which would lead to decreased plasma concentrations. Lansoprazole is not known to be an inducer of the CYP450 isoenzymes (A). If anything, it may be a weak inhibitor of CYP2C19; however, this inhibition would not have any effect on ketoconazole plasma concentrations. Lansoprazole does not bind to acidic drugs in the GI tract (C). Lansoprazole also does not have prokinetic effects in the GI tract (D); metoclopramide has these properties. Lansoprazole does not compete with ketoconazole for transport mechanisms in the GI tract (E).

6. **D, E**

Both metoclopramide (D) and ranitidine (E) are primarily excreted in the urine as unchanged drug. Therefore, the doses of these drugs need to be adjusted in patients with renal impairment. In fact, the dose of all H_2RAs needs to be adjusted in this patient population. None of the PPIs (C) needs to be dose adjusted in patients with renal impairment. Also, neither adalimumab (A) nor budesonide (B) needs to be dose-adjusted in these patients.

7. **A, C, D, E**

Sulfasalazine (Azulfidine) (B) is a sulfa derivative and should be avoided in patients with a history of anaphylaxis to sulfa products (e.g., trimethoprim/sulfamethoxazole). Mesalamine (Asacol HD) (A), olsalazine (Dipentum) (C), golimumab (Simponi) (D), and budesonide (Uceris) (E) are not sulfa derivatives and could be safely used in this patient with UC.

8. **A**

UC is more likely to be confined to the colon and rectum, whereas CD can affect anywhere in the GI tract from the mouth to the anus. Fistulas (B) are more likely to develop in patients with CD as opposed to those with UC. The inflammation in CD occurs in a segmented or cobblestone pattern (C), while it occurs in a more continuous fashion in UC. The mucosal lesions in UC are more superficial than those in CD, which are more transmural (D). Systemic complications can occur with either UC or CD (E).

9. **B**

Sulfasalazine can impair folate absorption. Therefore, patients taking chronic sulfasalazine therapy are at risk for developing folate deficiency and should supplement with folic acid to prevent this adverse effect. Sulfasalazine does not impair the absorption of calcium (A), iron (C), vitamin B_{12} (D), or vitamin C (E). Therefore, routine supplementation of these vitamins/minerals during sulfasalazine is not necessary.

10. **C**

Before starting therapy with certolizumab pegol, patients should be evaluated for tuberculosis risk factors and latent tuberculosis infection with a PPD. Cases of reactivation of tuberculosis or new tuberculosis infections have been reported in patients receiving therapy with TNF-inhibitors, including certolizumab pegol; patients who are receiving these drugs are at increased risk for developing serious infections. Certolizumab pegol has not been associated with PML (life-threatening), so there is no need to perform a brain MRI (A) before starting therapy with this drug; a baseline brain MRI should be performed prior to initiating therapy with natalizumab. Certolizumab pegol is not associated with hepatotoxicity or nephrotoxicity, so there is no need to monitor baseline LFTs (B) or SCr (D). Finally, certolizumab pegol does not affect uric acid levels, so this parameter does not need to be monitored at baseline.

Viral Hepatitis

This chapter covers the following diseases:

- **Hepatitis B**
- **Hepatitis C**

There are five different types of viral hepatitis: hepatitis A, hepatitis B, hepatitis C, hepatitis D, and hepatitis E. While all five of these viruses can cause acute hepatitis, hepatitis B, C, D are most likely to cause chronic hepatitis. Chronic viral hepatitis may lead to cirrhosis, which may result in complications such as end-stage liver disease and/or hepatocellular carcinoma. This overview will focus on hepatitis B and hepatitis C, as these are the most common types of viral hepatitis.

HEPATITIS B

Guidelines Summary

Preferred Regimens for Patients with Chronic HBV

Phase	HBeAg Status	HBV DNA	ALT	Treatment and Duration
Immune-tolerant	Positive	<1,000,000 IU/mL	Normal	No treatment; monitor ALT q4-6 mo
Immune-tolerant (>40 yo with liver biopsy showing significant necroinflammation or fibrosis)	Positive	>1,000,000 IU/mL	Normal	Peginterferon (peg-IFN) alfa-2a × 48 wk **OR** Entecavir **OR** Tenofovir
Immune-active	Positive or negative	>20,000 IU/mL	≥2 × ULN	Peginterferon (peg-IFN) alfa-2a × 48 wk **OR** Entecavir **OR** Tenofovir
Inactive carrier	Negative	≤2,000 IU/mL	Normal	Observe/monitor (no treatment)

Interferons

Generic • Brand • Dose/Dosage Forms	Contraindications	Primary Side Effects	Key Monitoring	Pertinent Drug Interactions	Med Pearl
Mechanism of action – induces the innate antiviral immune response					
Peginterferon alfa-2a • Pegasys • 180 mcg subcut 1 × /wk • Injection	• Autoimmune hepatitis • Hepatic decompensation before treatment • Neonates/infants (contains benzyl alcohol)	• Flu-like symptoms • Fatigue • Depression • Hallucinations • Aggression • Insomnia • Suicidal ideation • Neutropenia • Thrombocytopenia • Anemia • Hypo-/hyperthyroidism • Visual disturbances • Hepatic decompensation/failure • Hypersensitivity reactions • Hypotension • Arrhythmia • Tachycardia	• Liver function tests (LFTs) • Electrocardiogram (ECG) • Complete blood count (CBC) with differential • Thyroid function tests (TFTs) • Blood urea nitrogen (BUN)/serum creatinine (SCr) • CD4+ cell counts (in patients with HIV) • HBV RNA levels	• May ↑ theophylline and methadone levels • ↑ risk of bone marrow suppression with zidovudine	• Inject into abdomen or thigh • Adjust dose in renal impairment

Nucleoside/Nucleotide Analogs

Generic • Brand • Dose/Dosage Forms	Contraindications	Primary Side Effects	Key Monitoring	Pertinent Drug Interactions	Med Pearl
Mechanism of action – inhibit HBV replication by interfering with HBV viral DNA polymerase					
Adefovir • Hepsera • 10 mg PO daily • Tabs	None	• Renal impairment • Nausea/diarrhea • Headache • Lactic acidosis • Hepatomegaly with steatosis	• BUN/SCr • LFTs • HIV status • HBV DNA levels • HBeAg and anti-HBe	• ↑ risk of nephrotoxicity when used with amphotericin B, loop diuretics, tacrolimus, cyclosporine, or cisplatin • Not to be used with tenofovir-containing products	• Adjust dose in renal impairment • Considered 2nd-line oral therapy for HBV
Entecavir • Baraclude • Treatment-naïve: 0.5 mg PO daily • Lamivudine-resistant viremia (or known lamivudine- or telbivudine-resistant mutations): 1 mg PO daily • Decompensated liver disease: 1 mg PO daily • Solution, tabs	None	• Nausea • Headache • Fatigue • Dizziness • Lactic acidosis • Hepatomegaly with steatosis		Nephrotoxic drugs may ↑ levels	• Adjust dose in renal impairment • Give on an empty stomach (2 hr before or after a meal)
Lamivudine • Epivir HBV • 100 mg PO daily • Solution, tabs	None	• Diarrhea • Lactic acidosis • Hepatomegaly with steatosis		Not to be used with lamivudine- or emtricitabine-containing products	• Adjust dose in renal impairment • Lamivudine + tenofovir one of the preferred regimens in patients coinfected with HBV and HIV; cannot use Epivir HBV formulation for this use (must use Epivir 150 mg BID or 300 mg PO daily)

Nucleoside/Nucleotide Analogs   *(cont'd)*

Generic • Brand • Dose/Dosage Forms	Contraindications	Primary Side Effects	Key Monitoring	Pertinent Drug Interactions	Med Pearl
Tenofovir Viread (disoproxil fumarate) • 300 mg PO daily • Powder, tabs Vemlidy (alafenamide) • 25 mg PO daily • Tabs	Creatinine clearance (CrCl) <15 mL/min (alafenamide)	• Renal impairment (> with disoproxil fumarate) • Fanconi syndrome • ↓ bone mineral density (> with disoproxil fumarate) • Lactic acidosis • Hepatomegaly with steatosis	• BUN/SCr • Bone mineral density • LFTs • HIV status • HBV DNA levels • HBeAg and anti-HBe	• ↓ atazanavir levels • ↑ didanosine levels (↓ didanosine dose) • Lopinavir/ritonavir, atazanavir/ritonavir, darunavir/ritonavir, acyclovir, valacyclovir, ganciclovir, valganciclovir, aminoglycosides, ledipasvir/sofosbuvir, and nonsteroidal anti-inflammatory drugs ↑ levels • Not to be used with tenofovir-containing products	• Adjust dose of disoproxil fumarate in renal impairment • Oral powder can be used if patient unable to swallow tabs • Alafenamide is associated with ↓ risk of renal impairment and ↓ bone density • Lamivudine + tenofovir **OR** tenofovir + emtricitabine preferred regimens in patients coinfected with HBV and HIV

HEPATITIS C

Guidelines Summary

Recommended Regimens for Treatment-Naïve Patients with HCV

Genotype	Treatment and Duration	
	Without Cirrhosis	*With Cirrhosis*
1a	Elbasvir/grazoprevir × 12 wk **OR** Ledipasvir/sofosbuvir × 12 wk **OR** Ombitasvir/paritaprevir/ritonavir + dasabuvir + ribavirin (RBV) × 12 wk **OR** Simeprevir + sofosbuvir × 12 wk **OR** Sofosbuvir/velpatasvir × 12 wk **OR** Daclatasvir + sofosbuvir × 12 wk	Elbasvir/grazoprevir × 12 wk **OR** Ledipasvir/sofosbuvir × 12 wk **OR** Sofosbuvir/velpatasvir × 12 wk

Recommended Regimens for Treatment-Naïve Patients with HCV *(cont'd)*

Genotype	Treatment and Duration	
	Without Cirrhosis	*With Cirrhosis*
1b	Elbasvir/grazoprevir × 12 wk **OR** Ledipasvir/sofosbuvir × 12 wk **OR** Ombitasvir/paritaprevir/ritonavir + dasabuvir × 12 wk **OR** Simeprevir + sofosbuvir × 12 wk **OR** Sofosbuvir/velpatasvir × 12 wk **OR** Daclatasvir + sofosbuvir × 12 wk	Elbasvir/grazoprevir × 12 wk **OR** Ledipasvir/sofosbuvir × 12 wk **OR** Ombitasvir/paritaprevir/ritonavir + dasabuvir × 12 wk **OR** Sofosbuvir/velpatasvir × 12 wk
2	Sofosbuvir/velpatasvir × 12 wk	Sofosbuvir/velpatasvir × 12 wk
3	Daclatasvir + sofosbuvir × 12 wk **OR** Sofosbuvir/velpatasvir × 12 wk	Sofosbuvir/velpatasvir × 12 wk **OR** Daclatasvir + sofosbuvir +/− RBV × 24 wk
4	Ombitasvir/paritaprevir/ritonavir + RBV × 12 wk **OR** Sofosbuvir/velpatasvir × 12 wk **OR** Elbasvir/grazoprevir × 12 wk **OR** Ledipasvir/sofosbuvir × 12 wk	
5 or 6	Sofosbuvir/velpatasvir × 12 wk **OR** Ledipasvir/sofosbuvir × 12 wk	

Ribavirin

Generic • Brand • Dose/Dosage Forms	Contraindications	Primary Side Effects	Key Monitoring	Pertinent Drug Interactions	Med Pearl
Mechanism of action – inhibits replication of DNA (HBV) and RNA (HCV) viruses					
Ribavirin • Copegus (with peg-IFN alfa-2a), Rebetol (with peg-IFN alfa-2b) • Copegus: Genotypes 1, 4: <75 kg: 500 mg PO BID, ≥75 kg: 600 mg PO BID; Genotypes 2,3 or HIV coinfection: 400 mg PO BID • Rebetol: 800–1,400 mg/day (in divided doses, based on weight) • Caps, solution, tabs	• Pregnancy and men with partners who are pregnant • Hemoglobinopathy (including sickle-cell disease) • Concurrent use with didanosine • CrCl <50 mL/min (Rebetol only)	• Rash • Fatigue • Nausea/vomiting (N/V) • Anemia	• LFTs • CBC with differential • Pregnancy test	• ↑ risk of hepatic failure, peripheral neuropathy, and pancreatitis with didanosine (contraindicated) • ↑ risk of bone marrow suppression with azathioprine and zidovudine	• Patients must use ≥2 forms of contraception during treatment and for 6 mo after discontinuation • Adjust dose in renal impairment • Give with food

Protease Inhibitor

Generic • Brand • Dose/ Dosage Forms	Contraindications	Primary Side Effects	Key Monitoring	Pertinent Drug Interactions	Med Pearl
Mechanism of action – inhibits HCV replication by blocking the NS3/4A protease enzyme from cleaving the HCV polyprotein					
Simeprevir • Olysio • 150 mg PO daily • Caps	None	• Photosensitivity • Rash • Nausea • Myalgia • Dyspnea	• LFTs • HCV RNA levels • NS3 Q80K polymorphism (before treatment)	• Cytochrome P450 (CYP) 3A4 and P-glycoprotein (P-gp) substrate • CYP1A2 inhibitor • Concurrent use of simeprevir/sofosbuvir with amiodarone ↑ risk of bradycardia (avoid concurrent use)	• Must be used with other antiviral drugs (peg-IFN alfa/RBV or sofosbuvir) • ↓ efficacy in patients with NS3 Q80K polymorphism • Use with caution in patients with sulfa allergy • Discontinue simeprevir, peg-IFN alfa, and RBV if HCV RNA ≥25 IU/mL at wk 4 or wk 12; discontinue peg-IFN alfa and RBV if HCV RNA ≥25 IU/mL at wk 24

NS5A Inhibitor

Generic • Brand • Dose/Dosage Forms	Contraindications	Primary Side Effects	Key Monitoring	Pertinent Drug Interactions	Med Pearl
Mechanism of action – inhibits HCV replication by inhibiting the NS5A protein					
Daclatasvir • Daklinza • 60 mg PO daily • Concurrent use of strong CYP3A inhibitors: ↓ dose to 30 mg PO daily • Concurrent use of moderate CYP3A inducers: ↑ dose to 90 mg PO daily • Tabs	Concurrent use with phenytoin, carbamazepine, rifampin, or St. John's wort	• Headache • Fatigue • Nausea • Diarrhea	• LFTs • HCV RNA levels • NS5A polymorphism (before treatment in genotype 1a)	• CYP3A4 substrate • P-gp inhibitor • Concurrent use of daclatasvir/ sofosbuvir with amiodarone ↑ risk of bradycardia (avoid concurrent use)	Must be used with sofosbuvir

NS5B Inhibitor

Generic • Brand • Dose/Dosage Forms	Contraindications	Primary Side Effects	Key Monitoring	Pertinent Drug Interactions	Med Pearl
Mechanism of action – inhibits HCV replication by inhibiting HCV NS5B RNA-dependent RNA polymerase					
Sofosbuvir • Sovaldi • 400 mg PO daily • Tabs	None	• Fatigue • Headache • Nausea	• LFTs • HCV RNA levels	• P-gp substrate • Concurrent use with another HCV direct acting antiviral and amiodarone ↑ risk of bradycardia (avoid concurrent use)	Must be used with RBV or peg-IFN alfa + RBV

Combination Therapy

Generic • Brand • Dose/Dosage Forms	Pertinent Drug Interactions	Med Pearl
Elbasvir/grazoprevir • Zepatier • 1 tab = elbasvir 50 mg/grazoprevir 100 mg • 1 tab PO daily	• Elbasvir: CYP3A4 and P-gp substrate • Grazoprevir: CYP3A4 and P-gp substrate	• Elbasvir = NS5A inhibitor • Grazoprevir = protease inhibitor
Ledipasvir/sofosbuvir • Harvoni • 1 tab = ledipasvir 90 mg/sofosbuvir 400 mg • 1 tab PO daily	• Ledipasvir: P-gp substrate and inhibitor • Sofosbuvir: P-gp substrate • Concurrent use with amiodarone ↑ risk of bradycardia (avoid concurrent use)	• Ledipasvir = NS5A inhibitor • Sofosbuvir = NS5B inhibitor
Ombitasvir/paritaprevir/ritonavir • Technivie • 1 tab = ombitasvir 12.5 mg/paritaprevir 75 mg/ritonavir 50 mg • 2 tabs PO daily	• Ombitasvir: P-gp substrate • Paritaprevir: CYP3A4 and P-gp substrate; P-gp inhibitor • Ritonavir: CYP3A4 and P-gp substrate; CYP3A4 and P-gp inhibitor	• Ombitasvir = NS5A inhibitor • Paritaprevir = protease inhibitor • Ritonavir = CYP3A4 inhibitor • Give with food
Ombitasvir/paritaprevir/ritonavir + dasabuvir • Viekira Pak • Contains ombitasvir 12.5 mg/paritaprevir 75 mg/ritonavir 50 mg combination tablet + dasabuvir 250-mg tablet • 2 ombitasvir/paritaprevir/ritonavir tabs daily + 1 dasabuvir tab PO BID • Viekira XR • 1 tab = dasabuvir 200 mg/ombitasvir 8.33 mg/paritaprevir 50 mg/ritonavir 33.33 mg • 3 tabs PO daily	• Ombitasvir: P-gp substrate • Paritaprevir: CYP3A4 and P-gp substrate; P-gp inhibitor • Ritonavir: CYP3A4 and P-gp substrate; CYP3A4 and P-gp inhibitor • Dasabuvir: CYP2C8 substrate	• Ombitasvir = NS5A inhibitor • Paritaprevir = protease inhibitor • Ritonavir = CYP3A4 inhibitor • Dasabuvir = NS5B inhibitor • Give all tabs with food
Sofosbuvir/velpatasvir • Epclusa • 1 tab = sofosbuvir 400 mg/velpatasvir 100 mg • 1 tab PO daily	• Sofosbuvir: P-gp substrate • Velpatasvir: CYP2B6, CYP2C8, CYP3A4, and P-gp substrate • Concurrent use with amiodarone ↑ risk of bradycardia (avoid concurrent use)	• Sofosbuvir: NS5B inhibitor • Velpatasvir: NS5A inhibitor

Renal Disorders

This chapter covers the following:

- **Renal disorders**

RENAL DISORDERS

Guidelines Summary

- **Goals of therapy:**
  - Slow the progression of the disease, ↓ proteinuria, prevent complications, correct and manage reversible risk factors
  - Blood pressure (BP) <130/80 mmHg for CKD + any degree of proteinuria (A_2, A_3)
  - BP <140/90 mmHg for CKD with A_1 proteinuria (<30 mcg/mg)
- **Pharmacologic therapy for CKD**
  - CKD and hypertension
    - » Patients with any degree of proteinuria (A_2, A_3) should be initiated on an angiotensin-converting enzyme inhibitor (ACEI) or an angiotensin II receptor blocker (ARB).
    - » Patients with A_1 proteinuria (<30 mcg/mg) should be initiated on diuretic therapy (thiazide if creatinine clearance [CrCl] >30 mL/min or loop if <30 mL/min).
    - » Patients with BP that is elevated >20/10 mmHg above goal should be initiated on ACEI + diuretic.

- CKD without hypertension
  - » Patient with macroalbuminuria should be initiated on ACEI or ARB.
  - » Patient with microalbuminuria and diabetes mellitus (DM) should be initiated on ACEI or ARB.
  - » Patient with microalbuminuria without DM should not be initiated on pharmacologic therapy.
- With initiation of ACEI or ARB, up to 30% increase in serum creatinine is acceptable/expected.
- **Pharmacologic therapy for complications of CKD**
  - Edema: loop diuretics
  - Hyperkalemia: loop diuretics, sodium polystyrene sulfonate, calcium, regular insulin, dialysis
  - Anemia
    - » When hemoglobin falls below 10 g/dL, erythropoietin stimulating agents (ESAs) are indicated. Iron indices should also be monitored and appropriately supplemented.
  - Renal osteodystrophy
    - » Hyperphosphatemia (phosphate goals: 2.7–4.6 mg/dL for stages 3 and 4; 3.5–5.5 mg/dL for stage 5)
      - – Calcium-containing phosphate binders are the treatment of choice as long as corrected calcium <10.2 mg/dL and calcium phosphate product <55 mg^2/dL^2.
      - – Non–calcium containing phosphate binders such as sevelamer and lanthanum are appropriate for patients with corrected calcium >10.2 mg/dL or calcium phosphate product >55 mg^2/dL^2.
      - – Aluminum-containing phosphate binders are only indicated in severe hyperphosphatemia (serum phosphate >7 mg/dL) because they are associated with an ↑ risk for side effects.
    - » Secondary hyperparathyroidism (intact parathyroid hormone [iPTH] goals: 35–70 pg/mL for stage 3; 70–110 pg/mL for stage 4; and 150–300 pg/mL for stage 5)
      - – Phosphate should be at goal before treating elevated iPTH.
      - – Activated vitamin D analogs are paricalcitol, calcitriol, doxercalciferol.
    - » Vitamin D insufficiency/deficiency (goal 25(OH) vitamin D >30 ng/mL)
      - – Insufficiency 16–30 ng/mL
      - – Deficiency ≤15 ng/mL
      - – Treatment: loading dose (ergocalciferol) followed by maintenance dose
      - – Treatment timeframe determined by severity of deficiency

Medications for Chronic Kidney Disease

Generic • Brand • Dose/Dosage Forms	Contraindications	Primary Side Effects	Key Monitoring	Pertinent Drug Interactions	Med Pearl
Calcium-containing phosphate binders					
Calcium carbonate • Tums • 1,000 mg of elemental calcium/day (max should not exceed 2,000 mg/day)	Hypercalcemia	• Constipation • Flatulence • Hypercalcemia	• Serum calcium concentrations • Serum phosphorus concentrations • Intact parathyroid hormone (iPTH) concentrations	May ↓ absorption of tetracyclines, fluoroquinolones, levothyroxine, ketoconazole, and atazanavir (separate by 2–4 hr)	• For females ≥51 yr, recommended daily allowance is 1,200 mg of elemental calcium/day • Take with meals • Take in doses <500 mg of elemental calcium at a time for greatest absorption
Calcium acetate☆ • Eliphos, PhosLo, Phoslyra • Initial: 1,334 mg with each meal; can be ↑ every 2–3 wk to usual dose of 2,001–2,668 mg with each meal					Do not give additional calcium supplements
Non–calcium-containing phosphate binders					
Sevelamer • Renagel, Renvela • 800–1,600 mg TID with meals; initial dose may be based on serum phosphorus concentrations	Bowel obstruction	• Nausea/vomiting/diarrhea (N/V/D) • Dyspepsia • Abdominal pain • Constipation	• Serum calcium concentrations • Serum phosphorus concentrations • Bicarbonate concentrations • Chloride concentrations • iPTH concentrations	May ↓ absorption of ciprofloxacin and mycophenolate	Initial dose may be based on serum phosphorus
Lanthanum • Fosrenol • 500 mg TID with meals; can ↑ by up to 750 mg/day every 2–3 wk (max = 3,000 mg/day)	• Bowel obstruction • Fecal impaction • Ileus	• N/V • Abdominal pain • Constipation	• Serum calcium concentrations • Serum phosphorus concentrations • iPTH concentrations	May ↓ absorption of tetracyclines, fluoroquinolones, and levothyroxine, (separate by 2–4 hr)	• Do not swallow intact tablets (chew them) • Sprinkle oral powder over applesauce (not to be dissolved in liquid)

Medications for Chronic Kidney Disease   *(cont'd)*

Generic • Brand • Dose/Dosage Forms	Contraindications	Primary Side Effects	Key Monitoring	Pertinent Drug Interactions	Med Pearl
Ferric citrate • Auryxia • 2 tabs (420 mg ferric iron) TID with meals; adjust dose based on serum phosphorus concentrations (max = 12 tabs [2,520 mg ferric iron] daily)	Hemochromatosis	• N/V/D • Discolored stools	• Serum phosphorus concentrations • iPTH concentrations • Serum iron concentrations • Ferritin • Transferrin saturation	May ↓ absorption of doxycycline and ciprofloxacin (separate by 1–2 hr)	None
Sucroferric oxyhydroxide • Velphoro • 500 mg TID with meals; can ↑ by 500 mg every wk (max = 3,000 mg/day)	None	• N/D • Discolored stools	• Serum phosphorus concentrations • iPTH concentrations	May ↓ absorption of doxycycline and levothyroxine (separate from doxycycline by >1 hr; avoid use with levothyroxine)	Do not swallow intact tablets (chew them)
Aluminum-containing phosphate binders					
Aluminum hydroxide • 300–600 mg TID with meals	Hypersensitivity	• Hypomagnesemia • Hypophosphatemia • Constipation • Neurotoxicity	• Serum calcium concentrations • Serum phosphorus concentrations • Serum magnesium concentrations • iPTH concentrations	• May ↓ absorption of tetracyclines, fluoroquinolones, levothyroxine, ketoconazole, and atazanavir (separate by 2–4 hr)	
Calcimimetics					
Cinacalcet • Sensipar • Secondary hyperparathyroidism: initial: 30 mg daily; adjust dose based on iPTH concentration (max = 180 mg daily) • Parathyroid carcinoma or primary hyperparathyroidism: initial: 30 mg BID; adjust dose based on serum calcium concentrations (max = 90 mg 3–4 ×/day)	Hypocalcemia	• QTc interval prolongation • Seizures • Hypotension • Worsening heart failure • Bone fracture • N/V • Paresthesia	• Serum calcium concentrations • Serum phosphorus concentrations • iPTH concentrations • Electrocardiogram • Bone mineral density • BP	• CYP3A4 substrate • CYP2D6 inhibitor • CYP3A4 inhibitors may ↑ effects/toxicity • CYP3A4 inducers may ↓ effects • May ↑ effects/toxicity of CYP2D6 substrates	• For patients with secondary hyperparathyroidism on dialysis • Titrate every 2–4 wk • May require dosage adjustment if used with strong 3A4 inhibitors • Take with food • Do not crush, chew, or divide tabs

Medications for Chronic Kidney Disease *(cont'd)*

Generic • Brand • Dose/Dosage Forms	Contraindications	Primary Side Effects	Key Monitoring	Pertinent Drug Interactions	Med Pearl
Etelcalcetide • Parsabiv • 5 mg IV bolus 3 × /wk at the end of hemodialysis • Max: 15 mg 3 × /wk	Hypersensitivity to etelcalcetide or any component of the formulation	• Decreased serum calcium • Hypophosphatemia • N/D • Muscle spasm	• S/S of hypocalcemia, worsening heart failure, or GI bleeding/ulceration • QT interval in patients at risk for QT prolongation and ventricular arrhythmia • Corrected serum calcium and PTH levels	Cinecalcet may ↑ hypocalcemic effect of etelcalcetide	• Store intact vials in original carton to protect from light • Use within 7 days (if stored in original carton) or 4 hr (if removed from original carton) if removed from the refrigerator
Vitamin D Analogs					
Paricalcitol • Zemplar • Stages 3 and 4 CKD: iPTH ≤500 pg/mL: 1 mcg PO daily or 2 mcg PO 3 × /wk; iPTH >500 pg/mL: 2 mcg PO daily or 4 mcg PO 3 × /wk • Stage 5 CKD: 0.04-0.1 mcg/kg IV during dialysis	• Hypercalcemia • Vitamin D toxicity	• Hypercalcemia • Calciphylaxis • N/D • Edema	• Serum calcium concentrations • Serum phosphorus concentrations • Serum 25(OH)D concentrations • iPTH concentrations	• CYP3A4 substrate • CYP3A4 inhibitors may ↑ effects/toxicity • CYP3A4 inducers may ↓ effects • Thiazide diuretics may ↑ hypercalcemic effects	• Paricalcitol and doxercalciferol are synthetic forms of vitamin D that have less effect on calcium and phosphate • Calcitriol is active form of vitamin D (1,25-dihydroxyvitamin D) • Doxercalciferol needs to be metabolized to active form of vitamin D
Calcitriol☆ • Rocaltrol • Stages 3 and 4 CKD: 0.25−0.5 mcg PO daily • Stage 5 CKD: 0.5−1 mcg PO daily or 1−2 mcg IV 3 × /wk				Thiazide diuretics may ↑ hypercalcemic effects	
Doxercalciferol • Hectorol • Stages 3 and 4 CKD: 1−3.5 mcg PO daily • Stage 5 CKD: 10 mcg PO 3 × /wk or 4 mcg IV 3 × /wk					
Ergocalciferol • Calcidol, Calciferol, Drisdol • 50,000 units weekly for 8−12 wk	• Hypercalcemia • Malabsorption syndrome	• Constipation • Nausea/vomiting (N/V) • Hypercalcemia	• Serum calcium concentrations • Serum phosphorus concentrations • Serum 25(OH)D concentrations	Thiazide diuretics may ↑ hypercalcemic effects	• Dosing may differ depending on level of vitamin D deficiency • Needs to be converted into active form (1,25-dihydroxyvitamin D)

Medications for Chronic Kidney Disease   *(cont'd)*

Generic • Brand • Dose/Dosage Forms	Contraindications	Primary Side Effects	Key Monitoring	Pertinent Drug Interactions	Med Pearl
Calcifediol • Rayaldee • Stages 3 and 4 CKD: 30–60 mcg PO daily	None	• Hypercalcemia • ↑ serum creatinine • Dyspnea	• Serum calcium concentrations • Serum phosphorus concentrations • Serum 25(OH)D concentrations • iPTH concentrations	• CYP3A4 substrate • CYP3A4 inhibitors may ↑ effects/ toxicity • CYP3A4 inducers may ↓ effects • Thiazide diuretics may ↑ hypercalcemic effects	Synthetic form of vitamin D
Erythropoiesis stimulating agents					
Epoetin alfa • Epogen, Procrit • 50–100 U/kg IV or subcut 3 × /wk	• Hypersensitivity • Uncontrolled hypertension • Pure red cell aplasia	• Hypertension • Seizures • Anaphylaxis • Thromboembolism	• Hemoglobin/ hematocrit • Ferritin • Transferrin saturation • BP	None	• Boxed warning: ↑ risk of death, myocardial infarction, stroke, and thrombosis in patients with CKD • Initiate treatment with hemoglobin <10 g/dL • Do NOT exceed hemoglobin of 11 g/dL
Darbepoetin alfa • Aranesp • 0.45 mcg/kg IV or subcut weekly or 0.75 mcg/kg IV or subcut every 2 wk					

Dosing Considerations in Patients with CKD

Estimating Renal Clearance

As serum creatinine increases, renal function declines. The Cockcroft-Gault equation is the most commonly used method of estimating creatinine clearance (CrCl). The CrCl serves as an approximation of the GFR when considering the renal clearance of medications.

$$Creatinine\ clearance\ (female)(mL/min) = \frac{(140 - age) \times IBW \times 0.85}{72 \times serum\ creatinine}$$

$$Creatinine\ clearance\ (male)(mL/min) = \frac{(140 - age) \times IBW}{72 \times serum\ creatinine}$$

This formula is not ideal for use in the very elderly, very young, or in end stage renal disease (ESRD). IBW is ideal body weight.

Medications Requiring Dose Adjustment in CKD

Medications that are primarily eliminated via renal excretion often require dose and/or interval adjustment in advanced stages of renal disease. Reducing medication doses results in reduced peak concentrations while trough concentrations are maintained. Extending dosing intervals results in reduced trough concentrations while peak concentrations are maintained. Certain renally eliminated medications should be avoided in the setting of advanced renal disease due to the risk of serious side effects related to accumulation. Examples of commonly used medications that should be avoided and that require renal dose adjustment are provided in the following list.

Commonly Used Medications Requiring Dose/Interval Adjustment in CKD

- Acyclovir
- Allopurinol
- Aminoglycosides
- Amphotericin B
- Aztreonam
- Beta-lactam antibiotics
- Clarithromycin
- Colchicine
- Dabigatran
- Didanosine
- Digoxin
- Enoxaparin
- Ethambutol
- Famotidine
- Fluoroquinolones
- Gabapentin
- Ganciclovir
- Lamivudine
- Metoclopramide
- Penicillins
- Pregabalin
- Sulfamethoxazole/trimethoprim
- Tramadol
- Valacyclovir
- Vancomycin

- Venlafaxine
- Zidovudine
- Zoledronic acid

Commonly Used Medications That Should Be Avoided or Discontinued in Advanced CKD

- Alendronate
- Chlorpropamide
- Cidofovir
- Dabigatran
- Dofetilide
- Duloxetine
- Eplerenone
- Fondaparinux
- Foscarnet
- Glyburide
- Lithium
- Meperidine
- Metformin
- Nitrofurantoin
- NSAIDs
- Rivaroxaban
- Sotalol
- Spironolactone
- Tadalafil
- Tenofovir

Dosing Considerations in Dialysis

Patients with ESRD who require dialysis also require careful consideration of medication regimens to determine if medications are removed during dialysis and if replacement dosing is necessary post-dialysis. Some factors affecting removal of a drug via dialysis include the drug's volume of distribution, molecular size, and degree of protein binding as well as the type of dialysis membrane. Drugs with larger volume of distribution, larger molecular size, and higher degree of protein binding will be less effectively cleared via dialysis. High-flux dialysis membranes remove more medication than low- or medium-flux membranes.

PRACTICE QUESTIONS

1. A 66-year-old female (5′2″, 80 kg) has a stable serum creatinine of 1.5 mg/dL. Which is an accurate assessment of her renal function?

    (A) Stage 1 CKD
    (B) Stage 2 CKD
    (C) Stage 3 CKD
    (D) Stage 4 CKD

2. A 58-year-old man (5′10″, 92 kg) presents for routine follow-up. He has a medical history of hypertension. At last visit 4 months ago, BP was 148/96 mmHg, serum creatinine was 1.6 mg/dL, and urine albumin:creatinine was 10 mcg:mg. Data today includes BP 146/94 mmHg, HR 84 bpm, serum potassium 4.5 mEq/L, serum creatinine 1.5 mg/dL, and urine albumin:creatinine 10 mcg:mg. Which of the following is the BEST recommendation?

    (A) Initiate chlorthalidone
    (B) Initiate lisinopril
    (C) Initiate amlodipine
    (D) Non-pharmacological therapy only

3. A female patient with stage 3A CKD and hypertension presents for follow-up after a BP reading at last visit of 138/88 mmHg. She began non-pharmacological therapy for BP at that time. Vital signs today include BP 136/84 mmHg and HR 88 bpm. Serum labs include potassium 4.2 mEq/L, sCr 1.4 mg/dL, and urine albumin:creatinine ratio 100 mg:g. Which is the BEST recommendation?

    (A) Initiate chlorthalidone
    (B) Initiate lisinopril
    (C) Initiate amlodipine
    (D) Non-pharmacological therapy only

4. Which is the MOST appropriate therapy in a patient with stage 4 CKD and edema?

    (A) Indapamide
    (B) Spironolactone
    (C) Bumetanide
    (D) Chlorthalidone

5. A patient with stage 3B CKD presents for a routine follow-up and has the following serum lab results: 25(OH) vitamin D 40 ng/mL, PTH 115 pg/mL, phosphate 5.3 mg/dL, calcium 9.9 mg/dL, albumin 3 mg/dL. Which is the MOST appropriate therapy to recommend at this time?

    (A) Sevelamer
    (B) Calcitriol
    (C) Calcium carbonate
    (D) Ergocalciferol

6. A patient with stage 4 CKD presents for routine follow up with the following serum lab results: 25(OH) vitamin D 35 ng/mL, PTH 105 pg/mL, phosphate 5.3 mg/dL, calcium 9.2 mg/dL, albumin 3.8 mg/dL. Which is the MOST appropriate therapy to recommend?

    (A) Sevelamer
    (B) Calcitriol
    (C) Calcium carbonate
    (D) Ergocalciferol

ANSWERS AND EXPLANATIONS

1. **D**

$$\text{Creatinine clearance (female) (mL/min)} = \frac{(140 - \text{age}) \times \text{IBW} \times 0.85}{72 \times \text{serum creatinine}}$$

$$= \frac{(140 - 66) \times 50.1 \times 0.85}{72 \times 1.5} = 29\ \text{mL/min}$$

This patient has an estimated creatinine clearance of 29 mL/min calculated via the Cockcroft-Gault equation. Stage 4 CKD includes estimated GFR (calculated CrCl) of 15–29 mL/min.

2. **A**

This patient's estimated GFR (calculated CrCl) is 52 mL/min placing him into stage 3A CKD (45–59 mL/min). His urine protein assessment is below the range considered positive for A2 microalbuminuria (<30 mcg:mg). Patient's with non-proteinuric CKD have a BP goal of <140/90 mmHg and, therefore, pharmacotherapy is indicated making (D) incorrect. First line therapy per NKF is thiazide-type diuretic such as chlorthalidone (A). Lisinopril (B), an ACEI, would be an appropriate second line choice or would be appropriate first-line option for him if he had proteinuria. Calcium channel blockers are appropriate for add on therapy for hypertension.

3. **B**

Because this patient has CKD with A2 proteinuria, her evidence-based BP goal is <130/80 mmHg and her BP readings require treatment. Therefore, option (D) is incorrect. First line therapy for hypertension in patients with CKD and proteinuria is an ACEI such as lisinopril (B) or an ARB per National Kidney Foundation (NKF) guidelines. Thiazide diuretics such as chlorthalidone (A) are appropriate first line therapy in a patient with non-proteinuric CKD or as second line therapy in a patient with proteinuric CKD per the NKF. Calcium channel blockers such as amlodipine (C) are appropriate add-on agents for BP reduction but are not first line treatment.

4. **C**

Patients with stage 4 CKD have an estimated glomerular filtration rate (GFR) of <30 mL/min. In this setting, loop diuretics (e.g., [C] bumetanide) maintain efficacy, whereas thiazide diuretics such as (A) indapamide and (D) chlorthalidone do not. Additionally, loop diuretics are more effective in treating edema as compared to aldosterone antagonists (B) spironolactone and thiazide diuretics.

5. **A**

This patient has complications of CKD including hyperphosphatemia and secondary hyperparathyroidism. Before treating hyperparathyroidism, the phosphate should be brought into the goal range. Both sevelamer (A) and calcium carbonate (C) are phosphate binders. The calcium-containing phosphate binder, calcium carbonate, should be avoided because the patient's corrected calcium is >10.2 mg/dL and the calcium × phosphate product is >55 mg^2/dL^2. Ergocalciferol (D) is incorrect because patient's 25(OH) vitamin D level is at goal of >30 ng/mL.

6. **C**

This patient has hyperphosphatemia as a complication of CKD. Because the patient's corrected calcium is <10.2 mg/dL (9.4 mg/dL) and calcium × phosphate product is <55 mg^2/dL^2, a calcium-containing phosphate binder such as calcium carbonate (C) is the best recommendation. Sevelamer (A) is reserved for hyperphosphatemia in the setting of elevated corrected calcium (>10.2 mg/dL) or elevated calcium × phosphate product (>55 mg^2/dL^2). Calcitriol (B) would not be indicated as the patient's intact PTH is within the stage 4 CKD range of 70–110 pg/mL. Ergocalciferol (D) is not indicated because 25(OH) vitamin D level is at goal of >30 ng/mL.

Oncology

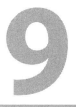

This chapter covers the following topics:

- **Cancer chemotherapy drugs**
- **Targeted and biologic agents**
- **Supportive care**

Many of the drugs used in chemotherapy are indicated for multiple types of cancer (e.g., lymphoma, leukemia, lung cancer, colorectal cancer, breast cancer, prostate cancer, ovarian cancer). Because cancer therapy is generally protocol-driven, your focus should be mostly on drug toxicities and on certain cases where a specific drug is indicated on the basis of cell-surface markers such as CD20 or HER-2 overexpression. Supportive care (antiemetic agents and colony-stimulating factors) is covered at the end of this chapter.

CANCER CHEMOTHERAPY DRUGS

Alkylating Agents

Generic • Brand • Dosage Forms	Contraindications	Primary Side Effects	Key Monitoring	Pertinent Drug Interactions	Med Pearl
Mechanism of action – alkylate DNA, making it more prone to breakage; most effective against rapidly dividing cells					
Cyclophospha-mide • Only available generically • Caps, injection (IV), tabs	Hypersensitivity to any alkylating agent	• Alopecia • Hemorrhagic cystitis • Infertility • Nausea, vomiting (N/V), mucositis, stomatitis • Bone marrow suppression	• Complete blood count (CBC) with differential • Blood urea nitrogen (BUN)/ serum creatinine (SCr) • Uric acid (UA)	Cytochrome P450 (CYP) 3A4 inducers may ↑ levels of active metabolite (acrolein)	• Maintain adequate hydration to avoid hemorrhagic cystitis; can also use mesna • High emetogenic potential
Chlorambucil • Leukeran • Tabs		• Bone marrow suppression • Infertility • Secondary leukemias • Seizures • Stevens-Johnson syndrome • Hepatotoxicity	• CBC with differential • Liver function tests (LFTs)	None	Take on empty stomach
Carmustine • BiCNU, Gliadel • Injection (IV), intracranial implant		• Bone marrow suppression • Pulmonary fibrosis • Severe N/V • Hypotension (IV) • Secondary leukemias (with long-term use) • Reversible elevation of LFTs	• CBC with differential • Pulmonary function tests • LFTs • Blood pressure (BP) (during IV administration)	IV solution contains ethanol; do not give aldehyde-dehydrogenase inhibitors	Very high emetogenic potential

Platinum-Based Agents

Generic • Brand • Dosage Forms	Contraindications	Primary Side Effects	Key Monitoring	Pertinent Drug Interactions	Med Pearl
Mechanism of action – crosslink DNA, causing it to break					
Cisplatin • Only available generically • Injection (IV)	• Hypersensitivity to any platinum-containing compounds • Renal impairment • Pre-existing hearing impairment (cisplatin)	• Anaphylaxis • Dose-related myelosuppression • N/V • Ototoxicity (cisplatin) • Nephrotoxicity with cumulative doses (esp. cisplatin) • Peripheral neuropathy • QT interval prolongation (oxaliplatin) • Rhabdomyolysis (oxaliplatin)	• BUN/SCr • Electrolytes • Neurologic exam • CBC with differential • Urine output	Administration with taxane derivatives may ↑ myelosuppression and ↓ efficacy of platinum agents	• Do not administer doses exceeding 100 mg/m^2 every 3 wk • High emetogenic potential
Carboplatin • Only available generically • Injection (IV)					• Moderate emetogenic potential • Dose often calculated by target AUC using Calvert formula (total dose [mg] = Target AUC × [GFR + 25]) • Adjust dose in renal impairment
Oxaliplatin • Eloxatin • Injection (IV)					• Moderate emetogenic potential • Warn patients to wear a scarf if being treated during cold weather • Adjust dose in renal impairment

Enzyme Inhibitors

Generic • Brand • Dosage Forms	Contraindications	Primary Side Effects	Key Monitoring	Pertinent Drug Interactions	Med Pearl
Mechanism of action – target enzymes responsible for DNA replication and repair					
Irinotecan • Camptosar • Injection (IV)	Concurrent therapy with strong CYP3A4 inhibitors	• Bone marrow suppression • Severe, life-threatening diarrhea	• CBC with differential • Electrolytes (esp. if diarrhea)	CYP3A4 substrate	• Diarrhea may be early or late onset • Moderate emetogenic potential • Atropine can be used to treat early-onset diarrhea; loperamide for late-onset diarrhea
Irinotecan liposomal • Onivyde • Injection (IV)	None	• Bone marrow suppression • Severe, life-threatening diarrhea • Interstitial lung disease (ILD) • Hypersensitivity reactions	• CBC with differential • Electrolytes (esp. if diarrhea) • S/S of ILD	CYP3A4 substrate	• Diarrhea may be early or late onset • Atropine can be used to treat early-onset diarrhea; loperamide for late-onset diarrhea

Enzyme Inhibitors *(cont'd)*

Generic • Brand • Dosage Forms	Contraindications	Primary Side Effects	Key Monitoring	Pertinent Drug Interactions	Med Pearl
Etoposide • Only available generically • Caps, injection (IV)	None	• Bone marrow suppression • Hypersensitivity reactions	• CBC with differential • LFTs • BUN/SCr	CYP3A4 substrate	• Do NOT give IV push (may cause hypotension) • Do NOT give IM (necrosis) • Adjust dose in renal impairment

Antimitotic Agents

Generic • Brand • Dosage Forms	Contraindications	Primary Side Effects	Key Monitoring	Pertinent Drug Interactions	Med Pearl
Mechanism of action – spindle poisons; interfere with mitotic spindle; prevent chromosome segregation and lead to cell death					
Vincristine • Only available generically • Injection (IV)	None	• Peripheral neuropathy (dose-limiting) • Constipation • Paralytic ileus (secondary to neurologic toxicity)	• Neurologic exam • Change in frequency of bowel movements	CYP3A4 substrate	• Do NOT give intra-thecally (IT) (fatal) • All patients should be on a prophylactic bowel management regimen • Avoid extravasation (vesicant) • Should NOT exceed 2 mg/dose
Vincristine liposomal • Marqibo • Injection (IV)	Demyelinating conditions	• Peripheral neuropathy (dose-limiting) • Bone marrow suppression • Constipation • Paralytic ileus (secondary to neurologic toxicity) • Hepatotoxicity	• Neurologic exam • Change in frequency of bowel movements • LFTs	CYP3A4 substrate	• NOT interchange-able with vincristine • Associated with less neurotoxicity than vincristine • Do NOT give IT (fatal) • Avoid extravasation (vesicant)
Vinblastine • Only available generically • Injection (IV)	None	• Peripheral neuropathy • Bone marrow suppression (dose-limiting)	• CBC with differential • Neurologic exam	CYP3A4 substrate	• Do not give IT (fatal) • Avoid extravasation (vesicant)

Antimitotic Agents   *(cont'd)*

Generic • Brand • Dosage Forms	Contraindications	Primary Side Effects	Key Monitoring	Pertinent Drug Interactions	Med Pearl
Paclitaxel • Only available generically • Injection (IV)	• Hypersensitivity to Cremophor • Baseline neutrophils <1,500/mm^3 (ovarian, lung, or breast cancer) • ANC <1,000/mm^3 (Kaposi's sarcoma)	• Bone marrow suppression (dose-limiting) • Hypersensitivity reactions • Peripheral neuropathy • Cardiac rhythm abnormalities • Mucositis, stomatitis (severe)	• CBC with differential • Electrocardiogram (ECG) • Neurologic exam	• CYP2C8 and CYP3A4 substrate • Administer prior to platinum derivatives to limit myelosuppression and enhance efficacy	• Premedicate with dexamethasone, diphenhydramine, and H$_2$-receptor antagonist • Adjust dose in hepatic impairment
Paclitaxel protein-bound particles • Abraxane • Injection (IV)	• Baseline neutrophils <1,500/mm^3				• No need for premedication • Adjust dose in hepatic impairment
Docetaxel • Taxotere, Docefrez • Injection (IV)	• Hypersensitivity to polysorbate 80 • Baseline neutrophils <1,500/mm^3 • Severe hepatic impairment	• Significant, dose-dependent fluid retention • Bone marrow suppression • Hypersensitivity reactions • Erythema (with edema) • Peripheral neuropathy	• CBC with differential • LFTs • Weight, signs of edema	CYP3A4 substrate	• Avoid doses >100 mg/m^2 • Premedicate with corticosteroids for 3 days (starting 1 day before docetaxel administration) to prevent fluid retention and hypersensitivity reactions • Contains ethanol • Adjust dose in hepatic impairment

Antimetabolites

Generic • Brand • Dosage Forms	Contraindications	Primary Side Effects	Key Monitoring	Pertinent Drug Interactions	Med Pearl
Mechanism of action – nucleoside analogs					
Cytarabine • Only available generically • Injection (IV)	None	• Severe bone marrow suppression • Cytarabine syndrome: myalgia, bone pain, rash, conjunctivitis, and fever • Sudden respiratory distress syndrome • Tumor lysis syndrome	• CBC with differential • BUN/SCr • Uric acid	None	• Premedicate with corticosteroid; may prevent cytarabine syndrome • May be administered IV, IT or subcut • Moderate emetogenic potential • Premedicate with antihyperuricemics and hydration in patients at ↑ risk for tumor lysis syndrome
Cytarabine liposomal • DepoCyt • Injection (IT)	Active meningeal infection	• Chemical arachnoiditis (N/V, headache, and fever) • Neurotoxicity	Monitor closely for signs of immediate reactions and neurotoxicity	None	• Coadminister dexamethasone to lessen chemical arachnoiditis • Moderate emetogenic potential
5-Fluorouracil • Only available generically • Injection (IV)	Dihydropyrimidine dehydrogenase (DPD) deficiency	• Hand-and-foot syndrome • N/V/D • Mucositis • Stomatitis • Bone marrow suppression	CBC with differential	• CYP2C9 inhibitor • May ↑ risk of bleeding with warfarin	Leucovorin ↑ effectiveness and toxicity; dose of fluorouracil may need to be ↓
Mechanism of action – folic acid antagonist					
Methotrexate☆ • Trexall (PO), Xatmep (PO) • Injection (IM, IT, IV), solution, tabs	None	• Nephrotoxicity • Bone marrow suppression • Stevens-Johnson syndrome • Severe diarrhea and ulcerative stomatitis • Neurotoxicity • Hepatotoxicity • Pneumonitis • Tumor lysis syndrome	• CBC with differential • BUN/SCr • Uric acid • LFTs • Chest x-ray	Diuretics and nonsteroidal anti-inflammatory drugs may ↑ risk of toxicity	• Give leucovorin rescue 24 hr after dosing to limit toxicity; do not administer concurrently • Premedicate with antihyperuricemics and hydration in patients at ↑ risk for tumor lysis syndrome • Can be given IT for leukemias • Also used subcut or PO as DMARD for rheumatoid arthritis

Anthracyclines

Generic • Brand • Dosage Forms	Contraindications	Primary Side Effects	Key Monitoring	Pertinent Drug Interactions	Med Pearl
Mechanism of action – intercalate DNA and generate reactive oxygen species					
Daunorubicin • Cerubidine • Injection (IV) Doxorubicin • Only available generically • Injection (IV) Doxorubicin liposomal • Doxil • Injection (IV)	• Pre-existing severe myocardial insufficiency or arrhythmia • Baseline neutrophils <1,500/mm^3 • Severe hepatic impairment	• Dose-related cardiotoxicity • Severe bone marrow suppression • Secondary leukemias • Red coloration of body fluids	• CBC with differential • ECG • Left ventricular ejection fraction (LVEF)	↑ risk of cardiotoxiocity with trastuzumab, pertuzumab, cyclophosphamide, and taxane derivatives	• Greatest risk of irreversible myocardial damage at cumulative dose >550 mg/m^2 • Moderate emetogenic potential • Avoid extravasation (vesicant) • Dexrazoxane indicated to prevent doxorubicin-induced cardiotoxicity or to treat anthracycline-induced extravasation • Liposomal doxorubicin indicated for Kaposi's sarcoma, multiple myeloma, and ovarian cancer

Hormonal Agents

Generic • Brand • Dosage Forms	Contraindications	Primary Side Effects	Key Monitoring	Pertinent Drug Interactions	Med Pearl
Mechanism of action – treat cancers in which growth is accelerated by hormones					
Leuprolide • Eligard, Lupron Depot • Injection (subcut, IM/subcut depot)	• Spinal cord compression • Undiagnosed abnormal vaginal bleeding	• Abnormal menses • Exacerbation of endometriosis • Hot flashes/ sweats • ↓ bone mineral density (if used >6 mo) • Spinal cord compression and urinary tract obstruction in prostate cancer • Tumor flare • Depression, mood disturbances	• Leutinizing hormone (LH) and follicle-stimulating hormone (FSH) levels • Serum testosterone (males), estradiol (females) • Bone mineral density	None	• Subcut injection administered daily • Rotate injection sites • Subcut/IM depot injection administered every 1–6 mo depending on dosage

Hormonal Agents   *(cont'd)*

Generic • Brand • Dosage Forms	Contraindications	Primary Side Effects	Key Monitoring	Pertinent Drug Interactions	Med Pearl
Tamoxifen☆ • Soltamox • Solution, tabs	• Concurrent warfarin therapy • History of deep vein thrombosis (DVT) or pulmonary embolism	• Thromboembolic events • ↑ risk of endometrial cancer • Hot flashes • Altered menses • Mood disturbances, depression • ↓ bone mineral density	Annual gynecologic exams	• CYP3A4 substrate • May ↑ risk of bleeding with warfarin • Selective serotonin reuptake inhibitors may ↓ effects	• Bone pain may indicate a good therapeutic response; manage with mild analgesia • Duration of treatment = 5–10 yr (depending on menopausal status)
Anastrozole☆ • Arimidex • Tabs	None	• ↓ bone mineral density • Hyperlipidemia • Mood disturbances • Hot flashes • Insomnia	• Bone mineral density • Low-density lipoprotein (LDL) and total cholesterol	None	• Aromatase inhibitor • Indicated for postmenopausal women with breast cancer • Duration of treatment = 5 yr
Exemestane • Aromasin • Tabs	None	• ↓ bone mineral density • Hot flashes • Insomnia	Bone mineral density	CYP3A4 substrate	• Aromatase inhibitor • Indicated for postmenopausal women with breast cancer • Duration of treatment = 5 yr
Letrozole • Femara • Tabs	None	• ↓ bone mineral density • Hyperlipidemia • Hot flashes	• Bone mineral density • LDL and total cholesterol	None	• Aromatase inhibitor • Indicated for postmenopausal women with breast cancer • Duration of treatment = 5 yr • Adjust dose in hepatic impairment

Chemotherapy Agents: Common Adverse Effects

- Cardiotoxicity
  - Doxorubicin
  - Daunorubicin
  - Idarubicin
  - Lapatinib
  - Mitoxantrone
  - Pertuzumab
  - Trastuzumab
- N/V
  - Cisplatin
  - Carboplatin
  - Cytarabine
  - Doxorubicin
  - Cyclophosphamide
- Mucositis
  - Cytarabine
  - Cyclophosphamide
  - 5-Fluorouracil
  - Methotrexate
- Neuropathy
  - Vincristine
  - Vinblastine
  - Oxaliplatin
  - Paclitaxel
- Renal impairment
  - Cisplatin
  - Cyclophosphamide
  - Ifosfamide
- Pulmonary fibrosis
  - Bleomycin
  - Busulfan
- Infusion reactions
  - Monoclonal antibodies
  - Paclitaxel

TARGETED AND BIOLOGIC AGENTS

Monoclonal Antibodies

Generic • Brand • Dosage Forms	Contraindications	Primary Side Effects	Key Monitoring	Pertinent Drug Interactions	Med Pearl
Mechanism of action – target the CD20 antigen					
Ibritumomab tiuxetan • Zevalin • Injection (IV)	None	• Infusion-related reactions • Myelosuppression (prolonged) • Secondary leukemia • Myelodysplastic syndrome • Rash (can be severe)	• CBC with differential • S/S of infusion reactions • S/S of dermatologic reactions	Do not administer live vaccines	• Indicated for CD20-positive, B-cell NHL • Linked to a radioisotope that targets B cells • Used in combination with rituximab as part of a 2-step process • Premedicate with diphenhydramine and acetaminophen (to prevent infusion reactions)
Obinutuzumab • Gazyva • Injection (IV)		• Infusion-related reactions • Tumor lysis syndrome • Myelosuppression (prolonged) • Infection (esp. bacterial, fungal, or hepatitis B virus [HBV] reactivation) • Progressive multifocal leuko-encephalopathy (PML)	• CBC with differential • BUN/SCr • Uric acid • S/S of infusion reactions • S/S of infection • S/S of PML		• Indicated for CLL • HBV screening should be done before initiating treatment • Premedicate with diphenhydramine, acetaminophen, and glucocorticoid (to prevent infusion reactions) • Premedicate with antihyper-uricemics and hydration in patients at ↑ risk for tumor lysis syndrome
Ofatumumab • Arzerra • Injection (IV)		• Infusion-related reactions • Tumor lysis syndrome • Myelosuppression (prolonged) • HBV reactivation • PML	• CBC with differential • BUN/SCr • Uric acid • S/S of infusion reactions • S/S of HBV • S/S of PML		

Monoclonal Antibodies *(cont'd)*

Generic • Brand • Dosage Forms	Contraindications	Primary Side Effects	Key Monitoring	Pertinent Drug Interactions	Med Pearl
Rituximab • Rituxan • Injection (IV)	None	• Infusion-related reactions • Tumor lysis syndrome • Rash (can be severe) • PML • Arrhythmias • Infection (esp. bacterial, fungal, or HBV reactivation) • Nephrotoxicity • Bowel obstruction/ perforation	• CBC with differential • S/S of infusion reactions • S/S of infection • S/S of PML • BUN/SCr • Electrolytes • Uric acid • ECG • S/S of abdominal pain • S/S of dermatologic reactions	Do not administer live vaccines	• Indicated for CD20-positive, B-cell NHL, and CD20-positive CLL • Also indicated for rheumatoid arthritis • HBV screening should be done before initiating treatment • Premedicate with diphenhydramine and acetaminophen (to prevent infusion reactions) • Premedicate with antihyperuricemics and hydration in patients at ↑ risk for tumor lysis syndrome

Epidermal Growth Factor Receptor (EGFR) Inhibitors

Generic • Brand • Dosage Forms	Contraindications	Primary Side Effects	Key Monitoring	Pertinent Drug Interactions	Med Pearl
Mechanism of action – prevent tumor growth by inhibiting the various EGFR receptors					
Afatinib • Gilotrif • Tabs	None	• Diarrhea • Rash (can be severe) • ILD • Hepatotoxicity • Keratitis	• EGFR mutation status • LFTs • BUN/SCr • S/S of dermatologic reactions • S/S of dehydration • Electrolytes • S/S of ILD • S/S of eye inflammation/ visual abnormalities	P-glycoprotein (P-gp) substrate	• Indicated for metastatic NSCLC with EGFR exon 19 deletions or exon 21 substitution mutations • Adjust dose in renal impairment • Take 1 hr before or 2 hr after a meal
Cetuximab • Erbitux • Injection (IV)	None	• Infusion-related reactions • Rash (can be severe) • ILD • Sudden cardiac death • Electrolyte abnormalities ($\downarrow Mg^{2+}$, $\downarrow K^+$, $\downarrow Ca^{2+}$)	• EGFR and *K-Ras* status (for colorectal cancer) • S/S of infusion reactions • S/S of dermatologic reactions • S/S of ILD • Electrolytes	None	• Indicated for squamous cell cancer of head and neck and *K-Ras* wild type, EGFR expressing colorectal cancer • Premedicate with diphenhydramine (to prevent infusion reactions)

Epidermal Growth Factor Receptor (EGFR) Inhibitors *(cont'd)*

Generic • Brand • Dosage Forms	Contraindications	Primary Side Effects	Key Monitoring	Pertinent Drug Interactions	Med Pearl
Erlotinib • Tarceva • Tabs	None	• Rash (can be severe) • Diarrhea • ILD • Renal failure • Hepatotoxicity • Gastrointestinal (GI) perforation • Myocardial ischemia/ infarction • Stroke • Keratitis	• EGFR mutation status • S/S of dermatologic reactions • S/S of dehydration • S/S of ILD • BUN/SCr • Electrolytes • LFTs • S/S of GI perforation • S/S of eye inflammation/ visual abnormalities	• CYP1A2 and CYP3A4 substrate • CYP3A4 inducers, CYP1A2 inducers, and cigarette smoking ↓ levels (↑ erlotinib dose) • May ↑ risk of bleeding with warfarin • H_2-antagonists, proton pump inhibitors (PPIs), and antacids may ↓ absorption (avoid use with PPIs; space apart from H_2-antagonists or antacids)	Indicated for locally advanced/ metastatic NSCLC with EGFR exon 19 deletions or exon 21 substitution mutations; or locally advanced, surgically unresectable, or metastatic pancreatic cancer
Gefitinib • Iressa • Tabs	None	• Rash (can be severe) • Diarrhea • ILD • Hepatotoxicity • GI perforation • Keratitis	• EGFR mutation status • S/S of dermatologic reactions • S/S of dehydration • BUN/SCr • Electrolytes • S/S of ILD • LFTs • S/S of GI perforation • S/S of eye inflammation/ visual abnormalities	• CYP3A4 substrate • Strong CYP3A4 inducers ↓ levels (↑ gefitinib dose) • May ↑ risk of bleeding with warfarin • H_2-antagonists, PPIs, and antacids may ↓ absorption (avoid concomitant use of PPIs; may use H_2-antagonists or antacids [need to space administration])	Indicated for metastatic NSCLC with EGFR exon 19 deletions or exon 21 substitution mutations
Lapatinib • Tykerb • Tabs	None	• Cardiotoxicity • Diarrhea • Hepatotoxicity • Rash (can be severe) • QT interval prolongation • ILD	• HER2 status • LVEF • S/S of dehydration • Electrolytes • LFTs • S/S of dermatologic reactions • ECG • S/S of ILD	• CYP3A4 and P-gp substrate • CYP2C8, CYP3A4, and P-gp inhibitor • Avoid concomitant use of strong CYP3A4 inhibitors and inducers • May ↑ digoxin levels • ↑ risk of torsade de pointes (TdP) with other drugs that prolong QT interval	• Indicated for HER2-positive metastatic breast cancer • Adjust dose in hepatic imparment
Necitumumab • Portrazza • Injection (IV)	None	• Cardiopulmo-nary arrest • ↓ Mg^{2+} • Thromboem-bolic events • Rash (can be severe) • Infusion-related reactions	• Electrolytes • S/S of thromboembolism • S/S of dermatologic reactions • S/S of infusion reactions	None	Indicated for metastatic NSCLC

Epidermal Growth Factor Receptor (EGFR) Inhibitors *(cont'd)*

Generic • Brand • Dosage Forms	Contraindications	Primary Side Effects	Key Monitoring	Pertinent Drug Interactions	Med Pearl
Osimertinib • Tagrisso • Tabs	None	• ILD • QT interval prolongation • Cardiotoxicity • Keratitis	• EGFR mutation status • S/S of ILD • ECG • LVEF	• CYP3A4 substrate and inhibitor • CYP1A2 and CYP3A4 inducer • Avoid concomitant use of strong CYP3A4 inhibitors and inducers • ↑ risk of TdP with other drugs that prolong QT interval	Indicated for metastatic NSCLC with EGFR T790M mutation
Panitumumab • Vectibix • Injection (IV)	None	• Diarrhea • Rash (can be severe) • Infusion-related reactions • ILD • Electrolyte abnormalities ($\downarrow$ Mg^{2+}, $\downarrow$ K$^+$, $\downarrow$ Ca^{2+}) • Keratitis • Photosensitivity	• *K-Ras* status • S/S of dehydration • Electrolytes • S/S of dermatologic reactions • S/S of infusion reactions • S/S of ILD • S/S of eye inflammation/visual abnormalities	None	• Indicated for wild-type *K-Ras* metastatic colorectal cancer • Advise patients to wear sunscreen
Pertuzumab • Perjeta • Injection (IV)	None	• Cardiotoxicity • Infusion-related reactions • Anaphylaxis	• HER2 status • LVEF • S/S of infusion reactions/anaphylaxis	↑ risk of cardiotoxicity with anthracyclines	Indicated for HER2-positive metastatic breast cancer
Trastuzumab • Herceptin • Injection (IV)	None	• Cardiotoxicity • Infusion-related reactions • Myelosuppression • ILD	• HER2 status • LVEF • S/S of infusion reactions • CBC with differential • S/S of ILD	↑ risk of cardiotoxicity with anthracyclines	Indicated for HER2-positive metastatic breast cancer and gastric cancer
Ado-trastuzumab emtansine • Kadcyla • Injection (IV)	None	• Hepatotoxicity • Cardiotoxicity • Infusion-related reactions • ILD • Myelosuppression • Peripheral neuropathy • Hemorrhage	• HER2 status • LFTs • LVEF • S/S of infusion reactions • S/S of ILD • CBC with differential • S/S of neuropathy • S/S of bleeding	• CYP3A4 substrate • Avoid concomitant use of strong CYP3A4 inhibitors or inducers • ↑ risk of cardiotoxicity with anthracyclines	Indicated for HER2-positive metastatic breast cancer

Vascular Endothelial Growth Factor (VEGF) Inhibitors

Generic • Brand • Dosage Forms	Contraindications	Primary Side Effects	Key Monitoring	Pertinent Drug Interactions	Med Pearl
Mechanism of action —block angiogenesis and tumor growth by inhibiting VEGF receptors					
Axitinib • Inlyta • Tabs	None	• Thromboembolic events • Hypertension • Hemorrhage • Heart failure • GI perforation/fistula formation • Hypo-/hyperthyroidism • Proteinuria • ↑ LFTs • Impaired wound healing • Reversible posterior leuko-encephalopathy syndrome (RPLS)	• S/S of thromboembolism • BP • S/S of bleeding • S/S of heart failure • Thyroid function tests (TFTs) • Urinalysis • LFTs • S/S of GI perforation/fistula formation • S/S of RPLS	• CYP3A4 substrate • Avoid concomitant use of strong CYP3A4 inhibitors or inducers	• Indicated for metastatic renal cell carcinoma • Adjust dose in hepatic impairment
Bevacizumab • Avastin • Injection (IV)	None	• Thromboembolic events • Hypertension • Hemorrhage • GI perforation/fistula formation • Proteinuria • ↑ LFTs • Impaired wound healing • Infusion-related reactions • RPLS	• S/S of thromboembolism • BP • S/S of bleeding • Urinalysis • LFTs • S/S of GI perforation/fistula formation • S/S of infusion reactions • S/S of RPLS	None	Indicated for metastatic colorectal cancer; locally advanced, recurrent, or metastatic nonsquamous NSCLC; glioblastoma; metastatic renal cell carcinoma; persistent, recurrent, or metastatic cervical cancer; or recurrent epithelial ovarian, fallopian tube, or primary peritoneal cancer
Cabozantinib • Cabometyx, Cometriq • Caps (Cometriq), tabs (Cabometyx)	None	• Thromboembolic events • Hypertension • Hemorrhage • GI perforation/fistula formation • Diarrhea • Palmar-plantar erythrodysesthesia syndrome • RPLS	• S/S of thromboembolism • BP • S/S of bleeding • S/S of GI perforation/fistula formation • S/S of dehydration • Electrolytes • S/S of RPLS	• CYP3A4 substrate • Avoid concomitant use of strong CYP3A4 inhibitors or inducers	• Indicated for advanced renal cell carcinoma (Cabometyx) or metastatic, medullary thyroid cancer (Cometriq) • Adjust dose in hepatic impairment

Vascular Endothelial Growth Factor (VEGF) Inhibitors   *(cont'd)*

Generic • Brand • Dosage Forms	Contraindications	Primary Side Effects	Key Monitoring	Pertinent Drug Interactions	Med Pearl
Ramucirumab • Cyramza • Injection (IV)	None	• Thromboembolic events • Hypertension • Hemorrhage • GI perforation • Hypo-/hyperthyroidism • Proteinuria • ↑ LFTs • Impaired wound healing • Infusion-related reactions • RPLS	• S/S of thromboembolism • BP • S/S of bleeding • TFTs • Urinalysis • LFTs • S/S of GI perforation • S/S of infusion reactions • S/S of RPLS	None	• Indicated for advanced gastric cancer; metastatic NSCLC; and metastatic colorectal cancer • Premedicate with diphenhydramine
Sorafenib • Nexavar • Tabs	None	• Myocardial ischemia/infarction • Hepatotoxicity • Diarrhea • Rash (can be severe) • Hand-foot syndrome • Hypertension • QT interval prolongation • Hemorrhage • Hypo-/hyperthyroidism • Impaired wound healing • GI perforation	• LFTs • S/S of dehydration • Electrolytes • S/S of dermatologic reactions • BP • ECG • S/S of bleeding • TFTs • S/S of GI perforation	• CYP3A4 substrate • Avoid concomitant use of strong CYP3A4 inducers • May ↑ risk of bleeding with warfarin • ↑ risk of TdP with other drugs that prolong QT interval	Indicated for advanced renal cell carcinoma; unresectable hepatocellular carcinoma; or locally recurrent or metastatic, progressive differentiated thyroid cancer
Sunitinib • Sutent • Caps	None	• Hepatotoxicity • Diarrhea • Rash (can be severe) • Hypertension • Heart failure • QT interval prolongation • Hemorrhage • Tumor lysis syndrome • Hypo-/hyperthyroidism • Proteinuria • Hypoglycemia • Impaired wound healing	• LFTs • S/S of dehydration • Electrolytes • S/S of dermatologic reactions • BP • LVEF • S/S of heart failure • ECG • S/S of bleeding • TFTs • Urinalysis • Glucose • BUN/SCr • Uric acid	• CYP3A4 substrate • Avoid concomitant use of strong CYP3A4 inhibitors or inducers	• Indicated for gastrointestinal stromal tumor (GIST); advanced renal cell carcinoma; or locally advanced unresectable or metastatic pancreatic neuroendocrine tumors • Premedicate with antihyperuricemics and hydration in patients at ↑ risk for tumor lysis syndrome

Tyrosine Kinase Inhibitors

Generic • Brand • Dosage Forms	Contraindications	Primary Side Effects	Key Monitoring	Pertinent Drug Interactions	Med Pearl
Mechanism of action – halt proliferation of tumor cells by inhibiting tyrosine kinase					
Bosutinib • Bosulif • Tabs	None	• N/V/D • Myelosuppression • Hepatotoxicity • Renal impairment • Fluid retention	• S/S of dehydration • Electrolytes • CBC with differential • LFTs • BUN/SCr • S/S of peripheral/ pulmonary edema	• CYP3A4 and P-gp substrate • P-gp inhibitor • Avoid concomitant use of strong or moderate CYP3A4 inhibitors or inducers • H_2-antagonists, PPIs, and antacids may ↓ absorption (avoid concomitant use of PPIs; may use H_2-antagonists or antacids [need to space administration])	• Indicated for Philadelphia-positive (Ph+) CML and Ph+ ALL • Adjust dose in hepatic or renal impairment
Dasatinib • Sprycel • Tabs	None	• Myelosuppression • Hemorrhage • Fluid retention • Pulmonary arterial hypertension • Rash (can be severe) • Tumor lysis syndrome • QT interval prolongation	• CBC with differential • BUN/SCr • Uric acid • S/S of bleeding • S/S of peripheral/ pulmonary edema • S/S of pulmonary arterial hypertension • S/S of dermatologic reactions • ECG	• CYP3A4 substrate and inhibitor • Avoid concomitant use of strong 3A4 inhibitors or inducers • H_2-antagonists, PPIs, and antacids may ↓ absorption (avoid concomitant use of H_2-antagonists and PPIs; may use antacids [need to space administration]) • ↑ risk of TdP with other drugs that prolong QT interval	• Indicated for Ph+ CML and Ph+ ALL • Premedicate with antihy-peruricemics and hydration in patients at ↑ risk for tumor lysis syndrome
Imatinib • Gleevec • Tabs	None	• Myelosuppression • Hemorrhage • Fluid retention • Rash (can be severe) • Tumor lysis syndrome • Heart failure • Hepatotoxicity • Hypothyroidism	• CBC with differential • BUN/SCr • Uric acid • S/S of bleeding • S/S of peripheral/ pulmonary edema • S/S of dermatologic reactions • S/S of heart failure • LFTs • TFTs	• CYP3A4 substrate and inhibitor • CYP2D6 inhibitor • Avoid concomitant use of strong CYP3A4 inhibitors or inducers	• Indicated for Ph+ CML, Ph+ ALL, Kit (CD117)-positive GIST, and a variety of other disorders • Adjust dose in hepatic or renal impairment • Premedicate with antihy-peruricemics and hydration in patients at ↑ risk for tumor lysis syndrome

Tyrosine Kinase Inhibitors   *(cont'd)*

Generic • Brand • Dosage Forms	Contraindications	Primary Side Effects	Key Monitoring	Pertinent Drug Interactions	Med Pearl
Lenvatinib • Lenvima • Caps	None	• Thromboembolic events • Hypertension • Hemorrhage • Heart failure • Hepatotoxicity • Proteinuria • Renal failure • GI perforation/fistula formation • QT interval prolongation • Hypocalcemia • RPLS • Hypothyroidism	• S/S of thromboembolism • BP • S/S of bleeding • LVEF • S/S of heart failure • LFTs • Urinalysis • BUN/SCr • S/S of GI perforation/ fistula formation • ECG • Electrolytes • S/S of RPLS • TFTs	↑ risk of TdP with other drugs that prolong QT interval	• Indicated for locally recurrent or metastatic, progressive radioactive iodine-refractory differentiated thyroid cancer and renal cell carcinoma • Adjust dose in hepatic or renal impairment
Nilotinib • Tasigna • Caps	• Hypokalemia • Hypomagnesemia • Long QT syndrome	• Myelosuppression • Hemorrhage • Fluid retention • QT interval prolongation • Cardiovascular events • Pancreatitis • Hepatotoxicity • Electrolyte abnormalities ($\downarrow PO_4$, $\downarrow/\uparrow K^+$, $\downarrow Na^+$) • Tumor lysis syndrome	• CBC with differential • BUN/SCr • Uric acid • S/S of bleeding • S/S of peripheral/ pulmonary edema • ECG • S/S of cardiovascular events • Amylase/lipase • Glucose • LFTs • Electrolytes	• CYP3A4 substrate and inhibitor • CYP2C8, CYP2C9, CYP2D6, and P-gp inhibitor • CYP2C9 inducer • Avoid concomitant use of strong CYP3A4 inhibitors or inducers • H$_2$-antagonists, PPIs, and antacids may ↓ absorption (avoid concomitant use of PPIs; may use antacids and H$_2$-antagonists [need to space administration]) • ↑ risk of TdP with other drugs that prolong QT interval	• Indicated for Ph+ CML • Take on empty stomach • Adjust dose in hepatic impairment • Premedicate with antihyperuricemics and hydration in patients at ↑ risk for tumor lysis syndrome

Anaplastic Lymphoma Kinase (ALK) Inhibitors

Generic • Brand • Dosage Forms	Contraindications	Primary Side Effects	Key Monitoring	Pertinent Drug Interactions	Med Pearl
Mechanism of action – reduce proliferation of tumor cells by inhibiting ALK					
Alectinib • Alecensa • Caps	None	• Hepatotoxicity • ILD • Bradycardia • Myalgias	• ALK status • S/S of ILD • ECG • Heart rate (HR) • Creatine kinase	None	Indicated for ALK-positive, metastatic NSCLC
Brigatinib • Alunbrig • Tabs	None	• ILD • Hypertension • Bradycardia • Visual disturbances • Myalgias • Hyperglycemia • Pancreatitis	• ALK status • S/S of ILD • BP • ECG • HR • Creatine kinase • Glucose • Amylase/lipase • Ophthalmologic examination	• CYP3A4 substrate and inducer • Avoid concomitant use of strong 3A4 inhibitors or inducers	Indicated for ALK-positive, metastatic NSCLC
Ceritinib • Zykadia • Caps	None	• N/V/D • Hepatotoxicity • ILD • QT interval prolongation • Hyperglycemia • Bradycardia • Pancreatitis	• ALK status • S/S of dehydration • Electrolytes • LFTs • S/S of ILD • ECG • Glucose • HR • Amylase/lipase	• CYP3A4 substrate • CYP2C9 and CYP3A4 inhibitor • Avoid concomitant use of strong 3A4 inhibitors or inducers	Indicated for ALK-positive, metastatic NSCLC
Crizotinib • Xalkori • Caps	None	• N/V/D • Hepatotoxicity • ILD • QT interval prolongation • Bradycardia • Vision loss	• ALK status • ROS-1 status • S/S of dehydration • Electrolytes • BUN/SCr • LFTs • S/S of ILD • ECG • HR	• CYP3A4 substrate and inhibitor • Avoid concomitant use of strong CYP3A4 inhibitors or inducers • Avoid concomitant use of CYP3A4 substrates with narrow therapeutic range • ↑ risk of TdP with other drugs that prolong QT interval	• Indicated for ALK-positive, metastatic NSCLC and ROS-1-positive NSCLC • Adjust dose in renal impairment

Platelet-Derived Growth Factor Receptor (PDGFR)-α Blocker

Generic • Brand • Dosage Forms	Contraindications	Primary Side Effects	Key Monitoring	Pertinent Drug Interactions	Med Pearl
Mechanism of action – monoclonal antibody that prevents binding of PDGF-AA, PDGF-BB, and PDGF-CC to PDGFR-α, which subsequently inhibits signaling to reduce cancer cell proliferation and metastasis					
Olaratumab • Lartruvo • Injection (IV)	None	• Infusion-related reactions • Myelosuppression	• CBC with differential • S/S of infusion reactions	None	• Indicated for soft tissue sarcoma • Should be used in combination with doxorubicin (for first 8 cycles) • Premedicate with diphenhydramine and dexamethasone (to prevent infusion reactions)

Poly (ADP-Ribose) Polymerase (PARP) Inhibitors

Generic • Brand • Dosage Forms	Contraindications	Primary Side Effects	Key Monitoring	Pertinent Drug Interactions	Med Pearl
Mechanism of action – inhibit PARP enzymes, resulting in $\uparrow$ formation of PARP-DNA complexes and subsequent DNA damage, apoptosis, and cell death					
Niraparib • Zejula • Caps	None	• Myelodysplastic syndrome/AML • Myelosuppression • Hypertension	• CBC with differential • BP	None	Indicated for recurrent epithelial ovarian, fallopian tube, or primary peritoneal cancer
Olaparib • Lynparza • Caps	None	• Myelodysplastic syndrome/AML • Pneumonitis	• *BRCA* mutation status • CBC with differential • BUN/SCr • S/S of pneumonitis	• CYP3A4 substrate • Avoid concomitant use of strong or moderate CYP3A4 inhibitors or inducers	• Indicated for deleterious *BRCA*-mutated advanced ovarian cancer • Adjust dose in renal impairment
Rucaparib • Rubraca • Tabs	None	• Myelodysplastic syndrome/AML • Anemia	• *BRCA* mutation status • CBC with differential	None	Indicated for deleterious *BRCA*-mutated advanced ovarian cancer

Programmed Death Ligand-1 (PD-L1) Inhibitor

Generic • Brand • Dosage Forms	Contraindications	Primary Side Effects	Key Monitoring	Pertinent Drug Interactions	Med Pearl
Mechanism of action – monoclonal antibody that prevents binding of PD-L1 to PD-1 and B7.1 receptors on T cells, which restores antitumor T cell function, resulting in ↓ tumor growth					
Atezolizumab • Tecentriq • Injection (IV)	None	• Infusion-related reactions • ILD • Hepatotoxicity • Colitis/diarrhea • Hypo-/ hyperthyroidism • Adrenal insuf- ficiency • Type 1 diabetes • Infection	• S/S of infusion reactions • S/S of ILD • LFTs • TFTs • Glucose • S/S of infection • Electrolytes (esp. if diarrhea)	None	Indicated for locally advanced or metastatic urothelial carcinoma and metastatic NSCLC

B-Cell Lymphoma-2 (BCL-2) Inhibitor

Generic • Brand • Dosage Form	Contraindications	Primary Side Effects	Key Monitoring	Pertinent Drug Interactions	Med Pearl
Mechanism of action – inhibits BCL-2, an anti-apoptotic protein, which subsequently restores the apoptotic process					
Venetoclax • Venclexta • Tabs	Concurrent therapy with strong CYP3A4 inhibitors during the ramp- up period (first 5 weeks)	• Tumor lysis syndrome • Myelosuppression	• 17p deletion status • CBC with differential • BUN/SCr • Uric acid	• CYP3A4 and P-gp substrate • Avoid concomitant use of strong or moderate CYP3A4 inhibitors or inducers or P-gp inhibitors	• Indicated for CLL with 17p deletion • Take with a meal • Premedicate with antihyperuricemics and hydration in patients at ↑ risk for tumor lysis syndrome

Cyclin-Dependent Kinase (CDK) Inhibitors

Generic • Brand • Dosage Forms	Contraindications	Primary Side Effects	Key Monitoring	Pertinent Drug Interactions	Med Pearl
Mechanism of action – inhibits CDK 4 and 6, which subsequently reduces cell cycle progression, cellular proliferation, and cell cycle progression					
Palbociclib • Ibrance • Caps	None	Myelosuppression	CBC with differential	• CYP3A4 substrate and inhibitor • Avoid concomitant use of strong CYP3A4 inhibitors or inducers	• Indicated for hormone-receptor positive, HER2-negative, advanced or metastatic breast cancer • Should be used with an aromatase inhibitor (in postmenopausal women) or fulvestrant
Ribociclib • Kisqali • Tabs	None	• QT interval prolongation • Hepatotoxicity • Myelosuppression	• ECG • Electrolytes • LFTs • CBC with differential	• CYP3A4 substrate and inhibitor • Avoid concomitant use of strong CYP3A4 inhibitors or inducers • ↑ risk of TdP with other drugs that prolong QT interval	• Indicated for postmenopausal women with hormone-receptor positive, HER2-negative, advanced or metastatic breast cancer • Should be used with an aromatase inhibitor • Adjust dose in hepatic impairment

SUPPORTIVE CARE

Nausea and Vomiting

About 55% of cancer patients experience nausea and vomiting during the first week of chemotherapy. $5HT_3$ antagonists are useful in most cases, but should be used only for prevention of nausea and vomiting. Corticosteroids should be given unless contraindicated, as they are synergistic with the $5HT_3$ antagonists; other drug therapies depend on the type of nausea and vomiting experienced.

- Benzodiazepines: Treatment of choice for anticipatory nausea and vomiting (caused by the sights and smells of the chemotherapy environment)
- Neurokinin-1 (NK-1) antagonist: Useful for delayed nausea and vomiting caused by drugs with high emetic potential (cisplatin, cyclophosphamide, doxorubicin)
- Prochlorperazine or metoclopramide: May be used in less severe cases

Management of Neutropenia and Anemia

Neutropenia and its major complication, neutropenic fever, are major concerns in many types of cancer. The nadir, or lowest, concentration of WBCs in the peripheral blood usually occurs 1–2 weeks following the administration of chemotherapy and is typically proportional to the dose. Subsequent chemotherapy is delayed until the ANC recovers, which explains the 3- to 4-week cycle length of most chemotherapy regimens. Classification of ANC is:

- Normal: 3,000–7,000 neutrophils/mm^3
- Mild neutropenia: 500–1,000/mm^3
- Moderate neutropenia: 100–500/mm^3
- Severe neutropenia: <100/mm^3

Colony-stimulating factors (CSF) such as filgrastim or PEG-filgrastim have been shown to shorten the duration of neutropenia, but they have little effect on mortality and are very expensive. CSFs do decrease hospitalizations, however, and clinical judgment should be used to determine which patients are most likely to benefit. Because infection leads to death in a large percentage of neutropenic patients (possibly up to 30%), anti-infective therapy is frequently needed. Broad-spectrum bactericidal antibiotics are generally used (third- and fourth-generation cephalosporins, carbapenems, or fluoroquinolones with or without aminoglycosides or β-lactams), with antipseudomonal activity being particularly important. If antifungal therapy is needed, amphotericin B is the drug of choice.

Anemia is also common in cancer patients. Treatment of anemia is currently the subject of much controversy; use of erythropoiesis-stimulating agents, including erythropoietin and darbepoetin, is no longer supported in myeloid malignancies (these agents have been associated with increase in mortality compared to patients not receiving erythropoietin). The hypothesis is that the drug may be stimulating cancer growth. These drugs should NOT be used in patients with myeloid malignancies who are receiving chemotherapy when the anticipated outcome is a cure. This finding may not apply to solid tumors; more information is needed. Refer to Chapter 8 for discussion of the erythropoiesis-stimulating agents.

Antiemetic Drugs

Generic • Brand • Dose • Dosage Forms	Contraindications	Primary Side Effects	Key Monitoring	Pertinent Drug Interactions	Med Pearl
Mechanism of action – 5HT$_3$ antagonists; prevent release of serotonin in GI mucosa					
Ondansetron ☆ • Zofran, Zuplenz • 16–24 mg PO or 8–12 mg IV • Films, injection (IV), orally disintegrating tabs, solution, tabs Granisetron • Sancuso, Sustol • 2 mg PO, 1 mg IV, or 10 mg subcut • Extended-release-injection (subcut), injection (IV), tabs, transdermal patch Dolasetron • Anzemet • 100 mg PO • Tabs Palonosetron • Aloxi • 0.25 mg IV • Injection (IV)	Current N/V (useful only for prevention)	• Headache • Constipation or diarrhea • Fatigue • Dry mouth • Transient ↑ LFTs • QT interval prolongation	None	• CYP3A4 substrates • Use with serotonergic agents may ↑ risk of serotonin syndrome • ↑ risk of TdP with other drugs that prolong QT interval	• Single dose prior to chemotherapy; repeat doses do not ↑ effect • Palonosetron effective in preventing acute and delayed N/V • Extended-release granisetron subcut injection should NOT be administered more frequently than every 7 days (every 14 days in renal impairment)

Antiemetic Drugs *(cont'd)*

Generic • **Brand** • **Dose** • **Dosage Forms**	Contraindications	Primary Side Effects	Key Monitoring	Pertinent Drug Interactions	Med Pearl
Mechanism of action – NK-1 antagonist; block substance P from NK-1 receptor					
Aprepitant • Emend • PO: 125 mg on day 1, then 80 mg daily on days 2 and 3 • IV: 150 mg on day 1 • Caps, injection (IV), suspension	None	• Asthenia • Fatigue • Diarrhea • Hiccups • Dizziness • Dehydration	Monitor levels of chemotherapy agents metabolized by CYP3A4	• CYP3A4 substrate and inhibitor • CYP2C9 inducer	• Use in combination with 5HT$_3$ antagonist and dexamethasone • Prevents acute and delayed N/V
Rolapitant • Varubi • 180 mg PO on day 1 • Tabs	Concurrent therapy with thioridazine	• Neutropenia • Hiccups • Anorexia • Dizziness • Dyspepsia	CBC with differential	CYP3A4 substrate and inhibitor	• Used in combination with 5HT$_3$ antagonist and dexamethasone • Prevents delayed N/V
Netupitant/palonosetron • Akynzeo • 1 capsule (300 mg netupitant/0.5 mg palonosetron) PO on day 1 • Caps	None	• Dyspepsia • Fatigue • Constipation • Headache • Asthenia	Monitor levels of chemotherapy agents metabolized by CYP3A4	• CYP3A4 substrate and inhibitor • Use with serotonergic agents may ↑ risk of serotonin syndrome	• Netupitant is NK-1 antagonist; palonosetron is 5HT$_3$ antagonist • Used in combination with dexamethasone • Prevents acute and delayed N/V
Mechanism of action – corticosteroids; potentiate antiemetic properties of 5HT$_3$ antagonists					
Dexamethasone • Decadron • 8–40 mg daily PO/IV • Injection, solution, tabs Methylprednisolone☆ • Solu-Medrol • 40–125 mg daily IV • Injection	Systemic fungal infections	• Hyperglycemia • Immunosuppression • Adrenal suppression • Insomnia • Mood changes, anxiety • GI irritation • Weight gain	• Hemoglobin/ hematocrit • Serum potassium • Glucose	CYP3A4 substrates	• Synergistic with 5HT$_3$ antagonists • Can use as single agents for mild chemotherapy-induced N/V
Mechanism of action – dopamine-2 antagonist					
Metoclopramide☆ • Reglan • 10–20 mg PO/IV q4–6h PRN • Injection, solution, tabs	Seizures	• Dizziness • Sedation • Diarrhea • Extrapyramidal symptoms (EPS)	EPS	Antipsychotic agents may ↑ risk of EPS	Should not drive or operate heavy machinery while taking this drug

Colony-Stimulating Factors

Generic • Brand • Dose	Contraindications	Primary Side Effects	Key Monitoring	Pertinent Drug Interactions	Med Pearl
Mechanism of action – stimulate production of WBCs					
Filgrastim • Granix, Neupogen, Zarxio • 5 mcg/kg subcut daily	Hypersensitivity to *E. coli*	• Bone pain • Hypertension • Swelling • Redness • Hypersensitivity reactions	CBC with differential	Use lithium with caution, as it can potentiate neutrophil release	• Requires daily administration • Neutrophil-specific
PEG-Filgrastim • Neulasta • 6 mg subcut with each chemotherapy cycle					• PEG unit ↑ half-life; can give once per chemotherapy cycle • Neutrophil-specific
Sargramostim • Leukine • 250–500 mcg/m^2/day subcut	• Hypersensitivity to yeast • Excessive leukemic myeloid blasts in bone marrow	• Fever, chills • Bone pain • Myalgia • Hypertension • Hypersensitivity reactions			• Requires daily administration • Stimulates formation of all WBCs except lymphocytes

PRACTICE QUESTIONS

1. Which of the following chemotherapeutic agents may cause left ventricular systolic dysfunction as a toxicity? (Select ALL that apply.)

    (A) Cetuximab
    (B) Cisplatin
    (C) Doxorubicin
    (D) Trastuzumab
    (E) Vincristine

2. Which of the following chemotherapeutic agents is associated with profound acute- and late-onset diarrhea?

    (A) Daunorubicin
    (B) Doxorubicin
    (C) Irinotecan
    (D) Methotrexate
    (E) Trastuzumab

3. The mechanism of action of Emend is

    (A) $5HT_3$ receptor antagonist.
    (B) neurokinin-1 receptor antagonist.
    (C) D_2 receptor antagonist.
    (D) benzodiazepine receptor agonist.
    (E) histamine receptor antagonist.

4. A patient with NHL is to be started on cyclophosphamide, doxorubicin, vincristine, and prednisone. Which of the following medications is MOST likely to be protective against the toxicity of doxorubicin?

    (A) Amifostine
    (B) Dexrazoxane
    (C) Folic acid
    (D) Leucovorin
    (E) Mesna

5. A patient receiving cancer chemotherapy presents to the emergency department complaining of an increase in urinary frequency and dysuria. No significant findings are apparent on physical examination. This patient's urinalysis reveals (−) WBC, (+) blood, (−) bacteria, (−) casts. If the symptoms experienced by the patient are related to the cancer chemotherapy, which of the following medications is MOST likely the cause?

   (A) Cyclophosphamide
   (B) Irinotecan
   (C) Methotrexate
   (D) Paclitaxel
   (E) Tamoxifen

6. Which of the following BEST describes the mechanism of action of Zofran?

   (A) It competes for the binding sites of serotonin receptors.
   (B) It inhibits the substance P/neurokinin-1 receptor.
   (C) It inhibits histamine H_1 receptors.
   (D) It stimulates dopamine-2 receptors.
   (E) It stimulates cannabinoid receptors.

7. Etoposide should NOT be administered via intravenous push because of the increased risk of which of the following adverse effects?

   (A) Diarrhea
   (B) Hepatotoxicity
   (C) Hypotension
   (D) Pulmonary fibrosis
   (E) Seizure

8. Pulmonary fibrosis is MOST likely to occur as a toxicity of which of the following chemotherapy drugs?

   (A) Bleomycin
   (B) Cisplatin
   (C) Daunorubicin
   (D) Trastuzumab
   (E) Vincristine

9. Which of the following antiemetic drugs is available as a transdermal patch?

   (A) Aprepitant
   (B) Dexamethasone
   (C) Granisetron
   (D) Metoclopramide
   (E) Prochlorperazine

10. Which of the following drugs is/are considered VEGF inhibitors? (Select ALL that apply.)

   (A) Bevacizumab
   (B) Ceritinib
   (C) Erlotinib
   (D) Rituximab
   (E) Trastuzumab

ANSWERS AND EXPLANATIONS

1. **C, D**

Cardiotoxicity is a major adverse effect associated with both doxorubicin (C) and trastuzumab (D). Cetuximab (A), cisplatin (B), and vincristine (E) do not cause cardiotoxicity. Instead, cetuximab is associated with severe rash and interstitial lung disease; cisplatin is associated with nephrotoxicity; ;and vincristine is associated with neurotoxicity.

2. **C**

Of the drugs listed, only irinotecan (C) exhibits major gastrointestinal adverse effects. The other drugs are more likely to lead to cardiomyopathy (trastuzumab [E], daunorubicin [A], and doxorubicin [B]) or neuro-, nephro-, and hepatotoxicity (methotrexate [D]).

3. **B**

Emend (aprepitant) is a highly selective emetogenic agent that works against the neurokinin-1 receptor. It has little to no affinity for the other receptor targets listed.

4. **B**

Dexrazoxane can be used to reduce the incidence and severity of cardiomyopathy associated with doxorubicin administration (cumulative doses >300 mg/m^2). Amifostine (A) is used to reduce the cumulative renal toxicity associated with repeated administration of cisplatin. The use of methotrexate can lead to folate deficiency; folic acid (C) can be administered to patients receiving methotrexate to prevent side effects. Leucovorin (D) can be given after administration of methotrexate to limit its toxicity. Mesna (E) is used to prevent hemorrhagic cystitis associated with cyclophosphamide or ifosfamide.

5. **A**

This patient is most likely exhibiting signs of chemotherapy-induced hemorrhagic cystitis. This adverse effect is most commonly associated with cyclophosphamide (A) and ifosfamide. The major toxicity associated with irinotecan (B) is diarrhea. Methotrexate (C) can cause numerous organ toxicities, including nephrotoxicity (acute renal failure), neurotoxicity, and hepatotoxicity. Paclitaxel (D) can be associated with peripheral neuropathy. The major adverse effect associated with tamoxifen (E) is thromboembolic events.

6. **A**

The antiemetic Zofran (ondansetron) is a selective serotonin (5HT$_3$) receptor antagonist. The antiemetics, aprepitant (Emend) and rolapitant (Varubi), inhibit the substance P/neurokinin-1 receptor (B). By inhibiting dopamine-2 receptors—not stimulating them (D)—metoclopramide (Reglan) also acts as an antiemetic.

7. **C**

Administering etoposide via intravenous (IV) push may lead to hypotension. Etoposide should be administered over 30–60 minutes to minimize the risk of this adverse effect.

8. **A**

Pulmonary fibrosis is a significant adverse effects associated with bleomycin (A) and busulfan. The major toxicity associated with cisplatin (B) is nephrotoxicity. Daunorubicin (C) and trastuzumab (D) are associated with cardiotoxicity. Vincristine (E) is associated with dose-limiting peripheral neuropathy.

9. **C**

Of the listed antiemetic drugs, only granisetron, a $5HT_3$ antagonist, is available as a transdermal patch (Sancuso). Aprepitant (A) is available as a capsule, oral suspension, and IV injection. Dexamethasone (B) is available as a tablet, oral solution, and IV injection. Metoclopramide (D) is available as a tablet, orally disintegrating tablet, oral solution, and IV injection. Prochlorperazine (E) is available as a tablet, rectal suppository, and IV injection.

10. **A**

Only bevacizumab (A) is considered a VEGF inhibitor. Ceritinib (B) is an anaplastic lymphoma kinase (ALK) inhibitor. Erlotinib (C) is an epidermal growth factor receptor (EGFR) inhibitor. Rituximab (D) is a monoclonal antibody directed against the CD20 antigen on B-lymphocytes. Trastuzumab (E) is a monoclonal antibody targeted against the HER2 receptor.

Psychiatric Disorders

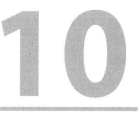

This chapter covers the following disease states:

- **Depression**
- **Anxiety**
- **Bipolar disorder**
- **Schizophrenia**
- **Sleep disorders**
- **Attention-deficit/hyperactivity disorder (ADHD)**

DEPRESSION

Guidelines Summary

- The primary goal of therapy is remission of symptoms.
- There are various antidepressant medications available. Clinical evidence indicates that, in general, efficacy is similar between classes.
- Initial choice of pharmacotherapy agent is based on anticipated side effects, tolerability of these side effects for an individual patient, co-morbid conditions, drug interactions, patient preference, quantity and quality of clinical evidence, and cost.
- First-line options for most patients include selective serotonin reuptake inhibitors (SSRIs), serotonin norepinephrine reuptake inhibitors (SNRIs), bupropion, and mirtazapine. Because of the potential for serious side effects and drug interactions, monoamine oxidase inhibitors (MAOIs) should be reserved for patients who do not respond to other therapies.
- An adequate therapy trial requires at least 4–8 weeks. Dose adjustments or treatment changes are made at 4- to 6-week intervals based upon response but may occur earlier if medications are not tolerated.

- There is significant interpatient variability in response to antidepressants. Patients may respond to classes/agents that have been effective in the past or that have been effective for family members.

- Bupropion has a lower incidence of sexual side effects and may be preferred in patients presenting with this complaint related to therapy.

- In 2005, the Food and Drug Administration required that all product labeling for antidepressants include a boxed warning regarding the potential for ↑ risk of clinical worsening and suicidality in children, adolescents, and young adults (<24 years old) taking these agents.

Antidepressants

Generic • Brand • Dose/Dosage Forms	Contraindications	Primary Side Effects	Key Monitoring Parameters	Pertinent Drug Interactions	Med Pearls
Mechanism of action – SSRIs: inhibit reuptake of serotonin, allowing more serotonin availability in synapses					
Citalopram☆ • Celexa • 10–40 mg daily • Age >60 yr: max = 20 mg daily • Solution, tabs	• Hypersensitivity • Use of MAOI within 2 wk • Concurrent use of pimozide • Concurrent use of linezolid or methylene blue • Congenital long QT syndrome • Use not recommended in patients with bradycardia, recent myocardial infarction (MI), uncompensated heart failure, hypokalemia, and hypomagnesemia	• Lightheadedness • Syncope • ↑ sweating • N/D • Xerostomia • Confusion • Dizziness • Somnolence • Insomia • Tremor • Ejaculation disorders • Impotence • Fatigue • Female sexual disorder • QT interval prolongation • Serotonin syndrome • Hyponatremia	• Reduction or resolution of symptoms • Withdrawal symptoms from abrupt discontinuation • Abnormal bleeding • Worsening of depression, suicidality, or unusual behavior at initiation of therapy or when changing dose • S/S of serotonin syndrome	• CYP2C19 and CYP3A4 substrate • CYP2C19 or CYP3A4 inhibitors may ↑ effects/toxicity; max dose = 20 mg/day when used with CYP2C19 inhibitors due to risk of QTc interval prolongation • CYP2C19 or CYP3A4 inducers may ↓ effects • ↑ risk of serotonin syndrome with MAOIs, SNRIs, triptans, tricyclic antidepressants (TCAs), amphetamines, fentanyl, lithium, dextromethorphan, meperidine, buspirone, linezolid, methylene blue, St. John's wort, and tramadol • ↑ risk of bleeding when used with aspirin, nonsteroidal anti-inflammatory drugs (NSAIDs), or anticoagulants	• Racemic mixture of R- and S- isomers • QTc interval prolongation, dose dependent risk, highest risk > 40 mg/day • Max dose of 20 mg/day in severe hepatic impairment
Escitalopram☆ • Lexapro • 10–20 mg daily • Solution, tabs	• Hypersensitivity • Use of MAOI within 2 wk • Concurrent use of pimozide • Concurrent use of linezolid or methylene blue				• Contains only the S-isomer of citalopram • Adjust dose in hepatic impairment

Antidepressants *(cont'd)*

Generic • Brand • Dose/Dosage Forms	Contraindications	Primary Side Effects	Key Monitoring Parameters	Pertinent Drug Interactions	Med Pearls
Fluoxetine ☆ • Prozac, Prozac Weekly, Sarafem • 20–80 mg daily or 90 mg weekly • Caps, ER caps, solution, tabs	• Hypersensitivity • Use of MAOI within 5 wk • Use of thioridazine within 5 wk • Concurrent use of pimozide • Concurrent use of linezolid or methylene blue	[Same as above]	[Same as above]	• CYP2C9 and CYP2D6 substrate • CYP2D6 inhibitor • CYP2C9 or CYP2D6 inhibitors may ↑ effects/toxicity • CYP2C9 inducers may ↓ effects • May ↑ effects/toxicity of CYP2D6 substrates • ↑ risk of serotonin syndrome with MAOIs, SNRIs, triptans, TCAs, amphetamines, fentanyl, lithium, dextromethorphan, meperidine, buspirone, linezolid, methylene blue, St. John's wort, and tramadol • ↑ risk of bleeding with used with aspirin, NSAIDs, or anticoagulants	• Allow 5 wk washout prior to using MAOI due to long half-life • Does not require taper due to long half-life • Also indicated for premenstrual dysphoric disorder (PMDD)
Fluvoxamine • Luvox • 50–300 mg daily • ER caps, tabs	• Hypersensitivity • Concurrent use of tizanidine, thioridazine, alosetron, or pimozide • Use of MAOI within 2 wk • Concurrent use of linezolid or methylene blue			• CYP1A2 and CYP2D6 substrate • CYP1A2 and CYP2C19 inhibitor • CYP1A2 or CYP2D6 inhibitors may ↑ effects/toxicity • CYP1A2 inducers may ↓ effects • May ↑ effects/toxicity of CYP1A2 or CYP2C19 substrates • ↑ risk of serotonin syndrome with MAOIs, SNRIs, triptans, TCAs, amphetamines, fentanyl, lithium, dextromethorphan, meperidine, buspirone, linezolid, methylene blue, St. John's wort, and tramadol • ↑ risk of bleeding when used with aspirin, NSAIDs, or anticoagulants	Only approved to treat obsessive-compulsive disorder (OCD)

Antidepressants *(cont'd)*

Generic • Brand • Dose/Dosage Forms	Contraindications	Primary Side Effects	Key Monitoring Parameters	Pertinent Drug Interactions	Med Pearls
Paroxetine ☆ • Paxil, Paxil CR, Pexeva • IR: 20–50 mg daily • ER: 25–62.5 mg daily • Suspension, tabs	• Hypersensitivity • Concurrent use of thioridazine or pimozide • Use of MAOI within 2 wk • Concurrent use of linezolid or methylene blue	[Same as above]	[Same as above]	• CYP2D6 substrate and inhibitor • CYP2D6 inhibitors may ↑ effects/toxicity • May ↑ effects/toxicity of CYP2D6 substrates • ↑ risk of serotonin syndrome with MAOIs, SNRIs, triptans, TCAs, amphetamines, fentanyl, lithium, dextromethorphan, meperidine, buspirone, linezolid, methylene blue, St. John's wort, and tramadol • ↑ risk of bleeding when used with aspirin, NSAIDs, or anticoagulants	• Short half-life may ↑ risk for discontinuation syndrome • Associated with more sedation, weight gain, sexual dysfunction, and anticholinerigc adverse events compared to other SSRIs • Brisdelle approved to treat vasomotor symptoms of menopause • Paxil CR also approved for PMDD • Adjust dose in renal impairment
Sertraline ☆ • Zoloft • 50–200 mg daily • Solution, tabs	• Hypersensitivity • Use of MAOI within 2 wk • Concurrent use of pimozide • Concurrent use of disulfiram-like products (oral concentrate contains alcohol) • Concurrent use of linezolid or methylene blue			• CYP2C19 and CYP2D6 substrate • CYP2D6 inhibitor • CYP2C19 or CYP2D6 inhibitors may ↑ effects/toxicity • CYP2C19 inducers may ↓ effects • May ↑ effects/toxicity of CYP2D6 substrates • ↑ risk of serotonin syndrome with MAOIs, SNRIs, triptans, TCAs, amphetamines, fentanyl, lithium, dextromethorphan, meperidine, buspirone, linezolid, methylene blue, St. John's wort, and tramadol • ↑ risk of bleeding when used with aspirin, NSAIDs, or anticoagulants	• Associated with high prevalence of nausea and diarrhea • Oral concentrate contains alcohol • Also indicated for PMDD

Antidepressants *(cont'd)*

Generic • Brand • Dose/Dosage Forms	Contraindications	Primary Side Effects	Key Monitoring Parameters	Pertinent Drug Interactions	Med Pearls
Mechanism of action – SSRI, 5-HT1A receptor agonist, 5-HT3 receptor antagonist					
Vortioxetine • Trintellix • 5–20 mg daily • Tabs	• Hypersensitivity • Use of MAOI within 2–3 wk • Concurrent use of linezolid or methylene blue	• N/V/D • Sexual dysfunction • Dizziness • Xerostomia • Constipation • Serotonin syndrome	• Reduction or resolution of symptoms • Withdrawal symptoms from abrupt discontinuation • Abnormal bleeding • Worsening of depression, suicidality, or unusual behavior at initiation of therapy or when changing dose • S/S of serotonin syndrome	• CYP2D6 and 3A4 substrate • CYP2D6 or CYP3A4 inhibitors may ↑ effects/toxicity; ↓ dose by 50% when used with strong CYP2D6 inhibitor • CYP3A4 inducers may ↓ effects • ↑ risk of serotonin syndrome with MAOIs, SNRIs, triptans, TCAs, amphetamines, fentanyl, lithium, dextromethorphan, meperidine, buspirone, linezolid, methylene blue, St. John's wort, and tramadol • ↑ risk of bleeding when used with aspirin, NSAIDs, or anticoagulants	Associated with high prevalence of nausea and diarrhea
Mechanism of action – SSRI, partial 5-HT1A receptor agonist					
Vilazodone • Viibryd • 10–40 mg daily • Tabs	Use of MAOI within 2 wk	• N/D • Xerostomia • Dizziness • Insomnia • Serotonin syndrome	• Reduction or resolution of symptoms • Withdrawal symptoms from abrupt discontinuation • Abnormal bleeding • Worsening of depression, suicidality, or unusual behavior at initiation of therapy or when changing dose • S/S of serotonin syndrome	• CYP3A4 substrate • CYP3A4 inhibitors may ↑ effects/toxicity; max dose = 20 mg/day when used with strong CYP3A4 inhibitors • CYP3A4 inducers may ↓ effects; consider ↑ dose when used with strong CYP3A4 inducers (max dose = 80 mg/day) • ↑ risk of serotonin syndrome with MAOIs, SNRIs, triptans, TCAs, amphetamines, fentanyl, lithium, dextromethorphan, meperidine, buspirone, linezolid, methylene blue, St. John's wort, and tramadol • ↑ risk of bleeding when used with aspirin, NSAIDs, or anticoagulants	• Take with food to enhance absorption • Associated with high prevalence of nausea and diarrhea

Antidepressants *(cont'd)*

Generic • Brand • Dose/Dosage Forms	Contraindications	Primary Side Effects	Key Monitoring Parameters	Pertinent Drug Interactions	Med Pearls
Mechanism of action – TCAs: ↑ synaptic concentration of norepinephrine and serotonin					
Amitriptyline☆ • Only available generically • 25–300 mg/day in 1–3 divided doses • Tabs Amoxapine • Only available generically • 50–600 mg/day in 2–3 divided doses • Tabs	• Hypersensitivity • Use of MAOI within 2 wk • Concurrent use of linezolid or methylene blue • Acute recovery period post-MI	• Anticholinergic symptoms • Weight gain • Bloating • Blurred vision • Xerostomia • Constipation • Dizziness • Somnolence • Headache • Fatigue • Serotonin syndrome	• Reduction or resolution of symptoms • Withdrawal symptoms from abrupt discontinuation • Worsening of depression, suicidality, or unusual behavior at initiation of therapy or when changing dose • Blood pressure (BP) • Electrocardiogram (ECG) (in patients with cardiac disease or hyperthyroidism) • Incidence of seizures due to seizure threshold lowering • S/S of serotonin syndrome • Therapeutic blood concentrations	• CYP2D6 substrate • CYP2D6 inhibitors may ↑ effects/toxicity • ↑ risk of serotonin syndrome with MAOIs, SSRIs, SNRIs, triptans, fentanyl, lithium, dextromethorphan, meperidine, buspirone, linezolid, methylene blue, St. John's wort, and tramadol	• Dangerous in overdose situations • Avoid in patients with high suicidality • Avoid dispensing large quantities • Also used for sleep disorders and for the treatment of neuropathic pain • Anticholinergic side effects may adversely effect older adults
Clomipramine • Anafranil • 25–250 mg/day in 3 divided doses • Caps					• Dangerous in overdose situations • Avoid in patients with high suicidality • Avoid dispensing large quantities • Indicated only for OCD
Desipramine • Norpramin • 25–300 mg/day in 1–2 divided doses • Tabs					• Dangerous in overdose situations • Avoid in patients with high suicidality • Avoid dispensing large quantities

Antidepressants   *(cont'd)*

Generic • Brand • Dose/Dosage Forms	Contraindications	Primary Side Effects	Key Monitoring Parameters	Pertinent Drug Interactions	Med Pearls
Doxepin ☆ • Silenor, Zonalon • 25–300 mg/day in 1–3 divided doses • Caps, solution, tabs, topical cream	[Same as above]	[Same as above]	[Same as above]	[Same as above]	• Dangerous in overdose situations • Avoid in patients with high suicidality • Avoid dispensing large quantities • Silenor approved for the treatment of insomnia • Zonalon approved for treatment of pruritus
Imipramine ☆ • Tofranil • 75–300 mg/day in 1–2 divided doses • Caps, tabs					• Dangerous in overdose situations • Avoid in patients with high suicidality • Avoid dispensing large quantities
Nortriptyline ☆ • Pamelor • 75–150 mg/day in 3–4 divided doses • Caps, solution					
Protriptyline • Vivactil • 10–60 mg/day in 3–4 divided doses • Tabs					
Trimipramine • Surmontil • 25–300 mg/day in 1–3 divided doses • Caps				• CYP2C19, CYP2D6, and CYP3A4 substrate • CYP2C19, CYP2D6, or CYP3A4 inhibitors may ↑ effects/toxicity • CYP2C19 or CYP3A4 inducers may ↓ effects • ↑ risk of serotonin syndrome with MAOIs, SSRIs, SNRIs, triptans, fentanyl, lithium, dextromethorphan, meperidine, buspirone, linezolid, methylene blue, St. John's wort, and tramadol	

Antidepressants   *(cont'd)*

Generic • Brand • Dose/Dosage Forms	Contraindications	Primary Side Effects	Key Monitoring Parameters	Pertinent Drug Interactions	Med Pearls
Mechanism of action – SNRIs: inhibit the reuptake of serotonin and norepinephrine to allow higher available synaptic concentrations					
Duloxetine ☆ • Cymbalta • 30–120 mg/day in 1–2 divided doses • DR caps	• Hypersensitivity • Use of MAOI within 2 wk • Concurrent use of linezolid or methylene blue • Hepatic impairment • Severe renal impairment (CrCl <30 mL/min)	• Hepatotoxicity • Orthostatic hypotension • Rash (Stevens-Johnson syndrome possible) • Palpitations • ↑ sweating • Constipation • ↓ appetite • N/D • Xerostomia • Asthenia • Dizziness • Insomnia or somnolence • Vertigo • Blurred vision • Polyuria • ↓ libido • Serotonin syndrome	• Liver function tests (LFTs) • BP • Reduction or resolution of symptoms • Withdrawal symptoms from abrupt discontinuation • Abnormal bleeding • Worsening of depression, suicidality, or unusual behavior at initiation of therapy or when changing dose • S/S of serotonin syndrome	• CYP1A2 and CYP2D6 substrate • CYP1A2 or CYP2D6 inhibitors may ↑ effects/toxicity; avoid concomitant use with strong CYP1A2 inhibitors • CYP1A2 inducers may ↓ effects • ↑ risk of serotonin syndrome with MAOIs, SSRIs, triptans, amphetamines, TCAs, fentanyl, lithium, dextromethorphan, meperidine, buspirone, linezolid, methylene blue, St. John's wort, and tramadol • ↑ risk of bleeding when used with aspirin, NSAIDs, or anticoagulants	• Doses >60 mg/day may not provide additional benefit • May also be used to treat neuropathic and musculoskeletal pain, fibromyalgia, and GAD
Venlafaxine ☆ • Effexor XR • IR: 37.5–225 mg/day in 2–3 divided doses • XR: 37.5–225 mg/day • ER caps/tabs, IR tabs		• Hypertension • ↑ sweating • Weight loss • Constipation • ↓ appetite • Nausea • Xerostomia • Insomnia or somnolence • Erectile dysfunction • Serotonin syndrome	• BP • Reduction or resolution of symptoms • Withdrawal symptoms from abrupt discontinuation • Abnormal bleeding • Worsening of depression, suicidality, or unusual behavior at initiation of therapy or when changing dose • S/S of serotonin syndrome	• CYP2D6 and CYP3A4 substrate • CYP2D6 or CYP3A4 inhibitors may ↑ effects/toxicity • CYP3A4 inducers may ↓ effects • ↑ risk of serotonin syndrome with MAOIs, SSRIs, triptans, amphetamines, TCAs, fentanyl, lithium, dextromethorphan, meperidine, buspirone, linezolid, methylene blue, St. John's wort, and tramadol • ↑ risk of bleeding when used with aspirin, NSAIDs, or anticoagulants	Adjust dose in renal or hepatic impairment

Antidepressants   *(cont'd)*

Generic • Brand • Dose/Dosage Forms	Contraindications	Primary Side Effects	Key Monitoring Parameters	Pertinent Drug Interactions	Med Pearls
Levomilnacipran • Fetzima • 20–120 mg daily • ER caps	[Same as above]	• Nausea • Orthostasis • Constipation • ↑ sweating • Tachycardia • Serotonin syndrome • Sexual dysfunction • Hypertension • Urinary retention	• BP • Heart rate • Renal function • Reduction or resolution of symptoms • Withdrawal symptoms from abrupt discontinuation • Abnormal bleeding • Worsening of depression, suicidality, or unusual behavior at initiation of therapy or when changing dose • S/S of serotonin syndrome	• CYP3A4 substrate • CYP3A4 inhibitors may ↑ effects/toxicity; max dose = 80 mg/day when used with strong CYP3A4 inhibitors • CYP3A4 inducers may ↓ effects • ↑ risk of serotonin syndrome with MAOIs, SSRIs, triptans, amphetamines, TCAs, fentanyl, lithium, dextromethorphan, meperidine, buspirone, linezolid, methylene blue, St. John's wort, and tramadol • ↑ risk of bleeding when used with aspirin, NSAIDs, or anticoagulants	Adjust dose in renal impairment
Milnacipran • Savella • 12.5–200 mg/day in 2 divided doses • Tabs		• N/V • Headache • Insomnia • Hot flashes • Constipation • Dizziness • Hypertension • Palpitations • ↑ sweating • Sexual dysfunction • Urinary retention		• ↑ risk of serotonin syndrome with MAOIs, SSRIs, triptans, amphetamines, TCAs, fentanyl, lithium, dextromethorphan, meperidine, buspirone, linezolid, methylene blue, St. John's wort, and tramadol • ↑ risk of bleeding when used with aspirin, NSAIDs, or anticoagulants	Indicated only for fibromyalgia
Desvenlafaxine☆ • Khedezla, Pristiq • 50 mg daily • ER tabs		• Hypertension • Nausea • Dizziness • Insomnia or somnolence • ↑ sweating • Constipation • ↓ appetite • Anxiety • Sexual dysfunction • Serotonin syndrome	• BP • Reduction or resolution of symptoms • Withdrawal symptoms from abrupt discontinuation • Abnormal bleeding • Worsening of depression, suicidality, or unusual behavior at initiation of therapy or when changing dose • S/S of serotonin syndrome	• ↑ risk of serotonin syndrome with MAOIs, SSRIs, triptans, amphetamines, TCAs, fentanyl, lithium, dextromethorphan, meperidine, buspirone, linezolid, methylene blue, St. John's wort, and tramadol • ↑ risk of bleeding when used with aspirin, NSAIDs, or anticoagulants	Adjust dose in renal or hepatic impairment

Antidepressants *(cont'd)*

Generic • Brand • Dose/Dosage Forms	Contraindications	Primary Side Effects	Key Monitoring Parameters	Pertinent Drug Interactions	Med Pearls
Mechanism of action – serotonin reuptake inhibitor/antagonist					
Trazodone • Only available generically • 25–600 mg/day • Tabs	• Hypersensitivity • Use of MAOI within 14 days • Concurrent use of linezolid or methylene blue	• Sedation • Headache • Dizziness • Fatigue • Constipation • Sexual dysfunction • Blurred vision • Serotonin syndrome	• LFTs • Worsening of depression, suicidality, or unusual behavior at initiation of therapy or when changing dose • S/S of serotonin syndrome	• CYP3A4 substrate • ↑ risk of serotonin syndrome with MAOIs, SSRIs, SNRIs, triptans, amphetamines, fentanyl, lithium, dextromethorphan, meperidine, buspirone, linezolid, methylene blue, St. John's wort, and tramadol • ↑ risk of bleeding when used with aspirin, NSAIDs, or anticoagulants	Mostly used for the treatment of insomnia
Nefazodone • Only available generically • 100–600 mg/day in 1–2 divided doses • Tabs	• Hypersensitivity • Previous nefazodone-induced hepatic damage • Hepatic impairment • Use of MAOI within 2 wk • Concurrent use with carbamazepine, triazolam, or pimozide	• Hepatotoxicity • Lightheadedness • Constipation • Nausea • Xerostomia • Urinary retention • Blurred vision • Confusion • Dizziness • Insomnia or somnolence • Sexual dysfunction • Serotonin syndrome	• LFTs • Reduction or resolution of symptoms • Withdrawal symptoms from abrupt discontinuation • Abnormal bleeding • Worsening of depression, suicidality, or unusual behavior at initiation of therapy or when changing dose • S/S of serotonin syndrome	• CYP2D6 and CYP3A4 substrate • CYP2D6 or CYP3A4 inhibitors may ↑ effects/toxicity • CYP3A4 inducers may ↓ effects • ↑ risk of serotonin syndrome with MAOIs, SSRIs, triptans, amphetamines, TCAs, fentanyl, lithium, dextromethorphan, meperidine, buspirone, linezolid, methylene blue, St. John's wort, and tramadol • ↑ risk of bleeding when used with aspirin, NSAIDs, or anticoagulants	Black box warning for hepatotoxicity

Antidepressants   *(cont'd)*

Generic • Brand • Dose/Dosage Forms	Contraindications	Primary Side Effects	Key Monitoring Parameters	Pertinent Drug Interactions	Med Pearls
Mechanism of action – MAOIs: ↑ epinephrine, norepinephrine, dopamine, and serotonin through inhibition of monoamine oxidase					
Isocarboxazid • Marplan • 10–60 mg/day in 2–4 divided doses • Tabs	• Hypersensitivity • Concurrent use of sympathomimetics, SSRIs, SNRIs, TCAs, central nervous system depressants, bupropion, meperidine, buspirone, dextromethorphan, anesthetics, or high-tyramine foods • Cardiovascular disease • Hypertension • Cerebrovascular disease • History of headache • Pheochromocytoma • Hepatic impairment • Severe renal impairment	• Weight gain • Orthostatic hypotension • Constipation • Xerostomia • Dizziness • Headache • Insomnia or somnolence • Blurred vision • Anxiety • Serotonin syndrome	• BP • LFTs • Reduction or resolution of symptoms • Withdrawal symptoms from abrupt discontinuation • Abnormal bleeding • Worsening of depression, suicidality, or unusual behavior at initiation of therapy or when changing dose • S/S of serotonin syndrome	• ↑ risk of serotonin syndrome with SSRIs, SNRIs, triptans, amphetamines, TCAs, fentanyl, lithium, dextromethorphan, meperidine, buspirone, linezolid, methylene blue, St. John's wort, and tramadol • ↑ risk of hypertensive crises with sympathomimetics and high-tyramine foods	Used very infrequently due to poor side effect profile and risk of drug and food interactions
Phenelzine Nardil • 45–90 mg daily (TID–QID) • Tabs	• Cardiovascular disease • Hypertension • Cerebrovascular disease • Concurrent administration of interacting medications • General anesthesia • History of headache • Hypersensitivity • Pheochromocytoma • Severe renal impairment				
Tranylcypromine • Parnate • 30–60 mg daily (divided doses) • Tabs					
Selegiline Emsam • 6–12 mg daily transdermal patch (max = 12 mg/ 24 hrs) • Transdermal patch	• Concurrent use of sympathomimetics, SSRIs, SNRIs, TCAs, bupropion, meperidine, tramadol, methadone, buspirone, dextromethorphan, carbamazepine, or high-tyramine foods • <12 yr old • Pheochromocytoma				• Apply patch once daily • Patch indicated for depression, not Parkinson's disease

Antidepressants *(cont'd)*

Generic • Brand • Dose/Dosage Forms	Contraindications	Primary Side Effects	Key Monitoring Parameters	Pertinent Drug Interactions	Med Pearls
Mechanism of action – weak inhibitor of dopamine and norepinephrine reuptake					
Bupropion☆ • Aplenzin, Forfivo XL, Wellbutrin SR, Wellbutrin XL • IR: 200–450 mg/day in 2–4 divided doses • SR: 150–400 mg in 2 divided doses • ER/XL: 150–450 mg daily • ER 12 hour tabs, ER/XL 24 hour tabs, IR tabs	• Hypersensitivity • Bulimia or anorexia • Abrupt discontinuation of alcohol, benzodiazepines, barbiturates, or AEDs • Seizure disorders • Use of MAOI within 2 wk • Concurrent use of linezolid or methylene blue	• Taste disturbance • Agitation • ↑ seizure activity • Hypertension • Psychotic symptoms • Anaphylaxis • Headache • Tachycardia • Weight loss	• Reduction or resolution of symptoms • Withdrawal symptoms from abrupt discontinuation • Worsening of depression, suicidality, or unusual behavior at initiation of therapy or when changing dose • Seizure activity	• CYP2B6 substrate • CYP2D6 inhibitor • CYP2B6 inhibitors may ↑ effects/toxicity • CYP2B6 inducers may ↓ effects • May ↑ effects/toxicity of CYP2D6 substrates • ↑ risk of hypertensive crises with MAOIs • May ↓ digoxin levels	Also used for smoking cessation (Zyban)
Mechanism of action – tetracyclic antidepressants: ↑ available synaptic concentrations of norepinephrine and/or serotonin					
Maprotiline • Only available generically • 25–225 mg/day in 2–3 divided doses • Tabs	• Hypersensitivity • Seizure disorder • Use of MAOI within 2 wk • Acute recovery period post-MI	• ↑ seizure activity • Somnolence • Constipation • Nausea • Xerostomia	• Reduction or resolution of symptoms • Withdrawal symptoms from abrupt discontinuation • Worsening of depression, suicidality, or unusual behavior at initiation of therapy or when changing dose • Seizure activity	• CYP2D6 substrate • CYP2D6 inhibitors may ↑ effects/toxicity	None
Mirtazapine☆ • Remeron, Remeron SolTab • 15–45 mg at bedtime • ODTs, tabs	• Hypersensitivity • Use of MAOI within 2 wk	• ↑ appetite • Hyperlipid-emia • Weight gain • Constipation • Somnolence • ↑ LFTs • Agranulocy-tosis • Serotonin syndrome	• Reduction or resolution of symptoms • Worsening of depression, suicidality, or unusual behavior at initiation of therapy or when changing dose • CBC • Weight • Lipid profile • Renal function • LFTs	• CYP1A2, CYP2D6, and CYP3A4 substrate • CYP1A2, CYP2D6, or CYP3A4 inhibitors may ↑ effects/toxicity • CYP1A2 or CYP3A4 inducers may ↓ effects	• Dosed at bedtime due to somnolence • Off-label use for appetite stimulation

ANXIETY

Summary of Treatment Recommendations

- Goals of therapy include improvement in overall functionality and quality of life through reduction of symptom frequency and intensity. Complete remission of illness is the long-term treatment goal.

- Treatment options are detailed in the medication charts and no consensus exists as to the preferred initial therapy or order of options thereafter. Not all medications are equivalent in the treatment of all anxiety disorders.

- Many clinicians prefer antidepressants (SSRIs, venlafaxine, duloxetine) as initial therapy due to their favorable side-effect profile as compared to other therapies. Benzodiazepines are commonly used, especially in acute situations. Although efficacious, these agents lend themselves to issues related to abuse/dependence, ↑ fall risk in the elderly, and potential for negative cognitive effects in general. Buspirone is a unique treatment option that is effective but requires 4 to 6 weeks to reach efficacy; thus, it is not useful in acute situations.

- Benzodiazepine selection should take into account varying pharmacokinetic profiles of agents. In elderly patients and those with hepatic impairment, preference is given to those agents that are shorter acting (less accumulation) and those metabolized by glucoronidation (e.g., lorazepam, oxazepam) versus oxidation (e.g., alprazolam, diazepam). Agents with a rapid onset and those with shorter half-lives have a greater potential for abuse.

Anxiolytics

Generic • Brand • Dose/Dosage Forms	Contraindications	Primary Side Effects	Key Monitoring Parameters	Pertinent Drug Interactions	Med Pearls
Mechanism of action – benzodiazepines: bind to GABA receptors, causing an influx of chloride which results in hyperpolarization and a less excitable state					
Alprazolam☆ • Xanax, Xanax XR • IR: 0.75–4 mg/day in 2–3 divided doses • ER: 0.5–6 mg daily • ER tabs, ODTs, solution, tabs	• Hypersensitivity • Narrow-angle glaucoma • Concurrent use with ketoconazole or itraconazole (alprazolam) • Significant hepatic impairment (clonazepam) • Myasthenia gravis, severe respiratory impairment, severe hepatic impairment, or sleep apnea (diazepam)	• Somnolence • Ataxia • Dizziness • Changes in appetite • ↓ libido • Confusion • Constipation • Blurred vision • Dependence	• BP • Excessive sedation • Signs of withdrawal • LFTs (for chronic therapy)	• CYP3A4 substrates • CYP3A4 inhibitors may ↑ effects/ toxicity • CYP3A4 inducers may ↓ effects • Other CNS depressants, including alcohol, may ↑ CNS depressant effects • Use with opioids may lead to sedation, respiratory depression, coma, or death	• Schedule IV controlled substance • Adjust dose in severe hepatic impairment • Avoid use in pregnancy • Smoking ↓ concentration by up to 50% • Rapid onset, short-acting
Chlordiazepoxide • Librium • 5–25 mg 3–4 × /day • Caps					• Schedule IV controlled substance • Avoid in elderly • Avoid use in pregnancy • Slower-onset, long-acting
Clonazepam☆ • Klonopin • 0.25–2 mg BID • ODTs, tabs					• Schedule IV controlled substance • Avoid use in pregnancy • Intermediate-onset, long-acting
Clorazepate • Tranxene T-Tab • 3.75–15 mg 2–4 ×/day • Tabs					• Schedule IV controlled substance • Avoid in elderly • Avoid use in pregnancy • Rapid-onset, long-acting
Diazepam☆ • Diastat, Valium • 2–10 mg PO 2–4 × /day • 2–10 mg IV/IM every 3–4 hr PRN • Injection, rectal gel, solution, tabs					• Schedule IV controlled substance • Avoid use in pregnancy • Rapid-onset, long-acting
Lorazepam☆ • Ativan • 0.5–2 mg 2–3 ×/day (max = 10 mg/day) • Injection, solution, tabs				• Hepatic conjugation • Not affected by CYP3A4 • Use with opioids may lead to sedation, respiratory depression, coma, or death	• Schedule IV controlled substance • Avoid use in pregnancy • Medium-onset, short-acting
Oxazepam • Only availably generically • 10–30 mg 3–4 ×/day • Caps					• Schedule IV controlled substance • Avoid use in pregnancy • Medium-onset, short-acting

Anxiolytics *(cont'd)*

Generic • Brand • Dose/Dosage Forms	Contraindications	Primary Side Effects	Key Monitoring Parameters	Pertinent Drug Interactions	Med Pearls
Mechanism of action – SSRIs: selectively inhibit the reuptake of serotonin by presynaptic neuronal membranes with little to no effect on norepinephrine or dopamine reuptake					
Citalopram☆ • Celexa • Details in antidepressants table	[See Antidepressants table]		Unlabeled use for panic disorder, GAD, posttraumatic stress disorder (PTSD), and OCD		
Escitalopram☆ • Lexapro • Details in antidepressants table			Indicated for GAD		
Fluoxetine☆ • Prozac, Sarafem • Details in antidepressants table			Indicated for OCD, panic disorder		
Paroxetine☆ • Paxil, Paxil CR • Details in antidepressants table			Indicated for panic disorder, PTSD, GAD, OCD, social anxiety disorder (SAD)		
Sertraline☆ • Zoloft • Details in antidepressants table			Indicated for OCD, panic disorder, SAD, PTSD		
Fluvoxamine • Luvox • Details in antidepressants table			Indicated for OCD		
Mechanism of action – nonselective β-adrenergic blocker which competitively blocks response to β_1- and β_2-adrenergic stimulation in the heart muscle, vascular smooth muscle, and bronchial muscles					
Propranolol☆ (nonselective) • Inderal, Inderal LA, InnoPran XL • 10–80 mg 1 hr prior to anxiogenic event	• Hypersensitivity • Severe bradycardia • Heart block • Acute decompensated heart failure • Severe chronic obstructive pulmonary disease (COPD) or asthma	• Dizziness • Fatigue • Bradycardia • Gastrointesinal upset • Hypotension	• HR • BP	Use with other negative chronotropes (e.g., digoxin, verapamil, diltiazem, clonidine, or ivabradine) may ↑ risk of bradycardia	Unlabeled use for situational anxiety or acute panic attack

Anxiolytics *(cont'd)*

Generic • Brand • Dose/Dosage Forms	Contraindications	Primary Side Effects	Key Monitoring Parameters	Pertinent Drug Interactions	Med Pearls
Mechanism of action – exact mechanism is unknown; high affinity for 5-HT$_{1A}$ and 5-HT$_2$ receptors, mild affinity for dopamine (D$_2$) receptors					
Buspirone☆ • Only available generically • 7.5–30 mg BID • Tabs	• Hypersensitivity • Concurrent use with MAOI	• Headache • Dizziness • Nausea • Hostility • Confusion • Drowsiness • Restlessness	• Mental status • Symptoms of anxiety • Pseudo-parkinsonism	• CYP3A4 substrate • CYP3A4 inhibitors may ↑ effects/ toxicity • CYP3A4 inducers may ↓ effects	• Avoid use in severe renal or hepatic impairment • Takes 2–3 wk to reach efficacy
Mechanism of action – SNRIs: inhibit reuptake of neuronal serotonin and norepinephrine; may have weak inhibitory effect on reuptake of dopamine					
Venlafaxine XR☆ • Effexor XR • Details in antidepressants table	[See Antidepressants table]		Indicated for GAD, panic disorder, SAD; unlabeled use for PTSD and OCD		
Duloxetine • Cymbalta • Details in antidepressants table			Indicated for GAD		
Mechanism of action – competes with histamine for H$_1$-receptor sites on effector cells in GI, blood vessels, and respiratory tract					
Hydroxyzine☆ • Vistaril • 50–100 mg PO • 4 ×/day • 50–100 mg IM every 4–6 hr PRN • Caps, injection, solution, tabs	• Hypersensitivity • Early pregnancy	• Dizziness • Drowsiness • Fatigue • Xerostomia • Blurry vision • Urinary retention	• BP • Mental status	Other CNS depressants, including alcohol, may ↑ CNS depressant effects	• Indicated for anxiety, pruritus, N/V, and as a perioperative adjunct • Use with caution in benign prostatic hyperplasia, respiratory disease, or glaucoma • Avoid in elderly • Adjust dose in renal impairment

BIPOLAR DISORDER

Guidelines Summary

- First-line treatment options for patient with acute manic episodes include lithium, divalproex, risperidone ER, paliperidone ER, olanzapine, quetiapine, aripiprazole, ziprasidone, and asenapine. Antipsychotic medications are detailed in medication charts later in the Schizophrenia section of this chapter.

- First-line treatment options for acute depressive episodes include lithium, lamotrigine or quetiapine monotherapy, olanzapine in combination with an SSRI, and lithium or divalproex plus SSRI/bupropion.

- First-line options for maintenance therapy include lithium, lamotrigine, valproate, olanzapine, quetiapine, aripiprazole, risperidone long-acting injection, and adjunctive ziprasidone.

Mood Stabilizers

Generic • Brand • Dose/Dosage Forms	Contraindications	Primary Side Effects	Key Monitoring Parameters	Med Pearls
Mechanism of action – altered sodium transport leads to a shift toward intraneuronal metabolism of catecholamines; the specific mechanism in mania is not fully understood				
Lithium ☆ • Lithobid • IR: 300–1,800 mg/day in 3–4 divided doses • ER: 450–900 mg BID • Caps, ER tabs, solution, tabs	• Severe renal or cardiovascular disease • Dehydration	• V/D • Drowsiness • Muscle weakness • Lack of coordination • Ataxia • Blurred vision • Tinnitus • Hypothyroidism	• Serum drug concentration 0.6–1.2 mEq/L • Renal function • Thyroid function tests • Serum Na+ concentrations	• Angiotensin-converting enzyme inhibitors, angiotensin II receptor blockers, diuretics, and nonsteroidal anti-inflammtory drugs may ↑ levels and risk of toxicity • Sodium depletion ↑ risk of toxicity
Mechanism of action – not fully understood; thought to ↑ GABA concentrations in the brain				
Valproic acid (divalproex sodium) ☆ • Depakote, Depakote ER, Depakene, Depacon • 10–60 mg/kg/day • Caps, delayed-release caps/tabs, ER tabs, injection, solution, sprinkle caps	[Specific drug details outlined in Epilepsy section of Neurological Disorders chapter]			
Mechanism of action – inhibits voltage-gated sodium channels, thereby depressing electrical transmission in the nucleus ventralis anterior of the thalamus				
Carbamazepine ☆ • Equetro • 200–1,600 mg/day in 2 divided doses • ER caps	[Specific drug details outlined in Epilepsy section of Neurological Disorders chapter]			
Mechanism of action – affects sodium channels stabilizing neuronal membranes; the exact mechanism in bipolar disorder is unknown				
Lamotrigine ☆ • Lamictal • 25–700 mg/day in 1–2 divided doses • Chewable tabs, ODTs, tabs	[Specific drug details outlined in Epilepsy section of Neurological Disorders chapter]			

SCHIZOPHRENIA

Guidelines Summary

For many years, atypical antipsychotics were considered the obvious first-line choice because of significantly reduced incidence of extrapyramidal side effects (EPS). Considerable controversy has surfaced, because of the ability of these medications to ↑ the risk of metabolic syndrome. Choice of either a typical or atypical antipsychotic is appropriate as first-line therapy. It should be considered, however, that atypical agents may have better efficacy in treating negative symptoms associated with schizophrenia.

- Goals of therapy include: Reduce or eliminate symptoms, minimize side effects of pharmacological treatment, and prevent relapse.

- Atypical and typical antipsychotics have similar efficacy profiles. Decision on first-line therapy is based on consideration of side-effect profiles, adherence issues, history of response, and cost.

- EPS are more likely to occur with typical antipsychotics but may be seen with atypical antipsychotics depending on the agent and dose. EPS include acute dystonic reactions, akathisia, parkinsonism, and tardive dyskinesia (TD).

- TD may occur at any time after taking an antipsychotic but generally occurs months to years after initiation. Symptoms include involuntary movements of the mouth, tongue, face, extremities, and trunk. TD may be irreversible; therefore, monitoring of abnormal involuntary movements in patients on antipsychotics is recommended. If TD occurs, the patient may be treated with with clonazepam or valbenazine.

- Neuroleptic malignant syndrome (NMS) is a rare side effect associated with antipsychotic use that presents in less than 1% of patients but may be life-threatening if left untreated. NMS is characterized by rigidity, hyperthermia, and autonomic instability; however, elevation of serum creatinine may also been seen. The onset of NMS is generally within a week of starting treatment with an antipsychotic but may also occur with an ↑ in dose of the antipsychotic. If NMS occurs, antipsychotics should be discontinued and supportive care can be implemented to target hydration as well as cardiovascular and renal symptoms.

- All antipsychotics carry a black box warning for use in patients with dementia-related psychosis due to an ↑ risk of death.

Antipsychotics

Generic • Brand • Dose/Dosage Forms	Contraindications	Primary Side Effects	Key Monitoring Parameters	Pertinent Drug Interactions	Med Pearls
Typical Antipsychotics					
Mechanism of action – phenothiazines: block postsynaptic mesolimbic dopaminergic receptors in the brain					
Chlorpromazine • Only available generically • 30–800 mg/day PO in 2–4 divided doses • 25–100 mg IM every 4–6 hr PRN • Injection, tabs	• Hypersensitivity • Severe CNS depression • Coma	• Orthostatic hypotension • Falls • Drowsiness • Xerostomia • Constipation • Nausea • Urinary retention • Blurred vision • Photosensitivity • EPS • NMS • QT interval prolongation • Neutropenia	• BP • HR • Mental status • Lipid profile • Fasting blood glucose • Severity of EPS • Complete blood count (CBC) • LFTs • Involuntary movement • S/S of NMS • ECG	• CYP2D6 substrate (all but trifluoperazine and prochlorperazine) • CYP2D6 inhibitors may ↑ effects/toxicity • CYP1A2 substrate (tripfluoperazine only) • CYP1A2 inhibitors may ↑ effects/toxicity • CYP1A2 inducers may ↓ effects • CYP2D6 inhibitor (thio-ridazine only) • May ↑ effects/toxicity of CYP2D6 substrates • All may ↑ risk of torsades de pointes (TdP) with other drugs that prolong QT interval	May produce false-positive phenylketonuria and pregnancy test results
Fluphenazine • Only available generically • 2.5–10 mg/day PO in 3–4 divided doses • 1.25–2.5 mg IM every 6–8 hr PRN • Decanoate (long-acting): 12.5–100 mg IM/subcut every 2–4 wk • Injection, injection (long-acting), solution, tabs	• Hypersensitivity • Severe CNS depression • Coma • Subcortical brain damage • Blood dyscrasias • Hepatic impairment				
Perphenazine • Only available generically • 4–16 mg 2–4 ×/day • Tabs					
Trifluoperazine • Only available generically • 2–20 mg BID • Tabs					May produce false-positive phenylketonuria test results
Prochlorperazine ☆ • Compro • 15–150 mg/day PO in 3–4 divided doses • 10–20 mg IM every 4–6 hr PRN • Injection, rectal suppository, tabs					May produce false-positive phenylketonuria and pregnancy test results

Antipsychotics *(cont'd)*

Generic • Brand • Dose/Dosage Forms	Contraindications	Primary Side Effects	Key Monitoring Parameters	Pertinent Drug Interactions	Med Pearls
Thioridazine • Only available generically • 300–800 mg/day in 2–4 divided doses • Tabs	[Same as above]	[Same as above]	[Same as above]	[Same as above]	May produce false-positive methadone and phencyclidine results
Mechanism of action – not well established; thought to block postsynaptic mesolimbic dopaminergic D$_2$ receptors in the brain					
Haloperidol☆ • Haldol, Haldol Deconoate • 0.5–5 mg PO 2–3 ×/day • 2–5 mg IM every 4–8 hr PRN • Decanoate (long-acting): 10–15 × the daily PO dose (max = 200 mg) IM every 4 wk • Injection, injection (long-acting), solution, tabs	• Hypersensitivity • Parkinson's disease • Severe CNS depression • Coma	• Xerostomia • Drowsiness • Constipation • Nausea • Urinary retention • Blurred vision • Orthostatic hypotension • Falls • EPS • Priapism • QT interval prolongation • NMS • Neutropenia	• BP • HR • CBC • Mental status • ECG • EPS • Involuntary movement • S/S of NMS • LFTs	• CYP2D6 and CYP3A4 substrate • CYP2D6 or CYP3A4 inhibitors may ↑ effects/toxicity • CYP3A4 inducers may ↓ effects • May ↑ risk of TdP with other drugs that prolong QT interval	• IM decanoate form uses sesame oil • Immediate-release injection may also be given IV in ICU setting for treatment of delirium
Mechanism of action – a potent, centrally acting dopamine-receptor antagonist					
Pimozide • Orap • 1–2 mg/day in divided doses (max = 0.2 mg/kg/day or 10 mg/day, whichever is less) • Tabs	• Severe CNS depression • Coma • History of arrhythmias • Congenital long QT syndrome • Concurrent use with other QT interval prolonging medications • Hypokalemia or hypomagnesemia • Concurrent use with 3A4 inhibitors • Concurrent use with citalopram, escitalopram, or sertraline	• Somnolence • Drowsiness • Rash • Xerostomia • Constipation • Diarrhea • ↑ appetite • Taste disturbance • Impotence • Weakness • Visual disturbances • Speech disorder • Hypotension • QT interval prolongation • EPS • NMS • Neutropenia	• BP • HR • CBC • Mental status • ECG • EPS • Involuntary movement • S/S of NMS • LFTs	• CYP1A2, CYP2D6, and CYP3A4 substrate • CYP1A2, CYP2D6 or CYP3A4 inhibitors may ↑ effects/toxicity • CYP1A2 or CYP3A4 inducers may ↓ effects • May ↑ risk of TdP with other drugs that prolong QT interval	Only indicated for Tourette's disorder

Antipsychotics *(cont'd)*

Generic • Brand • Dose/Dosage Forms	Contraindications	Primary Side Effects	Key Monitoring Parameters	Pertinent Drug Interactions	Med Pearls
Mechanism of action – blocks postsynaptic mesolimbic D_1 and D_2 receptors in the brain, and also possesses serotonin 5-HT$_2$ blocking activity					
Loxapine • Adasuve • 20–250 mg/day PO in 2–4 divided doses • 10 mg via inhalation daily • Caps, inhalation	*PO:* • Hypersensitivity • Severe CNS depression • Coma *Inhalation:* • Hypersensitivity • Asthma, COPD, or other bronchospastic disease • Acute wheezing	• Hypotension • Falls • N/V • Constipation • Xerostomia • Weakness • Sexual dysfunction • Dizziness • EPS • NMS • Seizures	• BP • HR • Mental status • EPS • S/S of NMS • CBC • Involuntary movement • S/S of bronchospasm (with inhalation)	No significant CYP450 interactions	May produce false-positive phenylketonuria test results
Mechanism of action – exerts effect on the ascending reticular activating system					
Molindone • Only available generically • 30–100 mg/day in 3–4 divided doses • Tabs	• Hypersensitivity • Severe CNS depression • Coma	• Drowsiness • Xerostomia • Constipation • Hypotension • Tachycardia • EPS • NMS	• BP • HR • Mental status • EPS • Involuntary movement • S/S of NMS • CBC	No significant CYP450 interactions	None
Mechanism of action – blocks postsynaptic dopamine receptors, resulting in inhibition of dopamine-mediated effects; also has alpha-adrenergic blocking activity					
Thiothixene • Only available generically • 6–60 mg/day in 2–3 divided doses • Caps	• Hypersensitivity • Severe CNS depression • Coma • Blood dyscrasias	• Hypotension • Dizziness • N/V • Constipation • Sexual dysfunction • Tachycardia • Insomnia • EPS • NMS	• BP • HR • CBC • Mental status • EPS • Involuntary movement • S/S of NMS	• CYP1A2 substrate • CYP1A2 inhibitors may ↑ effects/toxicity • CYP1A2 inducers may ↓ effects	May cause false-positive pregnancy test results

Antipsychotics *(cont'd)*

Generic • Brand • Dose/Dosage Forms	Contraindications	Primary Side Effects	Key Monitoring Parameters	Pertinent Drug Interactions	Med Pearls
Atypical Antipsychotics					
Mechanism of action – mixed and varied (per agent) D_2/5-HT_2 antagonist activity					
Aripiprazole☆ Abilify (PO): • 10–30 mg PO daily • ODTs, solution, tabs Abilify Maintena (ER IM injection): • 300–400 mg IM monthly (doses must be ≥26 days apart) Aristada (ER IM injection): • 441–882 mg IM every 4–6 wk	• Hypersensitivity • Severe hepatic impairment (asenapine)	• Weight gain • Constipation • N/V/D • Akathisia • Hyperglycemia • Hyperlipidemia • Anxiety • Sedation • QT interval prolongation • Orthostatic hypotension • Falls • Tachycardia • Neutropenia • Impulse control disorders • EPS (rare) • NMS	• Fasting plasma glucose • Fasting lipid panel • CBC • BP • HR • ECG • Weight/body mass index • Waist circumference • Mental status • EPS • S/S of NMS	Aripiprazole and brexpip-razole: • CYP2D6 and CYP3A4 substrates • ↓ dose with CYP2D6 or CYP3A4 inhibitors; may ↑ effects/toxicity • Avoid use with CYP3A4 inducers; may ↓ effects Olanzapine, asenapine, and clozapine: • CYP1A2 substrates • CYP1A2 inhibitors may ↑ effects/toxicity • CYP1A2 inducers may ↓ effects Quetiapine, lurasidone, and cariprazine: • CYP3A4 substrates • CYP3A4 inhibitors may ↑ effects/toxicity • CYP3A4 inducers may ↓ effects Iloperidone and risperi-done: • CYP2D6 substrates • CYP2D6 inhibitors may ↑ effects/toxicity • All may ↑ risk of TdP with other drugs that prolong QT interval	• Partial D_2 agonist • Among the lowest risk of metabolic syndrome • Also indicated to treat acute manic and mixed episodes as-sociated with bipolar I disorder, MDD (as adjunctive therapy), irritabilty with autistic disorder, and Tourette's disorder • Overlap oral antipsychotic for 21 days upon initiation of Aristada and 14 days upon initiation of Abilify Maintena
Olanzapine☆ Zyprexa (PO, immediate-release IM injection), Zyprexa Zydis (ODT): • 5–20 mg PO daily • 10–30 mg/dose IM • IM (immediate release), ODTs, tabs Zyprexa Relprevv (ER IM injection): • 150–405 mg IM (max = 300 mg every 2 wk or 405 mg every 4 wk)		• Weight gain • Constipation • N/V/D • Akathisia • Hyperglycemia • Hyperlipidemia • Anxiety • Sedation • QT interval prolongation • Orthostatic hypotension • Falls • Tachycardia • Neutropenia • Hyperprolac-tinemia (rare) • EPS (rare) • NMS			• Higher degree of weight gain than some other atypicals • Oral formulations also indicated to treat acute and chronic manic and mixed epi-sodes associated with bipolar I disorder • Immediate-release IM injection indicated to treat acute agita-tion associated with schizophrenia and bipolar I mania • Zyprexa Relprevv is associated with postinjection de-lirium/sedation

Antipsychotics *(cont'd)*

Generic • Brand • Dose/Dosage Forms	Contraindications	Primary Side Effects	Key Monitoring Parameters	Pertinent Drug Interactions	Med Pearls
Paliperidone ☆ Invega (ER tabs): • 3–12 mg PO daily Invega Sustenna (monthly ER IM injection): • 39–234 mg IM monthly Invega Trinza (every 3 mo ER IM injection): • 273–819 mg IM every 3 mo	[Same as above]	[Same as above]	[Same as above]	[Same as above]	• Major active metabolite of risperidone • Invega Trinza should only be used in patients who have been stabilized with Invega Sustenna for ≥4 mo • Also indicated for schizoaffective disorder
Quetiapine ☆ • Seroquel, Seroquel XR • IR: 50–750 mg/day in 2–3 divided doses • ER: 300–800 mg daily • ER tabs, tabs					• ER tabs usually dosed at bedtime due to somnolence • Also indicated for manic and depressive episodes associated with bipolar I disorder
Iloperidone • Fanapt • 1–12 mg BID • Tabs					• Lower risk of weight gain than many atypicals • Low risk of somnolence • May improve cognitive function
Asenapine • Saphris • 5–10 mg BID • SL tabs					• Very low incidence of EPS • Also indicated to treat acute manic and mixed episodes associated with bipolar I disorder

Antipsychotics (cont'd)

Generic • Brand • Dose/Dosage Forms	Contraindications	Primary Side Effects	Key Monitoring Parameters	Pertinent Drug Interactions	Med Pearls
Risperidone☆ Risperdal, Risperdal M-Tab: • 2–16 mg/day PO in 1–2 divided doses • ODTs, solution, tabs Risperdal Consta (ER IM injection) • 12.5–50 mg IM every 2 wk	[Same as above]	[Same as above]	[Same as above]	[Same as above]	• Sedation often leads to bedtime dosing • Oral formulations also indicated to treat acute manic and mixed episodes associated with bipolar I disorder and irritabilty with autistic disorder • ER IM injection also indicated for maintenance treatment of bipolar I disorder • Oral antipsychotic should be overlapped for 3 weeks upon initiation of Risperdal Consta
Ziprasidone☆ • Geodon • 20–100 mg PO BID • 10 mg IM every 2 hr or 20 mg IM every 4 hr • Caps, injection	• Hypersensitivity • Decompensated heart failure • Recent MI • History of QT interval prolongation • Concurrent use of QT interval prolonging medications				• Must be administered with at least 500 calories • Lower risk of metabolic syndrome when compared to other atypicals • Oral formulation also indicated to treat acute manic and mixed episodes associated with bipolar I disorder and for maintenance treatment of bipolar I disorder • IM injection indicated to treat acute agitation associated with schizophrenia
Lurasidone • Latuda • 40–160 mg daily • Tabs	• Hypersensitivity • Concurrent use with strong 3A4 inhibitors or inducers				• Must be administered with at least 350 calories • Also indicated for treatment of depressive episodes associated with bipolar I disorder
Brexpiprazole • Rexulti • 1–4 mg daily • Tabs	Hypersensitivity				• Partial D_2 agonist • Also indicated as adjunctive therapy for major depressive disorder

Antipsychotics   *(cont'd)*

Generic • Brand • Dose/Dosage Forms	Contraindications	Primary Side Effects	Key Monitoring Parameters	Pertinent Drug Interactions	Med Pearls
Cariprazine • Vraylar • 1.5–6 mg daily • Caps	[Same as above]	[Same as above]	[Same as above]	[Same as above]	• Partial D_2 agonist • Also indicated to treat acute manic and mixed episodes associated with bipolar I disorder
Clozapine ☆ • Clozaril, FazaClo, Versacloz • 12.5–900 mg/day in 1–3 divided doses • ODTs, suspension, tabs	• Hypersensitivity • Seizures • Myocarditis, cardiomyopathy, mitral valve incompetence • Severe neutropenia • Orthostatic hypotension, bradycardia, syncope	• Orthostatic hypotension • Bradycardia • QT interval prolongation • Hyperglycemia • Hyperlipidemia • Weight gain • Agranulocytosis • NMS • Seizures • Myocarditis	• Absolute neutrophil count weekly for 6 mo, then every 2 wk for 6 mo, then every 4 wk • Fasting plasma glucose • Fasting lipid panel • BP • HR • ECG • Weight/body mass index • Mental status • S/S of NMS		• Prescribers, patients, and pharmacies must enroll in the Clozapine REMs program • Used less frequently than other atypicals due to requirement for frequent monitoring • Effective in treatment of refractory cases and in patients at high risk for suicide

Tardive Dyskinesia Treatment

Generic • Brand • Dose/Dosage Forms	Contraindications	Primary Side Effects	Key Monitoring Parameters	Pertinent Drug Interactions	Med Pearl
Mechanism of action – exact mechanism is unknown; thought to reversibly inhibit VMAT2					
Valbenazine • Ingrezza • 40–80 mg daily • Caps	• Hypersensitivity	• Drowsiness • Fatigue • Sedation • Falls • Equilibrium disturbance • Abnormal gait • Akathisia • Vomiting	• AIMS scale • DISCUS scale • ECG	• CYP3A4 substrate • Avoid use with strong CYP3A4 inducers	• Indicated for the treatment of TD

SLEEP DISORDERS

Insomnia

Guidelines Summary

- Goals of therapy: Improve quality and quantity of sleep and improve daytime sleep-related impairment.

- All patients should be educated about good sleep hygiene. Nonpharmacological measures are the preferred initial treatment.

- Pharmacological therapy should be combined with behavioral therapy to achieve the best results. Medication selection is based upon the following patient-specific elements: (1) symptom pattern, (2) patient preference, (3) availability, (4) cost, (5) prior response, (6) comorbid conditions, (7) contraindications, (8) concurrent medications, (9) side effect profile, and (10) treatment goals.

- Pharmacological classes for insomnia include benzodiazepines, benzodiazepine receptor agonists (BzRA), melatonin receptor agonists, and sedating antidepressants.

- Short-intermediate acting BzRAs, benzodiazepines, or melatonin receptor agonists are first-line therapy options for most patients. BzRAs and benzodiazepines ideally should be limited to short-term use (7–10 days); however, there is limited evidence to support use extended to 6–12 months.

- Inadequate response after an initial trial of the above agents can be followed with a trial on a second agent from within these therapeutic class options.

- Third-line options include sedating antidepressants or off-label combination therapy or self-care therapies such as antihistamines.

Treatment Algorithm

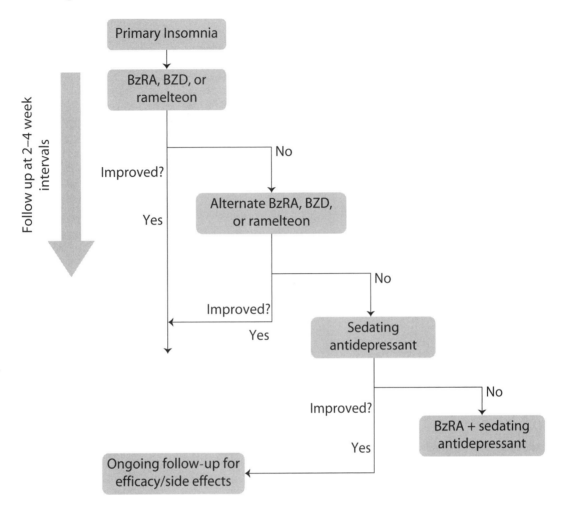

Medications for Insomnia

Generic • Brand • Dose/Dosage Forms	Contraindications	Primary Side Effects	Key Monitoring	Pertinent Drug Interactions	Med Pearl
Benzodiazepine receptor agonists (schedule IV controlled substances)					
Mechanism of action – enhances GABA through stimulation of the benzodiazepine 1 receptor, which results in hyperpolarization and a $\downarrow$ in neuronal excitabilty with sedative and hypnotic effects					
Eszopiclone☆ • Lunesta • 1–3 mg at bedtime • Tabs	Hypersensitivity	• Headache • Xerostomia • Dizziness • Nausea • Somnolence • Sleep-related activities: hazardous activities such as sleep-driving and cooking have been reported (rare), incidence $\uparrow$ with alcohol use or using above max doses • Behavior changes such as $\downarrow$ inhibition, aggression, agitation, hallucinations, and depersonalization (rare)	• Improvement in sleep quality/ quantity • Presence of side effects	• CYP3A4 substrate • CYP3A4 inhibitors may $\uparrow$ effects/toxicity • CYP3A4 inducers may $\downarrow$ effects • Other CNS depressants, including alcohol, may $\uparrow$ CNS depressant effects	• High-fat/heavy meal will delay absorption; administer on an empty stomach • Associated with taste disturbance
Zolpidem☆ • Ambien, Ambien CR, Zolpimist • IR or oral spray: 5–10 mg PO at bedtime (max = 5 mg for females) • CR: 6.25–12.5 mg PO at bedtime (max = 6.25 mg for females) • ER tabs, oral spray, tabs • Edluar, Intermezzo (SL tabs) • Edluar: 5–10 mg/night SL (max = 5 mg for females) • Intermezzo: 1.75–3.5 mg/ night SL (max = 1.75 mg for females)					• Take IR tabs, ER tabs, oral spray, and SL tabs (Edluar only) immediately before bedtime • SL tabs (Intermezzo only) helpful for nighttime awakenings; take in bed if patient wakes in the middle of the night (only if $\geq$4 hr remain before desired wake-up time) and there is difficulty in returning to sleep • Heavy/high-fat meal will delay absorption; administer on an empty stomach
Zaleplon • Sonata • 5–20 mg at bedtime • Caps					• Heavy/high-fat meal will delay absorption; administer on an empty stomach • Headache incidence = 30–40%

Medications for Insomnia   *(cont'd)*

Generic • Brand • Dose/Dosage Forms	Contraindications	Primary Side Effects	Key Monitoring	Pertinent Drug Interactions	Med Pearl
Benzodiazepines (schedule IV controlled substances)					
Mechanism of action – bind to GABA A receptors to enhance inhibitory effect of GABA on neuronal excitability					
Estazolam • Only available generically • 1–2 mg PO at bedtime • Tabs	• Pregnancy • Narrow-angle glaucoma • Concurrent use with itraconazole or ketoconazole	• Somnolence • Dizziness • Hypokinesia • Hangover effect • Abnormal coordination • Confusion • Xerostomia • Constipation	• Improvement in sleep quality/ quantity • Presence of side effects	• CYP3A4 substrate • CYP3A4 inhibitors may ↑ effects/ toxicity • CYP3A4 inducers may ↓ effects • Other CNS depressants, including alcohol, may ↑ CNS depressant effects	• Time to peak 0.5–6 hr; $T_{1/2}$ 10–24 hr • Administer on an empty stomach
Temazepam ☆ • Restoril • 7.5–30 mg PO at bedtime • Caps	• Pregnancy • Narrow-angle glaucoma				Time to peak 1.2–1.6 hr; $T_{1/2}$ 3.5–18 hr
Triazolam • Halcion • 0.125–0.5 mg PO at bedtime • Tabs	• Pregnancy • Narrow-angle glaucoma • Concurrent use with itraconazole, ketoconazole, nefazodone, or protease inhibitors				• Time to peak 1–2 hr; $T_{1/2}$ 1.5–5.5 hr • Administer on an empty stomach
Flurazepam • Only available generically • 15–30 mg PO at bedtime (max = 15 mg for females) • Caps	• Pregnancy • Narrow-angle glaucoma				Time to peak 3–6 hr; $T_{1/2}$ 2.5 hr (active metabolite ~70 hr)

Medications for Insomnia   *(cont'd)*

Generic • Brand • Dose/Dosage Forms	Contraindications	Primary Side Effects	Key Monitoring	Pertinent Drug Interactions	Med Pearl
Melatonin Receptor Agonists					
Mechanism of action – MT1 and MT2 receptor agonist					
Ramelteon • Rozerem • 8 mg within 30 min of bedtime • Tabs	• Angioedema with prior use • Concurrent use with fluvoxamine	• Anaphylaxis/angioedema • Dizziness • Fatigue • Depression • Sleep-related activities: hazardous activities such as sleep-driving and cooking have been reported (rare), incidence ↑ with alcohol use • Behavior changes such as agitation, hallucinations, and mania	• Improvement in sleep quality/quantity • Presence of side effects	• CYP1A2 substrate • CYP1A2 inhibitors may ↑ effects/toxicity • CYP1A2 inducers may ↓ effects • Other CNS depressants, including alcohol, may ↑ CNS depressant effects	• Not a scheduled/controlled substance • Heavy/high-fat meal will delay absorption; administer on an empty stomach
Tasimelteon • Hetlioz • 20 mg at bedtime • Caps	None	• Drowsiness • Headache • Abnormal dreams • ↑ LFTs	• Improvement in sleep quality/quantity • Presence of side effects • LFTs	• CYP1A2 and CYP3A4 substrate • CYP1A2 and CYP3A4 inhibitors may ↑ effects/toxicity • CYP1A2 and CYP3A4 inducers may ↓ effects • Other CNS depressants, including alcohol, may ↑ CNS depressant effects	• Indicated for non-24-hour sleep-wake disorder • Should be taken at the same time each night • Not a scheduled/controlled substance • May take weeks to months to see effect • Administer on an empty stomach

Medications for Insomnia *(cont'd)*

Generic • Brand • Dose/Dosage Forms	Contraindications	Primary Side Effects	Key Monitoring	Pertinent Drug Interactions	Med Pearl
Orexin Receptor Antagonist					
Mechanism of action – antagonizes OX1R and OX2R which blocks the binding of wake-promoting compounds orexin A and orexin B					
Suvorexant • Belsomra • 10–20 mg at bedtime • Tabs	Narcolepsy	• Drowsiness • Headache • Dizziness • Sleep-related activities: hazardous activities such as sleep-driving and cooking have been reported (rare), incidence ↑ with alcohol or other CNS depressant use or using above max doses • Depression • Abnormal dreams	• Improvement in sleep quality/ quantity • Presence of side effects	• CYP3A4 substrate • CYP3A4 inhibitors may ↑ effects/ toxicity • CYP3A4 inducers may ↓ effects • Other CNS depressants, including alcohol, may ↑ CNS depressant effects	• Schedule IV controlled substance • Should be taken with ≥7 hr remaining before planned time of awakening • Heavy/high-fat meal will delay absorption; administer on an empty stomach

Restless Leg Syndrome

Guidelines Summary

- First-line options for the treatment of RLS include ropinirole and pramipexole.
- Other treatment options include carbidopa/levodopa, opioids, gabapentin enacarbil, gabapentin, and pregabalin.

Drug Treatment

Please see the medication chart in the Parkinson's Disease section of the Neurological Disorders chapter for more specific information on ropinirole, pramipexole, and carbidopa/levodopa. Please see the medication chart in the Epilepsy section of the Neurological Disorders chapter for more specific information on gabapentin and pregabalin.

Narcolepsy

Guidelines Summary

- First-line treatment options for excessive daytime sedation include modafinil, sodium oxybate, stimulants (amphetamine, methamphetamine, dextroamphetamine, methylphenidate), and selegiline. For information on the stimulants, please see the Attention-Deficit Hyperactivity Disorder (ADHD) section in this chapter. For information on selegiline, please see the Parkinson's Disease section in the Neurological Disorders chapter.
- TCAs and fluoxetine may be used for the treatment of cataplexy. Please see the Depression section of this chapter for more information regarding these medications.
- Nonpharmacologic treatment includes scheduled naps.

Medications for Narcolepsy

Generic • Brand • Dose/Dosage Forms	Contraindications	Primary Side Effects	Key Monitoring	Pertinent Drug Interactions	Med Pearl
Mechanism of action – binds to the dopamine receptor, inhibiting dopamine reuptake					
Modafinil • Provigil • 200 mg daily • Tabs	Hypersensitivity	• Rash (Stevens-Johnson syndrome possible) • Angioedema • Headache • Nervousness • Anxiety • Dizziness • Insomnia • Hypertension • N/D	• Level of alertness • BP • Exacerbation of agitation, anxiety, depression	• CYP3A4 substrate and inducer • CYP2C19 inhibitor • CYP3A4 inhibitors may ↑ effects/toxicity • CYP3A4 inducers may ↓ effects • May ↑ effects/toxicity of CYP2C19 substrates • May ↓ effects of 3A4 substrates • May ↓ effects of hormonal contraceptives during and for 1 mo after discontinuing treatment	• Schedule IV controlled substance • If used for narcolepsy or obstructive sleep apnea/hypopnea, administer dose in the morning • If used for shift work sleep disorder, administer dose • 1 hr before work
Armodafinil • Nuvigil • 150–250 mg daily • Tabs					• R-enantiomer of modafinil • Schedule IV controlled substance • If used for narcolepsy or obstructive sleep apnea, administer dose in the morning • If used for shift work sleep disorder, administer dose • 1 hr before work
Mechanism of action – derivative of GABA that serves as an inhibitory transmitter					
Sodium oxybate • Xyrem • Initial: 2.25 g at bedtime after patient in bed, then 2.25 g 2.5–4 hr later; titrate dose to usual effective dose of 6–9 g per night • Solution	Concurrent use with alcohol or sedative hypnotic agents	• Dizziness • N/V • Somnolence • Enuresis • Tremor • Confusion • Anxiety • Sleepwalking • Depression	• Drug abuse • Depression or suicidality • Mental status	• CNS depressants, including alcohol, may ↑ CNS depressant effects • Divalproex sodium may ↑ effects/toxicity; ↓ sodium oxybate dose by 20%	• Schedule III controlled substance • 1.1 g Na+ in 6 g nightly dose • Administer on an empty stomach • Also effective for the treatment of cataplexy • REMS program

ATTENTION-DEFICIT/HYPERACTIVITY DISORDER (ADHD)

Guidelines Summary

- First-line pharmacologic therapy for ADHD includes stimulant medications. Approved options included methylphenidate, dexmethylphenidate, dextroamphetamine, dextroamphetamine + amphetamine, and lisdexamfetamine.

- Nonstimulant options approved for ADHD are generally reserved for one of the following: concerns related to abuse/diversion, strong family/patient preference for nonstimulant medications, or as adjunctive therapy to stimulants. Options include atomoxetine, guanfacine, and clonidine. Of these options, atomoxetine monotherapy is preferred to guanfacine and clonidine, which are generally reserved for adjunctive therapy.

- When selecting a stimulant, patient-specific factors such as ability to swallow tablets/capsules, affordability, number of daily doses required, and presence of a tic disorder are considerations.

- Interpatient variability in efficacy is recognized and alternate stimulant agents are recommended as second- and third-line options after appropriate titration to maximal effective/tolerated dose of initial stimulant selected.

Medications for Attention-Deficit/Hyperactivity Disorder

Generic • Brand • Dose & Max	Contraindications	Primary Side Effects	Key Monitoring	Pertinent Drug Interactions	Med Pearl
Stimulants					
Mechanism of action – block reuptake of norepinepherine and dopamine					
Methylphenidate IR☆ • Ritalin, Methylin • 10–60 mg/day in 2–3 divided doses • Chewable tabs, solution, tabs Methylphenidate ER • Aptensio XR: 10–60 mg daily • Concerta: 18–72 mg every morning • Metadate CD: 10–60 mg daily • Quillichew ER: 10–60 mg every morning • Quillivant XR: 10–60 mg every morning • Ritalin LA: 10–60 mg daily • Ritalin SR: 10–60 mg/day in 2–3 divided doses • ER caps, ER chewable tabs, ER suspension, ER tabs Methylphenidate transdermal patch • Daytrana • Initial: 10-mg patch daily; titrate to effect	• Anxiety • Tension • Agitation • Glaucoma • Motor tics • Recent MAOI, linezolid, or methylene blue use (within 14 days) • Family history or diagnosis of Tourette's syndrome • Advanced arteriosclerosis • Moderate to severe HTN • Symptomatic cardiac disease	General • Anorexia • Nausea • Weight loss • Insomnia • Dizziness • Lightheadedness • Irritability • ↑ sweating • Blurred vision • Priapism • Growth suppression • Peripheral vasculopathy (Raynaud's) • Dependence Cardiovascular • ↑ BP • Tachycardia Psychiatric • May exacerbate anxiety, mania, aggression, hostility, or depression • Use with caution in patients with pre-existing psychiatric conditions	• Resolution of symptoms • BP • HR • Height/weight • ECG at baseline and if chest pain or syncope • Signs of misuse/abuse	• MAOIs require 14-day washout period prior to stimulant initiation • ↑ risk of serotonin syndrome with MAOIs, SSRIs, SNRIs, triptans, tricyclic anti-depressants (TCAs), fentanyl, lithium, dextromethorphan, meperidine, buspirone, linezolid, methylene blue, St. John's wort	• Schedule II controlled substance • Black box: Potential for dependency • Generally taken every morning to avoid insomnia • Remove patch after 9 hr of wear; alternate application site (hips) • Withdrawal potential; titrate slowly and taper upon discontinuation • Also indicated for narcolepsy
Dexmethylphenidate IR • Focalin, Focalin XR • IR: 2.5–10 mg BID • ER: 5–40 mg every morning • ER caps, tabs					• Schedule II controlled substance • Black box: Potential for dependency • ER generally taken q A.M. to avoid insomnia • For IR, 1st dose given q A.M., 2nd dose given at least 4 hr later • Withdrawal potential; titrate slowly and taper upon discontinuation • D-enantiomer of methylphenidate

Medications for Attention-Deficit/Hyperactivity Disorder *(cont'd)*

Generic • Brand • Dose & Max	Contraindications	Primary Side Effects	Key Monitoring	Pertinent Drug Interactions	Med Pearl
Mechanism of action – promote the release of catecholamines					
Dextroamphetamine and amphetamine ☆ • IR only available generically, Adderall XR • IR: 5–40 mg/day in 1–3 divided doses • ER: 5–30 mg every morning • ER caps, tabs	• Anxiety • Tension • Agitation • Glaucoma • Motor tics • Recent MAOI, linezolid, or methylene blue use (within 14 days) • Family history or diagnosis of Tourette's syndrome • Advanced arteriosclerosis • Moderate to severe HTN • Symptomatic cardiac disease	General • Anorexia • Nausea • Weight loss • Insomnia • Dizziness • Lightheadedness • Irritability • ↑ sweating • Blurred vision • Priapism • Growth suppression • Peripheral vasculopathy (Raynaud's) • Dependence Cardiovascular • ↑ BP • Tachycardia Psychiatric • May exacerbate anxiety, mania, aggression, hostility, or depression • Use with caution in patients with pre-existing psychiatric conditions	• Resolution of symptoms • BP • HR • Height/weight • ECG at baseline and if chest pain or syncope • Signs of misuse/abuse	• MAOIs require 14-day washout period prior to stimulant initiation • ↑ risk of serotonin syndrome with MAOIs, SSRIs, SNRIs, triptans, tricyclic antidepressants (TCAs), fentanyl, lithium, dextromethorphan, meperidine, buspirone, linezolid, methylene blue, St. John's wort	• Schedule II controlled substance • Black box: Potential for dependency • ER generally taken q A.M. to avoid insomnia • Withdrawal potential; titrate slowly and taper upon discontinuation • IR also indicated for narcolepsy
Dextroamphetamine • IR only available generically, Dexedrine Spansules (ER) • IR: 2.5–40 mg/day in 1–2 divided doses • ER: 5–40 mg/day in 1–2 divided doses • ER caps, solution, tabs					• Schedule II controlled substance • Black box: Potential for dependency • ER generally taken q A.M. to avoid insomnia • For IR, 1st dose given q A.M., 2nd dose given 4–6 hr later • Withdrawal potential; titrate slowly and taper upon discontinuation • Also indicated for narcolepsy

Medications for Attention-Deficit/Hyperactivity Disorder *(cont'd)*

Generic • Brand • Dose & Max	Contraindications	Primary Side Effects	Key Monitoring	Pertinent Drug Interactions	Med Pearl
Lisdexamfetamine☆ • Vyvanse • 30–70 mg every morning • Caps, chewable tabs	[Same as above]	[Same as above]	[Same as above]	[Same as above]	• Schedule II controlled substance • Black box: Potential for dependency • Prodrug of dextroamphetamine; rapid effect muted if injected or snorted (designed to decrease abuse potential) • Contents can be mixed with water—drink immediately • Withdrawal potential; titrate slowly and taper upon discontinuation • Also indicated for binge eating disorder
Amphetamine • Adzensys XR-ODT, Dynavel XR, Evekeo • 2.5–20 mg/day • ER suspension, ER-ODT tabs, tabs					May use doses up to 30 mg/day for obesity or 60 mg/day for narcolepsy
Nonstimulants					
Mechanism of action – selectively inhibits norepinephrine reuptake					
Atomoxetine☆ • Strattera • 40–100 mg/day in 1–2 divided doses • Caps	• Narrow-angle glaucoma • Pheochromocytoma • Recent MAOI use (within 14 days) • Cardiovascular conditions that may worsen with ↑ BP or HR	• Headache • Insomnia • Nausea • Anorexia • Somnolence • Xerostomia • Menstrual changes • Orthostasis • Urinary hesitancy/retention • Growth suppression • Can exacerbate pre-existing psychiatric illness, including hallucinations/mania • Priapism • Suicidal ideation • Liver injury (rare)	• Resolution of symptoms • S/S liver injury (fatigue, abdominal pain, yellowed skin, darkened urine) • LFTs • BP • HR • Height/weight • ECG at baseline and if chest pain or syncope • Signs of misuse/abuse	• CYP2D6 substrate • CYP2D6 inhibitors may ↑ effects/toxicity; ↓ dose in patients who are CYP2D6 poor metabolizers if taking strong CYP2D6 inhibitor (paroxetine, fluoxetine, quinidine) • MAOIs require 14-day washout period prior to stimulant initiation	• Risk of suicidal ideation in children • Capsules cannot be opened

Medications for Attention-Deficit/Hyperactivity Disorder *(cont'd)*

Generic • Brand • Dose & Max	Contraindications	Primary Side Effects	Key Monitoring	Pertinent Drug Interactions	Med Pearl
Mechanism of action – selective alpha$_{2A}$ receptor agonist that reduces sympathetic outflow					
Guanfacine ☆ • Intuniv • 1–7 mg daily • ER tabs	Hypersensitivity	• Dizziness • Fatigue • Somnolence • Nausea • Xerostomia • Constipation • Bradycardia • Atrioventricular block • Headache • Hypotension • Syncope	• Resolution of symptoms • BP • HR • ECG	• CYP3A4 substrate • ↓ daily dose by 50% if used with strong or moderate CYP3A4 inhibitors; double daily dose if used with strong or moderate CYP3A4 inducers • Additive CNS depressant effects with other CNS depressants • Additive BP lowering with other antihypertensives	• High-fat meals ↑ medication absorption; administer on an empty stomach • Can be used as monotherapy or as adjunctive to stimulant therapy • Also used for hypertension (formulations not interchangeable) • Do not crush • Do not stop abruptly due to risk of rebound HTN
Mechanism of action – alpha$_2$ receptor agonist that results in reduced sympathetic outflow					
Clonidine • Kapvay • 0.1–0.4 mg at bedtime • ER tabs	Hypersensitivity	• Headache • Irritability • Nightmares • Insomnia • Constipation • Xerostomia • Somnolence • Bradycardia • Atrioventricular block • Hypotension • Rebound hypertension (if abruptly discontinued)	• Resolution of symptoms • BP • HR • ECG	• Additive CNS depressant effects with other CNS depressants • Additive BP lowering with other antihypertensives	• Do not crush • Do not stop abruptly due to risk of rebound HTN

PRACTICE QUESTIONS

1. Which of the following is first-line in the treatment of acute depressive episode in a patient with bipolar disorder? (Select ALL that apply.)

   (A) Lithium
   (B) Divalproex
   (C) Oxcarbazepine
   (D) Lamotrigine

2. A 48-year-old woman is newly diagnosed with depression. She has a medical history significant for type 2 diabetes and hypertension. Current medications include metformin 1,000 mg PO BID and lisinopril 40 mg PO daily. Her blood pressure remains elevated at today's visit. Which antidepressant has the greatest potential to worsen this patient's hypertension?

   (A) Citalopram
   (B) Desipramine
   (C) Venlafaxine
   (D) Vilazodone

3. To avoid withdrawal symptoms, most antidepressants require tapering upon discontinuation. Which SSRI does not require a taper upon discontinuation due to its long elimination half-life?

   (A) Escitalopram
   (B) Fluoxetine
   (C) Paroxetine
   (D) Sertraline

4. Antidepressants with serotonergic activity should be avoided in combination with which of the following antibiotics due to the clinically significant risk of serotonin syndrome?

   (A) Cefazolin
   (B) Meropenem
   (C) Vancomycin
   (D) Linezolid

5. A 36-year-old woman with bipolar disorder is on lithium 300 mg PO TID with a serum drug concentration of 0.9 mEq/L. She is diagnosed with hypertension and her physician is considering therapy initiation. Which of the following medications would result in a significant drug interaction with the patient's lithium, increasing the risk for lithium toxicity? (Select ALL that apply.)

   (A) Chlorthalidone
   (B) Metoprolol
   (C) Lisinopril
   (D) Amlodipine

6. Which of the following antipsychotics would have the greatest risk of extrapyramidal side effects?

   (A) Olanzapine
   (B) Risperidone
   (C) Clozapine
   (D) Asenapine

7. Coadministration with a high-fat meal would result in delayed absorption of which of the following medications?

   (A) Eszopiclone
   (B) Triazolam
   (C) Ramelteon
   (D) Melatonin

8. HC is a 34-year-old man recently diagnosed with GAD. Given HC's past history of substance abuse, which of the following medications would be BEST to treat his GAD?

   (A) Buspirone
   (B) Diazepam
   (C) Chlordiazepoxide
   (D) Alprazolam

9. Which of the following is indicated to treat non-24-hour sleep-wake cycle disorder?

    (A) Belsomra
    (B) Hetlioz
    (C) Ambien
    (D) Sonata

10. An 11-year-old boy is diagnosed with attention-deficit/hyperactivity disorder (ADHD). He has an older brother (age 18 years) with ADHD and opioid dependence. The patient's family wants to avoid pharmacological treatment options with potential for dependency. Which of the following would be the MOST appropriate first-line pharmacological therapy for this patient's ADHD?

    (A) Methylphenidate
    (B) Atomoxetine
    (C) Guanfacine
    (D) Clonidine

ANSWERS AND EXPLANATIONS

1. **A, D**

According to the guidelines, first-line treatment options for acute depression episodes include lithium, lamotrigine, or quetiapine as monotherapy; olanzapine in combination with an SSRI; and lithium or divalproex plus an SSRI or bupropion, or in combination with antimania agents. Divalproex (B) is used as a first-line treatment option for acute manic episodes. Oxcarbazepine (C) is a third-line agent for the treatment of acute manic episodes.

2. **C**

Serotonin, norepinephrine reuptake inhibitors, specifically venlafaxine, can increase blood pressure due the impact on norepinephrine. Citalopram (A) and vilazodone (D) are not associated with increasing blood pressure. Tricyclic antidepressants such as desipramine (B) can result in orthostatic hypotension due to anticholinergic side effects.

3. **B**

Fluoxetine's terminal half-life is measured in days (4–16) rather than hours; this pharmacokinetic principle allows the medication to slowly eliminate thereby diminishing the need for tapering upon discontinuation. The other drugs' half-lives are escitalopram (A) about 28 hours, paroxetine (C) 21 hours, and sertraline (D) 26 hours.

4. **D**

Linezolid is a reversible, nonselective inhibitor of monoamine oxidase, and coadministration with serotonergic agents such as SSRIs should be avoided due to the significant risk of serotonin syndrome.

5. **A, C**

Both thiazide diuretics such as chlorthalidone (A) and ACEIs such as lisinopril (C) decrease the clearance of lithium and increase the risk of lithium toxicity. Although these medications may be used in combination with lithium, the concomitant administration should be monitored very closely. Beta blockers such as metoprolol (B) and calcium channel blockers such as amlodipine (D) do not interact with lithium.

6. **B**

Risperidone has a relatively low risk of EPS compared with the first-generation (typical) antipsychotics. Its risk is greater, however, compared with the atypical antipsychotics such as olanzapine (A), asenapine (C), and clozapine (D).

7. **A**

BzRAs such as eszopiclone have demonstrated delayed absorption when co-administered with high-fat/heavy meals. The same precaution does not apply to benzodiazepines such as triazolam (B), melatonin receptor agonists such as ramelteon (C), or melatonin (D).

8. **A**

Buspirone would be the best choice as it is not a controlled substance and can be used to treat GAD. Diazepam (B), chlordiazepoxide (C), and alprazolam (D) are all benzodiazepines and could place a patient at risk for substance abuse.

9. **B**

Hetlioz (tasimelteon) is a melatonin receptor agonist used to treat non-24-hour sleep-wake disorder, which affects primarily patients with total blindness. Belsomra (suvorexant) (A) is an orexin receptor antagonist used to treat insomnia. Ambien (zolpidem) (C) and Sonata (zaleplon) (D) are nonbenzodiazepine benzodiazepine receptor agonists that are used in the treatment of insomnia.

10. **B**

Atomoxetine is a nonstimulant option that is not a scheduled/controlled substance. Methylphenidate (A) is a stimulant option and would not address the family's concerns related to dependence. For those with concerns regarding dependence, atomoxetine is considered the first-line option, while other nonstimulants such as guanfacine (C) and clonidine (D) are reserved for second-line/adjunctive therapy.

Pain Management

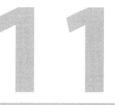

This chapter covers the following drug classes:

- **Nonsteroidal anti-inflammatory drugs (NSAIDs)**
- **Nonopioid pain management**
- **Opioid pain management**

The text also provides an overview of basic treatment and management of pain.

PAIN MANAGEMENT

Guidelines Summary

- Drug therapy is the mainstay of management for acute pain. The drugs discussed in this review are classified into three categories: Nonopioid analgesics, including acetaminophen and nonsteroidal anti-inflammatory drugs (NSAIDs); opioid pain management; and co-analgesics. The drug classes can be used in monotherapy and combination for pain.
- As the pain ↑, so does the dose of medications, the migration to stronger medications, and the use of combinations of medications with different mechanisms of actions.
- Acetaminophen and NSAIDs are useful for acute and chronic pain arising from a variety of causes, including surgery, trauma, arthritis, and cancer.
- NSAIDs are indicated for pain involving inflammation because acetaminophen lacks clinically effective anti-inflammatory properties.
- Major differences between NSAIDs and opioid analgesics:
  - NSAIDs are both analgesics and anti-inflammatory in nature and have some antipyretic effect.
  - NSAIDs have a dose ceiling of effect in relationship with adverse effects.
  - NSAIDs do not produce physical or psychological dependence.

- Initiation of opioid analgesics should be based on a pain-directed history and physical that includes repeated pain assessment.
  - Opioid analgesics should be added to nonopioids to manage acute pain and cancer-related pain that does not respond to nonopioids alone.
  - There is enormous variability in doses of opioids required to provide pain relief, even among opioid-naïve patients.
  - It is important to give each analgesic an adequate trial. As a result, a clinician may ↑ the opioid dose to establish analgesia or until unacceptable side effects appear before changing to another opioid.
  - It is recommended to administer analgesics on a regular schedule if pain is present most of the day. This approach allows the patient to stay ahead of the pain.
    - » For chronic pain, consider having a scheduled long-acting agent on board and a short-acting agent for times of breakthrough pain.
- Summary of Centers for Disease Control (CDC) guidelines for prescribing opioids for chronic pain:
  - Nonopioids and nonpharmacologic treatment options are preferred for the treatment of chronic pain.
  - Goals of treatment, risks, expected benefits, and patient and clinician responsibilities should be discussed before opioids are started.
  - When starting treatment, start with immediate-release (IR) opioids at the lowest effective dose.
  - Use caution with doses >50 morphine milligram equivalents (MME)/day. Doses >90 MME/day should be avoided if possible or justified for chronic use.
  - For acute pain, provide only the quantity of opioids needed for the expected duration. A quantity for ≤3 days is often sufficient and patients will rarely need >7 days of opioids.
  - After starting opioids, reassess risks and benefits within 1–4 weeks. For chronic therapy, reassess risks and benefits every 3 months. Discontinue therapy if the risks outweigh the benefits.
- Patient-controlled analgesia (PCA) using an intravenous (IV) opioid for acute pain is a commonly used technique for pain control.
  - PCA is used with a computerized-controlled infusion pump.
  - PCA is most often used for the IV administration of opioids for acute pain and allows patients considerable control over the treatment of pain.
  - PCA is not recommended in situations in which oral opioids could readily manage pain or in patients with altered cognition.

- Skeletal muscle relaxants (SMRs) are classified as either antispastic agents (baclofen, dantrolene, tizanidine), which are used to treat cerebral palsy or multiple sclerosis, or as antispasmodic agents (carisoprodol, chlorzoxazone, cyclobenzaprine, metaxolone, methocarbamol, orphenadrine), which are used for the treatment of musculoskeletal conditions such as lower back pain.

  - SMRs should not be used as first-line agents in the treatment of musculoskeletal pain. SMRs should be used only for the short-term treatment of acute low back pain if the patient is unable to tolerate or is unresponsive to NSAIDs or acetaminophen.

Nonnarcotic Oral and Nonsteroidal Anti-Inflammatory Drugs (NSAIDs)

Generic • Brand • Dose & Max mg (frequency)	Contraindications	Primary Side Effects	Key Monitoring Parameters	Pertinent Drug Interactions	Med Pearls
Mechanism of action – ↓ pain through inhibition of central cyclooxygenase, which in turn inhibits prostaglandin synthesis					
Acetaminophen (APAP) • Tylenol, Ofirmev (injection) • Oral: 325–1,000 mg TID–QID (max = 4,000 mg/day) • IV: < 50 kg: 15 mg/kg every 6 hr (max = 3.75 g/day) ≥50 kg: 1,000 mg every 6 hr (max = 4,000 mg/day)	• Hepatic disease • Alcoholism	Hepatotoxicity	Pain relief	Alcohol may ↑ risk of hepatotoxicity	• Oral is over-the-counter (OTC) • Best if taken on scheduled basis vs. as needed (PRN)
Mechanism of action – NSAIDs: ↓ pain and inflammation by inhibition of prostaglandin synthesis through inhibition of cyclooxygenase enzymes					
Aspirin • Various • IR: 325–3,600 mg/day in 4–6 divided doses • Extended release (ER): 650–1,300 mg TID (max = 5.4 g/day)	• Allergy to aspirin or NSAIDs • Active bleeding • Age <16 years	• Gastrointestinal (GI) (dyspepsia, GI ulceration) • Bleeding	• Pain relief • GI symptoms	May ↑ risk of bleeding with anticoagulants, other antiplatelets, and NSAIDs	• OTC • Anti-inflammatory only at high doses (>3 g/day)
Nonacetylated Salicylates					
Salsalate • Only available generically • 500–3,000 mg/day in 2–3 divided doses (max = 3 g/day)	• Hypersensitivity • Allergy to aspirin or NSAIDs	• GI (upset stomach, bleeding) • Rash • Diminished renal function • Edema	• Pain relief • GI symptoms • Renal function	May ↑ risk of bleeding with anticoagulants, antiplatelets, and NSAIDs	Monitor serum salicylate levels with chronic use or very high doses (desired range = 10–30 mg/dL)
Diflunisal • Only available generically • 250–750 mg BID	Hypersensitivity				Administer with food

Nonnarcotic Oral and Nonsteroidal Anti-Inflammatory Drugs (NSAIDs)   *(cont'd)*

Generic • Brand • Dose & Max mg (frequency)	Contraindications	Primary Side Effects	Key Monitoring Parameters	Pertinent Drug Interactions	Med Pearls
Acetic Acids					
Etodolac • Only available generically • 200–1,200 mg/day in 3–4 divided doses	Hypersensitivity	• GI (upset stomach, bleeding) • Rash • Diminished renal function • ↑ BP • Edema	• Pain relief • GI symptoms • Renal function • BP	• May ↑ risk of bleeding with anticoagulants, antiplatelets, and NSAIDs • May ↑ risk of lithium toxicity	Administer with food
Diclofenac☆ • Tabs: Only available generically • IR: 50–150 mg/day in 2–3 divided doses • ER: 100 mg daily • Caps: • Zipsor: 25 mg 4 × /day • Zorvolex: 18–35 mg TID • Oral solution: Cambia • 50 mg at onset of migraine • Transdermal patch: Flector • Apply 1 patch BID • Topical gel: Voltaren (1%) • Apply 2–4 g 4 × /day • Topical solution: Pennsaid (2%) • Apply 2 sprays BID • IV: Dyloject • 37.5 mg IV every 6 hr					• Administer with food • Cambia packet should be mixed in 1–2 oz of water
Indomethacin☆ • Indocin • IR: 25–200 mg/day in 2–3 divided doses • ER: 75 mg BID • Tivorbex • 20–40 mg TID		• GI (upset stomach, bleeding) • Rash • Diminished renal function • ↑ BP • Edema • CNS disturbances			• Most commonly used for treatment of gout • Fat-soluble, crosses blood-brain barrier • Administer with food
Ketorolac • PO/IV/IM: Only available generically • 10 mg PO every 4–6 hr • 30 mg IV/IM every 6 hr • Nasal spray: Sprix • 1 spray in each nostril every 6–8 hr	• Active peptic ulcer disease (PUD) or bleeding • History of GI bleeding • Severe renal impairment • Labor and delivery	• GI (upset stomach, bleeding) • Rash • Diminished renal function • ↑ BP			• Only approved for moderate–severe pain for ≤5 days' duration, due to risk of renal and GI dysfunction • Administer PO with food
Nabumetone • Only available generically • 500–2,000 mg/day in 1–2 divided doses	Hypersensitivity				Administer with food

Nonnarcotic Oral and Nonsteroidal Anti-Inflammatory Drugs (NSAIDs) *(cont'd)*

Generic • Brand • Dose & Max mg (frequency)	Contraindications	Primary Side Effects	Key Monitoring Parameters	Pertinent Drug Interactions	Med Pearls
Propionic Acids					
Fenoprofen • Nalfon • 200–3,200 mg/day in 3–4 divided doses	Hypersensitivity	• GI (upset stomach, bleeding) • Rash • Diminished renal function • ↑ BP	• Pain relief • GI symptoms • Renal function • BP	• May ↑ risk of bleeding with anticoagulants, antiplatelets, and NSAIDs • May ↑ risk of lithium toxicity	Administer with food
Flurbiprofen • Only available generically • 50–300 mg/day in 2–4 divided doses					Administer with food
Ibuprofen ☆ • PO: Motrin, Advil • 200–3,200 mg/day in 3–4 divided doses • IV: Caldolor • 400–800 mg IV every • 6 hr PRN					• Available OTC and Rx (400–800 mg tabs) • Administer with food • Available in pediatric preparations • Ibuprofen lysine (Neoprofen) indicated for closure of patent ductus arteriosus in premature infants
Ketoprofen • Only available generically • IR: 50–300 mg/day in 3–4 divided doses • ER: 200 mg daily					Administer with food
Naproxen ☆ • Naprosyn, Naprelan • IR: 1,000 mg/day in 2–3 divided doses • ER: 750–1,500 mg daily					• Available OTC and Rx • Administer with food
Naproxen sodium ☆ • Anaprox, Anaprox DS, Aleve • OTC: 200 mg every 8–12 hr • Rx: 275–550 mg BID					• Available OTC and Rx • Administer with food
Oxaprozin • Daypro • 600–1,200 mg daily					Administer with food

Nonnarcotic Oral and Nonsteroidal Anti-Inflammatory Drugs (NSAIDs)   *(cont'd)*

Generic • Brand • Dose & Max mg (frequency)	Contraindications	Primary Side Effects	Key Monitoring Parameters	Pertinent Drug Interactions	Med Pearls
Fenamates					
Meclofenamate • Only available generically • 50–400 mg/day in • 4–6 divided doses	Hypersensitivity	• GI (upset stomach, bleeding) • Rash • Diminished renal function • ↑ BP	• Pain relief • GI symptoms • Renal function • BP	• May ↑ risk of bleeding with anticoagulants, antiplatelets, and NSAIDs • May ↑ risk of lithium toxicity	Administer with food
Oxicams					
Piroxicam ☆ • Feldene • 10–20 mg/day in 1–2 divided doses Meloxicam ☆ • Mobic, Vivlodex • Mobic: 7.5–15 mg daily • Vivlodex: 5–10 mg daily	Hypersensitivity	• GI (upset stomach, bleeding) • Rash • Diminished renal function • ↑ BP	• Pain relief • GI symptoms • Renal function • BP	• May ↑ risk of bleeding with anticoagulants, antiplatelets, and NSAIDs • May ↑ risk of lithium toxicity	• More COX -2 selectivity than traditional NSAIDs • Slightly less GI symptoms
Selective COX -2 Inhibitors					
Celecoxib ☆ • Celebrex • 50–200 mg/day in • 1–2 divided doses	• Hypersensitivity • Sulfa allergy	• GI (upset stomach, bleeding; less than other NSAIDs) • Rash • Diminished renal function • ↑ BP • Edema	• Pain relief • GI symptoms • Renal function • BP	• May ↑ risk of bleeding with anticoagulants, antiplatelets, and NSAIDs • May ↑ risk of lithium toxicity	• Lower incidence of GI toxicity than with NSAIDs • Concern about cardiovascular adverse effects prompted withdrawal of similar drug from market (rofecoxib)

Opioid Analgesics

Generic • Brand • Dose/Dosage Forms	Contraindications	Primary Side Effects	Key Monitoring Parameters	Pertinent Drug Interactions	Med Pearls
Mechanism of action – stimulate opioid receptors in the brain					
Hydrocodone • Hysingla ER, Zohydro ER • Initial: 10 mg every 12 hr • ER caps, ER tabs Hydrocodone/ APAP ☆ • Norco • 5–10 mg/325 mg APAP every 4–6 hr • Dose is limited by APAP component • Do not exceed 4 g/ day of APAP • Tabs	• Hypersensitivity • Respiratory depression • Paralytic ileus • Severe or acute asthma • GI obstruction	• Constipation • Nausea/vomiting (N/V) • CNS depression • Confusion • Sedation • Respiratory depression • Hypotension • Bradycardia	• Pain relief • Respiratory rate (RR) • BP • Heart rate (HR) • Constipation • Mental status • Signs of abuse or misuse • State prescription drug monitoring plan (PDMP) data	• Hydrocodone is CYP3A4 substrate • CYP3A4 inhibitors may ↑ effects/ toxicity • CYP3A4 inducers may ↓ effects • Other CNS depressants, including alcohol, may ↑ CNS depressant effects • Monoamine oxidase inhibitors (MAOIs) may ↑ effects; avoid use if MAOIs have been used within past 2 wk	• Schedule II controlled substance • May take with food if nausea occurs • Adjust dose of hydrocodone ER in renal or hepatic impairment • Often need a laxative for constipation • High abuse potential • Hysingla ER and Zohydro ER are abuse deterrent formulations
Codeine ☆ • Only available generically • 15–60 mg every 4 hr (max = 360 mg/day) • Tabs Codeine/APAP • Tylenol with Codeine #3, Tylenol with Codeine #4 • 15–60 mg codeine every 4–6 hr (max = 360 mg/day of codeine and 4 g/ day of APAP) • Tabs	• Hypersensitivity • Respiratory depression • Acute or severe bronchial asthma • Paralytic ileus			• Codeine is CYP2D6 substrate • CYP2D6 inhibitors may ↓ effects • Other CNS depressants, including alcohol, may ↑ CNS depressant effects • MAOIs may ↑ effects; avoid use if MAOIs have been used within past 2 wk	• Schedule II controlled substance • Codeine has good antitussive properties • Must be metabolized by CYP2D6 to morphine for analgesic effect

Opioid Analgesics   *(cont'd)*

Generic • Brand • Dose/Dosage Forms	Contraindications	Primary Side Effects	Key Monitoring Parameters	Pertinent Drug Interactions	Med Pearls
Morphine ☆ • Astramorph, Duramorph, Infumorph, Kadian, Morphabond ER, MS Contin, Arymo ER • IR: 10–30 mg every 4 hr • IV: 2.5–5 mg every 3–4 hr • IV continuous infusion: 0.8–10 mg/hr • Rectal: 10–20 mg every 3–4 hr • Max dose of ER capsules = 1,600 mg/day • ER caps, ER tabs, injection (IV, IT, epidural), rectal suppository, solution, tabs	[Same as above]	[Same as above]	[Same as above]	• Other CNS depressants, including alcohol, may ↑ CNS depressant effects • MAOIs may ↑ effects; avoid use if MAOIs have been used within past 2 wk	• Schedule II controlled substance • May take with food if nausea occurs • Often need a laxative for constipation • High abuse potential • Most often started on IR then switched to ER • Kadian administered every 12 hr or every 24 hr • MS Contin and Arymo ER administered every 8 hr or every 12 hr • Morphabond ER administered every 12 hr • Generic ER caps administered every 24 hr • Arymo ER and Morphabond ER are abuse deterrent formulations
Morphine sulfate/ Naltrexone • Embeda • 20 mg/0.8 mg– 100 mg/4 mg daily • ER caps					• Schedule II controlled substance • Abuse deterrent formulation

Opioid Analgesics   *(cont'd)*

Generic • Brand • Dose/Dosage Forms	Contraindications	Primary Side Effects	Key Monitoring Parameters	Pertinent Drug Interactions	Med Pearls
Oxycodone☆ • Oxaydo, OxyContin, Roxicodone, Xtampza ER, Roxybond • IR: 5–15 mg every 4–6 hr • ER: Initiate oxycodone ER at a dose of 50% of the total daily oral oxycodone daily dose (mg/day) and administer every 12 hr • No max dose • Caps, ER caps, ER tabs, solution, tabs	• Hypersensitivity • Respiratory depression • Paralytic ileus • Severe or acute asthma • GI obstruction	[Same as above]	[Same as above]	• Oxycodone is CYP3A4 substrate • CYP3A4 inhibitors may ↑ effects/toxicity • CYP3A4 inducers may ↓ effects • Other CNS depressants, including alcohol, may ↑ CNS depressant effects • MAOIs may ↑ effects; avoid use if MAOIs have been used within past 2 wk	• Schedule II controlled substance • Oxaydo, OxyContin, and Xtampza ER are abuse deterrent formulations • May take with food if nausea occurs • ER caps should be administered with food and may be administered via nasogastric or gastric tube • Often need a laxative for constipation • High abuse potential • ER oxycodone caps are NOT bioequivalent to ER oxycodone tabs
Oxycodone/APAP☆ • Endocet, Percocet, Roxicet, Xartemis XR • IR: 2.5–10 mg/ 325 mg APAP every 6 hr • ER: 15 mg/650 mg APAP every 12 hr • Dose is limited by APAP component • Do not exceed 4 g/ day of APAP • ER tabs, solution, tabs					
Oxycodone/Naltrexone • Troxyca ER • 10 mg/1.2 mg– 80 mg/9.6 mg every 12 hr • ER tabs					• Schedule II controlled substance • Abuse deterrent formulation
Oxycodone/Naloxone • Targiniq ER • 10 mg/5 mg– 40 mg/20 mg every 12 hr • Max dose 80 mg/ 40 mg daily					• Schedule II controlled substance • Abuse deterrent formulation

Opioid Analgesics   *(cont'd)*

Generic • Brand • Dose/Dosage Forms	Contraindications	Primary Side Effects	Key Monitoring Parameters	Pertinent Drug Interactions	Med Pearls
Fentanyl☆ • Duragesic (transdermal patch) • 25–100 mcg/hr applied every 72 hr • Actiq (transmucosal lozenge) • 200 mcg per episode (limit to ≤4 units/day) • Fentora (buccal tab) • 100–200 mcg per episode (limit to ≤4 units/day) • Subsys (sublingual spray) • 100 mcg per episode (limit to ≤4 units/day) • Abstral (sublingual tablet) • 100–200 mcg per episode (limit to ≤4 units/day) • Lazanda (nasal spray) • 100–200 mcg per episode (limit to ≤4 episodes/day) • IV: 25–35 mcg every 1–2 hr • IV continuous infusion: 50–700 mcg/hr	• Hypersensitivity • Respiratory depression • Paralytic ileus • Severe or acute asthma • GI obstruction • Short-term treatment • Opioid-nontolerant patients	[Same as above]	[Same as above]	• CYP3A4 substrate • CYP3A4 inhibitors may ↑ effects/toxicity • CYP3A4 inducers may ↓ effects • Other CNS depressants, including alcohol, may ↑ CNS depressant effects • MAOIs may ↑ effects; avoid use if MAOIs have been used within past 2 wk	• Schedule II controlled substance • Patch takes 24 hr to begin working • Fentanyl remains in patch at 72 hr; fold in half to avoid diversion • Actiq, Fentora, Lazanda, Abstral, and Subsys should only be used for breakthrough pain; they are not interchangeable • Transdermal patch used to treat chronic, NOT acute pain • High potential for abuse

Opioid Analgesics   *(cont'd)*

Generic • Brand • Dose/Dosage Forms	Contraindications	Primary Side Effects	Key Monitoring Parameters	Pertinent Drug Interactions	Med Pearls
Hydromorphone☆ • Dilaudid, Dilaudid-HP, Exalgo • IR: 2–4 mg every 4–6 hr (tabs) or 2.5–10 mg every 3–6 hr (solution) • IV: 0.2–1 mg every 2–3 hr • IV continuous infusion: 0.5–3 mg/hr • Rectal: 3 mg every 6–8 hr • ER: Initiate hydromorphone ER at the same total daily dose of oral hydromorphone and administer every 24 hr • No max dose • ER tabs, injection (IV, epidural), rectal suppository, solution, tabs	• Hypersensitivity • Respiratory depression • Paralytic ileus • Severe or acute asthma • GI obstruction • Opioid-nontolerant patients	[Same as above]	[Same as above]	• Other CNS depressants, including alcohol, may ↑ CNS depressant effects • MAOIs may ↑ effects; avoid use if MAOIs have been used within past 2 wk	• Schedule II controlled substance • High potential for abuse • Dilaudid-HP is highly concentrated • Exalgo is an abuse deterrent formulation
Oxymorphone • Opana, Opana ER • IR: 5–10 mg every 4–6 hrs • Tab, ER tab, injection (IV, IM, subcut)	• Hypersensitivity • Respiratory depression • Acute or severe asthma • GI obstruction • Paralytic ileus • Moderate and severe hepatic impairment			• Other CNS depressants, including alcohol, may ↑ CNS depressant effects • MAOIs may ↑ effects; avoid use if MAOIs have been used within past 2 wk	• Schedule II controlled substance • Opana ER is an abuse deterrent formulation

Opioid Analgesics   *(cont'd)*

Generic • Brand • Dose/Dosage Forms	Contraindications	Primary Side Effects	Key Monitoring Parameters	Pertinent Drug Interactions	Med Pearls
Meperidine • Demerol • 50–150 mg PO/IM/subcut every 3–4 hr • Injection, solution, tabs	• Hypersensitivity • Use of MAOI within 2 wk • Respiratory depression	• Constipation • N/V • CNS depression • Confusion • Sedation • Respiratory depression • Hypotension • Bradycardia • Seizures	• Pain relief • RR • BP • HR • Seizures • S/S of serotonin syndrome	• Other CNS depressants, including alcohol, may ↑ CNS depressant effects • ↑ risk of serotonin syndrome with MAOIs, selective serotonin reuptake inhibitors (SSRIs) serotonin norepinephrine reuptake inhibitors (SNRIs), triptans, tricyclic antidepressants (TCAs), lithium, dextromethorphan, buspirone, linezolid, methylene blue, St. John's wort, and tramadol	• Schedule II controlled substance • NOT recommended as an analgesic • Accumulation of active metabolite, normeperidine, can ↑ risk of seizures • Renal or hepatic impairment can lead to accumulation of normeperidine • Treatment duration should be limited to ≤48 hr and doses should not exceed 600 mg/day
Methadone☆ • Dolophine, Methadose • Initial (opioid naïve): 2.5 mg PO every 8–12 hr or 2.5–10 mg IV every 8–12 hr • Injection, solution, tabs	• Hypersensitivity • Respiratory depression • Paralytic ileus • Severe or acute asthma	• Constipation • N/V • CNS depression • Confusion • Sedation • Respiratory depression • Hypotension • Bradycardia • QT interval prolongation	• Pain relief • RR • BP • HR • Constipation • Mental status • Signs of abuse or misuse • State PDMP data • Electrocardiogram (ECG)	• CYP3A4 substrate • CYP3A4 inhibitors may ↑ effects/toxicity • CYP3A4 inducers may ↓ effects • Other CNS depressants, including alcohol, may ↑ CNS depressant effects • MAOIs may ↑ effects; avoid use if MAOIs have been used within past 2 wk • May ↑ risk of torsades de pointes with other drugs that prolong QT interval	• Schedule II controlled substance • Long half-life and difficult to titrate • NOT to be used for acute pain

Opioid Analgesics *(cont'd)*

Generic • Brand • Dose/Dosage Forms	Contraindications	Primary Side Effects	Key Monitoring Parameters	Pertinent Drug Interactions	Med Pearls
Mechanism of action – binds to μ-opiate receptors in the CNS and inhibits the reuptake of norepinephrine					
Tapentadol • Nucynta, Nucynta ER • IR: 50–100 mg every 4–6 hr (max = 600 mg/day) • ER: Initiate tapentadol ER at the same total daily dose of oral tapentadol but divide into 2 doses and administer every 12 hr (max = 500 mg/day) • ER tabs, solution, tabs	• Hypersensitivity • Respiratory depression • Paralytic ileus • Severe or acute asthma • Use of MAOI within 2 wk	• Constipation • N/V • CNS depression • Confusion • Dizziness • Sedation • Respiratory depression • Hypotension • Bradycardia • Serotonin syndrome	• Pain relief • RR • BP • HR • Constipation • Mental status • Signs of abuse or misuse • State PDMP data • S/S of serotonin syndrome	• Other CNS depressants, including alcohol, may ↑ CNS depressant effects • MAOIs may ↑ effects; avoid use if MAOIs have been used within past 2 wk • ↑ risk of serotonin syndrome with MAOIs, SSRIs, SNRIs, triptans, TCAs, meperidine, lithium, dextromethorphan, buspirone, linezolid, methylene blue, St. John's wort, and tramadol	• Schedule II controlled substance • Avoid use in severe renal impairment
Mechanism of action – binds to μ-opiate receptors in the CNS, causing inhibition of ascending pain pathways					
Tramadol ☆ • Conzip, Ultram • IR: 50–100 mg every 4–6 hr (max = 400 mg/day) • ER: 100–300 mg daily • ER caps, ER tabs, tabs Tramadol/APAP • Ultracet • 2 tabs (tramadol 75 mg/APAP 650 mg) every 4–6 hr • Max = 8 tablets/day • Treatment duration should not exceed 5 days • Tabs	Hypersensitivity	• Confusion • Sedation • Suicidal thoughts • Rash • Nausea • Orthostatic hypotension • Seizures • Serotonin syndrome	• Pain relief • BP • Mental status • Signs of abuse or misuse • State PDMP data • Suicidality • S/S of serotonin syndrome	• Tramadol is CYP2D6 and CYP3A4 substrate • CYP2D6 or CYP3A4 inhibitors may ↑ effects/toxicity • CYP3A4 inducers may ↓ effects • ↑ risk of serotonin syndrome with MAOIs, SSRIs, SNRIs, triptans, TCAs, fentanyl, lithium, dextromethorphan, meperidine, buspirone, linezolid, methylene blue, and St. John's wort • Other CNS depressants, including alcohol, may ↑ CNS depressant effects	• Schedule IV controlled substance • Adjust dose in renal impairment

Opioid Analgesics   *(cont'd)*

Generic • Brand • Dose/Dosage Forms	Contraindications	Primary Side Effects	Key Monitoring Parameters	Pertinent Drug Interactions	Med Pearls
Mechanism of action – partial μ-opiate receptor agonist and weak K-receptor antagonist					
Buprenorphine • Belbuca, Buprenex, Butrans, Probuphine Implant • IM or IV: 0.3 mg every 6–8 hr • Buccal film: 75–900 mcg every 12 hr • Transdermal patch: 5–20 mcg/hr applied weekly • Buccal film, injection, subcut implant, sublingual tab, transdermal patch	• Hypersensitivity • Opioid allergy	• ↑ BP • Hypotension • Confusion • Respiratory depression • Withdrawal syndrome • Fatigue • Depression • Dizziness • N/V/D • Constipation • Abdominal pain • Xerostomia • Headache • Insomnia • Hepatotoxicity • Pruritus (implant) • Erythema (implant)	• Pain relief • RR • BP • Mental status • LFTs • State PDMP data • Signs of addiction, misuse, or abuse	• Buprenorphine is CYP3A4 substrate • Avoid opioids • CYP3A4 inhibitors may ↑ effects/toxicity • CYP3A4 inducers may ↓ effects • Other CNS depressants, including alcohol, may ↑ CNS depressant effects	• Schedule II controlled substance • Implant or sublingual tablet indicated for treatment of opioid dependence • Injection or buccal film used to treat pain
Buprenorphine/ Naloxone • Bunavail, Suboxone, Zubsolv • Buccal film, sublingual film, sublingual tab • Buccal film usual dose range: 2.1–12.6 mg/ 0.3–2.1 mg daily • Sublingual film usual dose range: 4–24 mg/ 1–6 mg daily • Sublingual tablet usual dose range: 2.9– 17.2 mg/0.71–4.2 mg daily		• Hypotension • Respiratory depression • Confusion • Headache • Withdrawal syndrome • Pain • Diaphoresis • Hepatotoxicity • Glossodynia (film) • Oral hypoesthesia (film) • Vomiting	• LFTs • RR • BP • Mental status • S/S of withdrawal • Signs of addiction, abuse, misuse		• Schedule III controlled substance • Indicated for the treatment of opioid dependence • Not recommended for heroin or opioid dependency induction treatment

Analgesic Adjuncts

Generic • Brand • Dose/Dosage Forms	Contraindications	Primary Side Effects	Key Monitoring Parameters	Pertinent Drug Interactions	Med Pearls
Mechanism of action – ↑ synaptic concentration of norepinephrine, desensitization of adenyl cyclase, and downregulation of serotonin receptors					
Desipramine • Norpramin • Initial: 10–25 mg/day (max = 300 mg/day) • Tabs Amitriptyline☆ • Only available generically • Initial: 25–50 mg/day (max = 150 mg) • Tabs	• Hypersensitivity • Use of MAOI within 2 wk • Concurrent use of linezolid or methylene blue • Acute recovery period post-myocardial infarction (MI)	• Anticholinergic symptoms • Weight gain • Bloating • Blurred vision • Xerostomia • Constipation • Dizziness • Somnolence • Headache • Fatigue • Serotonin syndrome	• Pain relief • Withdrawal symptoms from abrupt discontinuation • Suicidality • BP • ECG (in patients with cardiac disease or hyperthyroidism) • S/S of serotonin syndrome	• CYP2D6 substrate • CYP2D6 inhibitors may ↑ effects/toxicity • ↑ risk of serotonin syndrome with MAOIs, SSRIs, SNRIs, triptans, fentanyl, lithium, dextromethorphan, meperidine, buspirone, linezolid, methylene blue, St. John's wort, and tramadol	• Dangerous in over-dose situations • Avoid in patients with high suicidality • Avoid dispensing large quantities • Neuropathic pain is an unlabeled indication • Taper off when medication is discontinued
Mechanism of action – structurally related to GABA, modulates the release of excitatory neurotransmitters through voltage-gated calcium channels					
Gabapentin☆ • Neurontin • Initial 300 mg TID (max = 3,600 mg/day) • Caps, solution, tabs • Gralise • 300 mg daily on Day 1, then 600 mg daily on Day 2, then 900 mg daily on Days 3–6, then 1,200 mg daily on Days 7–10, then 1,500 mg daily on Days 11–14, then 1,800 mg daily • ER tabs • Horizant • 600 mg in A.M × 3 days, then 600 mg every 12 hr • ER tabs	Hypersensitivity	• Dizziness • Fatigue • Somnolence • Ataxia • Weight gain • Angioedema • Behavioral disturbances (aggression, agitation, anger, anxiety, depression, hostility, nervousness) • Difficulty concentrating • Restlessness	• Pain relief • Suicidality	Other CNS depressants, including alcohol, may ↑ CNS depressant effects	• Adjust dose in renal impairment • Chronic neuropathic pain is not a labeled indication for IR product • Neurontin, Gralise, and Horizant indicated to treat post-herpetic neuralgia • Gralise and Horizant are NOT inter-changeable with other gabapentin products

Analgesic Adjuncts   *(cont'd)*

Generic • Brand • Dose/Dosage Forms	Contraindications	Primary Side Effects	Key Monitoring Parameters	Pertinent Drug Interactions	Med Pearls
Mechanism of action – modulates influx of calcium by binding to the alpha2-delta subunit on voltage-gated calcium channels					
Pregabalin ☆ • Lyrica • Initial: 150 mg/day in 2–3 divided doses (max = 300–600 mg/day based on indication) • Caps, solution	Hypersensitivity	• Angioedema • Somnolence • Dizziness • Peripheral edema	• Pain relief • Suicidality	[Same as above]	• Schedule V controlled substance • Adjust dose in renal impairment • Indicated for neuropathic pain associated with diabetes or spinal cord injury, fibromyalgia, and postherpetic neuralgia
Mechanism of action – SNRIs: inhibit the reuptake of serotonin and norepinephrine to allow higher available synaptic concentrations					
Duloxetine ☆ • Cymbalta • 30–60 mg/day in 1–2 divided doses (max = 60 mg/day) • ER caps	• Hypersensitivity • Use of MAOI within 2 wk • Concurrent use of linezolid or methylene blue • Hepatic impairment • Severe renal impairment (CrCl <30 mL/min)	• Hepatotoxicity • Orthostatic hypotension • Rash (Stevens-Johnson syndrome possible) • Palpitations • Diaphoresis • Constipation • ↓ appetite • N/D • Xerostomia • Asthenia • Dizziness • Insomnia or somnolence • Vertigo • Blurred vision • Polyuria • ↓ libido • Serotonin syndrome	• Pain relief • LFTs • BP • Withdrawal symptoms from abrupt discontinuation • Abnormal bleeding • Suicidality • S/S of serotonin syndrome	• CYP1A2 and CYP2D6 substrate • CYP1A2 or CYP2D6 inhibitors may ↑ effects/toxicity; avoid concomitant use with strong CYP1A2 inhibitors • CYP1A2 inducers may ↓ effects • ↑ risk of serotonin syndrome with MAOIs, SSRIs, triptans, TCAs, fentanyl, amphetamines, lithium, dextromethorphan, meperidine, buspirone, linezolid, methylene blue, St. John's wort, and tramadol • ↑ risk of bleeding when used with aspirin, NSAIDs, or anticoagulants	Indicated to treat diabetic neuropathy, fibromyalgia, and chronic musculo-skeletal pain
Mechanism of action – induces the release of substance P, the principal chemomediator of pain impulses from the periphery					
Capsaicin • Salonpas, Zostrix-HP • Cream, gel, lotion: 0.025–0.1% applied 3–4 × daily • Patch: apply to affected area 3–4 × /day	Do not apply to wounds or damaged skin	Localized stinging	Pain relief	None	• OTC • Must be used regularly for ≥2 wk for maximal efficacy

Skeletal Muscle Relaxants

Generic • Brand • Dose & Max mg (frequency)	Contraindications	Primary Side Effects	Key Monitoring Parameters	Pertinent Drug Interactions	Med Pearls
Mechanism of action – inhibits reflexes at the level of the spinal cord by hyperpolarization of afferent fibers					
Baclofen • Gablofen, Lioresal • 5–20 mg PO TID–QID (max = 80 mg/day) • IT administration via infusion/implanted pump: 300–800 mcg/day	• Hypersensitivity • IV, IM, subcut, or epidural adminsi-tration (for IT use)	• Hypotonia • Drowsiness • Confusion • Headache • N/V • Hypotension • Seizures • Dizziness	• Pain relief • Mental status	Other CNS depressants, including alcohol, may ↑ CNS depressant effects	Antispastic agent
Mechanism of action – depresses polysynaptic neuronal transmission in the spinal cord and reticular formation					
Carisoprodol • Soma • 250–350 mg 4 × /day • Tabs	• Hypersensitivity • Acute intermittent porphyria	• Drowsiness • Dizziness • Headache	• Pain relief • Mental status • Signs of abuse/misuse/ addiction	• CYP2C19 substrate • CYP2C19 inhibitors may ↑ effects/toxicity • CYP2C19 inducers may ↓ effects • Other CNS depressants, including alcohol, may ↑ CNS depressant effects	• Schedule IV con-trolled substance • Antispasmodic agent • Metabolized to meprobamate
Mechanism of action – inhibits polysynaptic reflexes					
Chlorzoxazone • Only available generically • 250–750 mg 3–4 × /day • Tabs	Hypersensitivity	• Dizziness • Drowsiness • N/V/D • Urine discoloration • Hepatotoxicity	• Pain relief • LFTs	Other CNS depressants, including alcohol, may ↑ CNS depressant effects	Antispasmodic agent

Skeletal Muscle Relaxants   *(cont'd)*

Generic • Brand • Dose & Max mg (frequency)	Contraindications	Primary Side Effects	Key Monitoring Parameters	Pertinent Drug Interactions	Med Pearls
Mechanism of action – reduces tonic somatic motor activity by altering alpha and gamma motor neurons					
Cyclobenzaprine • Amrix • IR: 5–10 mg TID • ER: 15–30 mg daily • ER caps, tabs	• Hypersensitivity • Use of MAOI within 2 wk • Hyperthyroidism • Heart failure • Arrhythmias • Atrioventricular block or conduction disturbance • Acute recovery of MI	• Drowsiness • Dizziness • Xerostomia • Fatigue • Constipation • Confusion • Weakness • Blurred vision • Irritabilty • Serotonin syndrome	• Pain relief • Mental status • S/S of serotonin syndrome	• CYP1A2 substrate • CYP1A2 inhibitors may ↑ effects/toxicity • CYP1A2 inducers may ↓ effects • Other CNS depressants, including alcohol, may ↑ CNS depressant effects • ↑ risk of serotonin syndrome with MAOIs, SSRIs, SNRIs, triptans, TCAs, fentanyl, lithium, dextromethorphan, meperidine, buspirone, linezolid, methylene blue, St. John's wort, and tramadol	• Antispasmodic agent • ER formulation should not be used in older adults (>65 yr) or patients with hepatic impairment
Mechanism of action – inhibits the release of calcium from sarcoplasmic reticulum					
Dantrolene • Dantrium • 25 mg daily × 7 days, then 25 mg TID × 7 days, then 50 mg TID × 7 days, then 100 mg TID (max = 400 mg/day) • Caps	• Hypersensitivity • Active liver disease • If spasticity is used to maintain upright posture/ balance or function	• Hepatotoxicity • Drowsiness • Dizziness • Headache • Weakness • Diarrhea	• Pain relief • LFTs	• CYP3A4 substrate • CYP3A4 inhibitors may ↑ effects/toxicity • CYP3A4 inducers may ↓ effects • Concurrent use with estrogen may ↑ risk of hepatotoxicity • Other CNS depressants, including alcohol, may ↑ CNS depressant effects	• Antispastic agent • Females and patients >35 yr at ↑ risk for hepatotoxicity • IV formulation can also be used to treat malignant hyperthermia
Mechanism of action – general depression of the CNS					
Metaxalone • Skelaxin • 800 mg 3–4 × /day • Tabs	• Hypersensitivity • Severe renal or hepatic impairment • Predisposition to drug-induced, hemolytic, or other anemias	• Dizziness • Drowsiness • Headache • N/V • Hemolytic anemia • Jaundice • Rash	• Pain relief • Complete blood count	Other CNS depressants, including alcohol, may ↑ CNS depressant effects	Antispasmodic agent

Skeletal Muscle Relaxants   *(cont'd)*

Generic • Brand • Dose & Max mg (frequency)	Contraindications	Primary Side Effects	Key Monitoring Parameters	Pertinent Drug Interactions	Med Pearls
Mechanism of action — general depression of the CNS					
Methocarbamol • Robaxin • 4–6 g/day PO in 3–6 divided doses • 1 g IV/IM every 8 hr for no more than 3 consecutive days • Injection, tabs	• Hypersensitivity • Renal impairment (IV use because of polyethylene glycol in vehicle)	• Confusion • Impaired coordination • Headache • Sedation	• Pain relief • Presence of side effects	Other CNS depressants, including alcohol, may ↑ CNS depressant effects	Antispasmodic agent
Mechanism of action — central atropine-like effects for indirect skeletal muscle relaxation					
Orphenadrine • Only available generically • 100 mg PO BID • 60 mg IV/IM every 12 hr • ER tabs, injection	• Hypersensitivity • Glaucoma • GI obstruction • Peptic ulcer disease • Benign prostatic hyperplasia • Bladder obstruction • Megaesophagus • Myasthenia gravis	• Tachycardia • Palpitation • Dizziness • Syncope • Anaphylaxis • Drowsiness • Confusion • Constipation • N/V • Xerostomia • Urinary retention • Tremor • Blurred vision	• Pain relief • HR	• Additive effects with other anticholinergic medications • Other CNS depressants, including alcohol, may ↑ CNS depressant effects	Antispasmodic agent
Mechanism of action — alpha-2 receptor agonist					
Tizanidine • Zanaflex • 2–12 mg TID • Caps, tabs	Concurrent use with strong CYP1A2 inhibitors	• Somnolence • Hypotension • Syncope • Hepatotoxicity • Hallucinations • Anaphylaxis • Xerostomia • Weakness • Dizziness	• Pain relief • LFTs • BP	• CYP1A2 substrate • CYP1A2 inhibitors may ↑ effects/toxicity • CYP1A2 inducers may ↓ effects • Oral contraceptives may ↑ effects/toxicity • Concurrent use with clonidine may ↑ risk of hypotension • Other CNS depressants, including alcohol, may ↑ CNS depressant effects	Antispastic agent

PRACTICE QUESTIONS

1. Which of the following is a caution with the use of tramadol?

    (A) Bradycardia
    (B) GI bleed
    (C) HTN
    (D) Hyperglycemia
    (E) Seizures

2. Which of the following is a common effect of narcotic or opioid analgesics?

    (A) Constipation
    (B) Diarrhea
    (C) Hypertension
    (D) Tachypnea

3. Which of the following medications is contraindicated in a patient with a sulfa allergy?

    (A) Amitriptyline
    (B) Celecoxib
    (C) Gabapentin
    (D) Hydromorphone

4. Which of the following is TRUE regarding meperidine or the metabolite, norme-peridine?

    (A) May be used for long-term analgesia
    (B) Normeperidine may cause seizures
    (C) Only available in oral formulation
    (D) Preferred agent for use in renal failure
    (E) Recommended first line for analgesia

5. Which of the following should be avoided in PUD? (Select ALL that apply.)

    (A) Ibuprofen
    (B) Indomethacin
    (C) Ketorolac
    (D) Naproxen
    (E) Cyclobenzaprine

6. Which of the following can be used to treat neuropathic pain?

   (A) Acetaminophen
   (B) Capsaicin
   (C) Gabapentin
   (D) Ibuprofen
   (E) Ketorolac

7. Which of the following formulations are available for oxycodone? (Select ALL that apply.)

   (A) ER tablet
   (B) IR tablet
   (C) IV injection
   (D) Oral solution

8. Which of the following is FDA approved for the treatment of fibromyalgia?

   (A) Gabapentin
   (B) Ketorolac
   (C) Morphine
   (D) Pregabalin

9. Which of the following NSAIDs is available as an IM injection formulation?

   (A) Celecoxib
   (B) Ibuprofen
   (C) Ketorolac
   (D) Naproxen

10. Which of the following is associated with methadone use?

    (A) Diarrhea
    (B) GI bleeding
    (C) Hyperkalemia
    (D) Hypertension
    (E) QTc prolongation

ANSWERS AND EXPLANATIONS

1. **E**

Tramadol is associated with a risk of seizures and should be used with caution in patients with epilepsy or a history of a seizure disorder. The risk of seizures is increased if given concomitantly with other agents that may lower the seizure threshold.

2. **A**

Constipation is a common side effect associated with opioid analgesics, which often needs to be treated with stimulant laxatives to provide relief to the patient. Opioid analgesics may also be associated with hypotension and bradypnea.

3. **B**

Use of celecoxib is contraindicated in a patient with a sulfa allergy. Amitriptyline (A), gabapentin (C), and hydromorphone (D) can all be used in a patient with a sulfa allergy.

4. **B**

Normeperidine is a toxic metabolite of meperidine that is known to cause seizures. Meperidine should not be used for >48 hours (A) and should be avoided in renal failure to prevent the accumulation of normeperidine (D). Meperidine is available in oral and IV formulations (C). Meperidine should not be used as a first-line agent (E) due to the risk associated with the medication.

5. **A, B, C, D**

A, B, C and D are NSAIDs and should not be used if a patient has PUD or a history of GI bleeding. If an NSAID must be used in a patient with PUD or a history of GI bleeding, a COX-2 selective inhibitor such as celecoxib would be preferred. E, cyclobenzaprine is a SMR and can be used in the presence of PUD.

6. **C**

Gabapentin may be used to treat neuropathic pain. Neuropathic pain does not respond well to acetaminophen (A) or NSAIDs such as ibuprofen (D) or ketorolac (E).

7. **A, B, D**

Oxycodone is available in IR and ER tablet formulations as well as a solution and oral concentrate. It is not available for IV, IM, or subcutaneous injection.

8. **D**

Pregabalin (Lyrica) is FDA approved for the treatment of fibromyalgia. Other FDA-approved medications for the treatment of fibromyalgia include duloxetine (Cymbalta) and milnacipran (Savella). Fibromyalgia is also treated off-label with various other agents.

9. **C**

Ketorolac is available as an IM formulation. It is also available in IV and oral formulations. Celecoxib (A) is available only in an oral formulation. Ibuprofen (B) is available in oral tablet, capsule, solution, suspension, and IV formulations, as well as a cream. Naproxen (D) is available as an oral tablet, a capsule, an oral suspension, and a topical cream.

10. **E**

Methadone is known to prolong the QTc interval and should not be used with other agents that prolong the QTc interval. Methadone is associated with constipation (not diarrhea, A), hypokalemia (not hyperkalemia, C), and hypotension (not hypertension, D). It is also not known to cause GI bleeding (B).

Bone and Joint Disorders

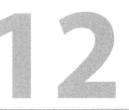

This chapter covers the following disease states:

- **Osteoarthritis**
- **Rheumatoid arthritis**
- **Osteoporosis**
- **Gout**

OSTEOARTHRITIS

Guidelines Summary

The goals of therapy are to ↓ pain and stiffness, maintain/improve joint mobility and limit functional impairment, and ↑ quality of life.

- OA of the hand:
  - First-line options: Topical capsaicin, topical nonsteroidal anti-inflammatory drugs (NSAIDs), oral NSAIDs, tramadol
  - Topical NSAIDs preferred over oral NSAIDs in patients ≥75 years of age
- OA of the knee or hip:
  - First-line option: Acetaminophen (scheduled, up to maximum of 4 g/day)
  - Second-line options: Topical or oral NSAIDs (topical preferred in patients ≥75 years of age) or intra-articular corticosteroid injections
  - Third-line options: Duloxetine, tramadol, or intra-articular hyaluronan injections

Treatment Algorithm

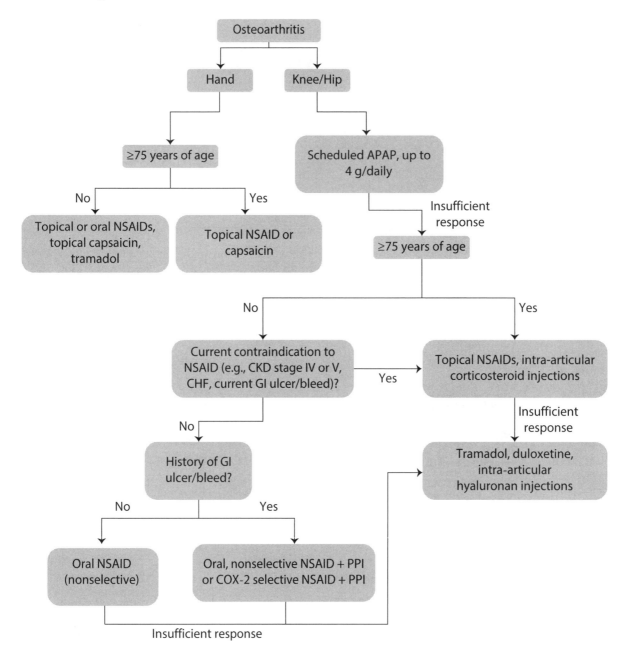

Drugs for Osteoarthritis

Acetaminophen and NSAIDs are reviewed in drug tables in the Pain Management chapter.

Generic • Brand • Dose/Dosage Forms	Contraindications	Primary Side Effects	Key Monitoring Parameters	Pertinent Drug Interactions	Med Pearls
Adjunctive Therapies/Nutritional Supplements					
Glucosamine sulfate • Various • 500–1,500 mg/day in 1–2 divided doses daily	Unknown	• Itching • Gastrointestinal (GI) upset	• Pain relief • Presence of side effects	Unknown	• Nutritional supplement • Available OTC • Conflicting clinical trial data
Intra-Articular Injections					
Mechanism of action – serves as a lubricant for joint tissue					
Hyaluronate and derivates • Synvisc, Synvisc-One • Synvisc: Inject 16 mg (2 mL) once weekly for 3 wk (total of 3 injections) • Sinvisc-One: Inject 48 mg (6 mL) once per knee	Hypersensitivity	• Injection site reaction • Bruising • Erythema • Lumps • Pain • Swelling • Pruritus • Skin discoloration • Arthralgia • Infection	S/S of inflammation or infection	No known significant drug interactions	None

RHEUMATOID ARTHRITIS

Guidelines Summary

- Goals of therapy include achieving low disease activity or remission.

- A disease-modifying antirheumatic drug (DMARD) should be initiated within 3 months of diagnosis to retard disease progression.

- Leflunomide, sulfasalazine, hydroxychloroquine, and methotrexate are first-line DMARD options.

- In patients with moderate to severe disease activity, combination therapy may be considered initially.

- NSAIDs are useful for symptomatic relief during onset of DMARD and then can be used as needed otherwise. NSAIDs do not alter disease progression in RA.

- Corticosteroids are used as adjunctive therapy in patient with refractory symptoms.

- Biologic agents are used generally when initial DMARD therapy has been demonstrated to be ineffective as monotherapy. Additional DMARDs may be tried prior to use of biologics.

- Biologic therapies ↑ the risk of serious infections and should not be initiated in a patient with an active infection or in combination with live vaccines.

Treatment Algorithm

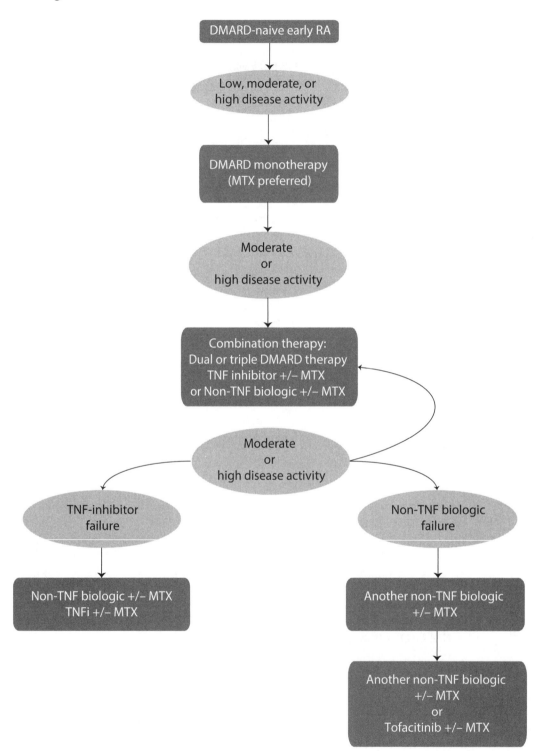

Medications for Rheumatoid Arthritis

Generic • Brand • Dose/Dosage Forms	Contraindications	Primary Side Effects	Key Monitoring Parameters	Pertinent Drug Interactions	Med Pearls
Mechanism of action – corticosteroids: exert anti-inflammatory and immunosuppressive effects by inhibiting prostaglandins and leukotrienes, which results in ↓ inflammation, ↓ pain, and a potential ↓ in joint destruction					
Prednisone ☆ • Only available generically • 5–60 mg daily initially; individualized • Solution, tabs	• Systemic fungal infection • Hypersensitivity	• Hyperglycemia • ↑ blood pressure (BP) • ↓ bone mineral density (BMD) • Fluid retention • Impaired wound healing • Infection • Hyperglycemia • ↑ appetite • Irritability • Insomnia • Weight gain	• Blood sugar • BP • Electrolytes • BMD • Presence of edema/weight	May ↑ anticoagulant effect of warfarin	Side effects generally present with chronic and/or long-term use
DMARDs					
Mechanism of action – inhibit cytokine production, inhibit purine biosynthesis, thereby ↓ inflammation in affected joints					
Methotrexate ☆ • Otrexup, Rasuvo, Rheumatrex, Trexall • 7.5 mg PO/subcut/IM weekly • Injection, tabs	• Hypersensitivity • Alcoholism • Liver disease • Immunodeficiency • Significant blood dyscrasias • Pregnancy • Lactation	• GI upset (nausea, diarrhea, abdominal pain) • Stomatitis • Thrombocytopenia • Leukopenia • Anemia • ↑ liver function tests (LFTs) • Interstitial lung disease • Rash (Stevens-Johnson syndrome possible) • Malaise • Fatigue • Fever/chills • Infection	• Pain relief • LFTs • Complete blood count (CBC) with differential • Folate concentrations • S/S of infection	• NSAIDs and salicylates ↑ risk of toxicity • Penicillins, sulfonamides, and tetracyclines may ↑ risk of toxicity	• May supplement with folic acid to ↓ side effects and prevent folate deficiency • Myelosuppression is biggest concern • Should be taken with food
Mechanism of action – not fully understood; thought to be related to immunosuppressant properties					
Hydroxychloroquine ☆ • Plaquenil • 200–600 mg/day in 1–2 divided doses • Tabs	• Hypersensitivity • Retinal changes with agent in past • Children	• Macular damage • Corneal deposits • Retinopathy • Rash • Nausea • Diarrhea • Neutropenia • Thrombocytopenia • Anemia	• Ocular exams every 3 mo • CBC with differential	May ↑ serum digoxin concentrations	Hemolysis can occur in patients with glucose-6-phosphate dehydrogenase deficiency

Medications for Rheumatoid Arthritis   *(cont'd)*

Generic • Brand • Dose/Dosage Forms	Contraindications	Primary Side Effects	Key Monitoring Parameters	Pertinent Drug Interactions	Med Pearls
Mechanism of action – inhibits pyrimidine synthesis, thereby ↓ lymphocyte proliferation and inflammation					
Leflunomide • Arava • 100 mg daily × 3 days, then 20 mg daily • Tabs	• Hypersensitivity • Severe hepatic impairment • Pregnancy	• Diarrhea • Hepatotoxicity • Alopecia • Rash (Stevens-Johnson syndrome possible) • Peripheral neuropathy • Interstitial lung disease • ↑ BP • Neutropenia • Thrombocytopenia • Anemia • Infection	• LFTs (monthly × 6 mo, then every 6–8 wk) • CBC with differential (monthly × 6 mo, then every 6–8 wk) • Pregnancy test (before therapy begins) • BP • S/S of infection	• CYP2C8 inhibitor • May ↑ effects/ toxicity of CYP2C8 substrates • May ↓ effects of warfarin • May ↑ toxicity of rosuvastatin (max dose of rosuvastatin = 10 mg/day)	• Highly teratogenic • Appropriate contraception should be used • After stopping therapy, accelerated drug elimination procedure should be used to rapidly ↓ concentrations of active metabolite (comprised of cholestyramine or activated charcoal)
Mechanism of action – not fully understood; related to anti-inflammatory properties					
Sulfasalazine • Azulfidine, Azulfidine EN-tabs • 500–3,000 mg/day in 2 divided doses • ER tabs, tabs	• Hypersensitivity to any sulfa-containing drug or salicylates • Intestinal or urinary obstruction • Porphyria	• N/V/D • Rash (Stevens-Johnson syndrome possible) • Photosensitivity • Neutropenia • Anemia • Hepatotoxicity • Renal impairment • Alopecia • Stomatitis • Infection	• CBC with differential (every other wk × 3 mo, then every mo × 3 mo, then every 3 mo) • LFTs (every other wk × 3 mo, then every mo × 3 mo, then every 3 mo) • Renal function • Folate concentrations	• May ↑ effects of warfarin • May ↓ serum digoxin concentrations	• May supplement with folic acid to ↓ side effects and prevent folate deficiency • Preferred option in pregnant patients
Biologics					
Mechanism of action – binds to and inhibits the cytokine tumor necrosis factor (TNF), thereby inhibiting the subsequent inflammatory cascade					
Etanercept • Enbrel • 50 mg subcut weekly • Injection	Sepsis	• Injection site reactions • Anaphylaxis • Infection (especially latent tuberculosis [TB] reactivation, fungal infections and hepatitis B virus [HBV] reactivation) • Lymphoma • Leukemia • Skin cancer • Heart failure (HF) exacerbation • Bone marrow suppression • Lupus-like syndrome • Demyelinating disorders	• PPD and HBV screening before initiating treatment • S/S of infection • S/S of heart failure • CBC with differential	• Not to be given with live vaccines	• Store in refrigerator • Use within 14 days once at room temp • Discontinue if serious infection occurs • Use with caution in patients with HF • Can be self-administered • Can be used alone or in combination with methotrexate

Medications for Rheumatoid Arthritis   *(cont'd)*

Generic • Brand • Dose/Dosage Forms	Contraindications	Primary Side Effects	Key Monitoring Parameters	Pertinent Drug Interactions	Med Pearls
Infliximab • Inflectra, Remicade • 3 mg/kg IV infusion at initiation, wk 2 and wk 6, then every 8 wk • Injection	• Hypersensitivity • Doses >5 mg/kg in moderate-severe HF	• Infusion reactions (hypotension, dyspnea, urticaria) • Delayed hypersensitivity reactions (fever, rash, myalgia, headache, sore throat, hand/facial edema, dysphagia, arthralgias) • Infection (especially latent TB reactivation, fungal infections, or HBV reactivation) • HF exacerbation • Bone marrow suppression • Lymphoma • Leukemia • Skin cancer • Hepatotoxicity	• PPD and HBV screening before initiating treatment • BP • LFTs • S/S of infection • S/S of HF • CBC with differential	[Same as above]	• Delayed hypersensitivity reaction may occur as early as after 2nd dose • Premedicate with H₁ antagonist, H₂ antagonist, acetaminophen, and/or corticosteroid • Dose limited to • ≤5 mg/kg in patients with HF • Discontinue if serious infection occurs • Indicated for use in combination with methotrexate
Golimumab • Simponi, Simponi Aria • 50 mg subcut monthly or 2 mg/kg IV infusion at initiation and wk 4, then every 8 wk • Injection	None	• Injection site reactions • Anaphylaxis • Infection (especially latent TB reactivation, fungal infections and HBV reactivation) • Lymphoma • Leukemia • Skin cancer • HF exacerbation • Bone marrow suppression • Lupus-like syndrome • Demyelinating disorders	• PPD and HBV screening before initiating treatment • S/S of infection • S/S of HF • CBC with differential		• Use with caution in patients with HF • Discontinue if serious infection occurs • Subcut injection can be self-administered • Store subcut injection in refrigerator • Indicated for use in combination with methotrexate
Adalimumab • Humira • 40 mg subcut every other wk (if not taking methotrexate, may give weekly) • Injection					• Use with caution in patients with HF • Discontinue if serious infection occurs • Can be self-administered • Store in refrigerator • Use within 14 days once at room temp • Can be used alone or in combination with methotrexate or other non-biological DMARDs

Medications for Rheumatoid Arthritis *(cont'd)*

Generic • Brand • Dose/Dosage Forms	Contraindications	Primary Side Effects	Key Monitoring Parameters	Pertinent Drug Interactions	Med Pearls
Certolizumab pegol • Cimzia • 400 mg subcut at initiation, wk 2, and wk 4, then 200 mg subcut every other wk • Injection	[Same as above]	[Same as above]	[Same as above]	[Same as above]	• Use with caution in patients with HF • Discontinue if serious infection occurs • Can be self-administered • Store in refrigerator • Can be used alone or in combination with methotrexate or other non-biological DMARDs
Mechanism of action – interleukin-6 (IL-6) receptor antagonist					
Sarilumab • Kevzara • 200 mg subcut every 2 wk	• Absolute neutrophil count $<2,000/mm^3$ • Platelets $<150,000/mm^3$ • ALT or AST $>1.5\times$ the upper limit of normal	• ↑ LFTs • Pruritus at injection site • Infections (upper respiratory, pneumonia, urinary tract) • Hypertriglyceridemia	• PPD screening before initiating treatment • CBC with differential (prior to therapy, 4–8 wk after initiation, then every 3 mo) • LFTs (prior to therapy, 4–8 wk after initiation, then every 3 mo) • S/S of infection • Lipid panel • (4–8 wk after initiation)	Not to be given with live vaccines	• Indicated for moderate–severe disease that has not responded to >1 DMARD • Can be self-administered • Store in refrigerator • Use within 14 days once at room temp • Can be used alone or in combination with methotrexate or other non-biological DMARDs
Mechanism of action – binds to interleukin-1 (IL-1) receptors on target cells, thereby preventing release of chemotactic factors and adhesion molecules and subsequently ↓ inflammation and connective tissue damage					
Anakinra • Kineret • 100 mg subcut daily • Injection	Hypersensitivity	• Injection-site reactions (inflammation, ecchymosis) • Infection (including latent TB reactivation) • Neutropenia • Anaphylaxis	• PPD screening before initiating treatment • CBC with differential • S/S of infection	• Not to be given with TNF inhibitors • Not to be given with live vaccines	• Indicated for moderate–severe disease that has not responded to >1 DMARD • Can be self-administered • Store in refrigerator • Can be used alone or in combination with other non-biological DMARDs

Medications for Rheumatoid Arthritis   *(cont'd)*

Generic • Brand • Dose/Dosage Forms	Contraindications	Primary Side Effects	Key Monitoring Parameters	Pertinent Drug Interactions	Med Pearls
Mechanism of action – IL-6 receptor antagonist					
Tocilizumab • Actemra • IV: 4 mg/kg IV infusion every 4 wk; may be ↑ to 8 mg/kg based on clinical response (max = 800 mg per infusion) • Subcut: <100 kg: 162 mg subcut every other wk (may be ↑ to every wk based on clinical response); ≥100 kg: 162 mg subcut weekly • Injection	• Hypersensitivity • Absolute neutrophil count <2,000/mm³ • Platelets <150,000/mm³ • ALT or AST >1.5× the upper limit of normal	• Infection (especially latent TB reactivation, fungal infections and viral reactivation) • GI perforation • Neutropenia • Thrombocytopenia • ↑ LFTs • Dyslipidemia • Anaphylaxis • Demyelinating disorders	• PPD screening before initiating treatment • S/S of infection • CBC with differential • Lipid panel • LFTs	• Not to be given with TNF inhibitors • Not to be given with live vaccines	• Indicated for moderate–severe disease that has not responded to >1 DMARD • Discontinue if serious infection occurs • Subcut injection can be self-administered • Store subcut injection in refrigerator • Can be used alone or in combination with methotrexate or other non-biological DMARDs
Mechanism of action – selective costimulation modulator; inhibits T-cell activation					
Abatacept • Orencia • IV infusion administered at initiation, wk 2, and wk 4, then every 4 wk • IV weight-based dose: <60 kg: 500 mg; 60–100 kg: 750 mg; >100 kg: 1,000 mg • Subcut: 125 mg subcut weekly (may be initiated with or without an IV loading dose)	None	• Anaphylaxis • Infection (especially latent TB reactivation, fungal infections and HBV reactivation) • Chronic obstructive pulmonary disease (COPD) exacerbations • Headache • Nausea	• PPD and HBV screening before initiating treatment • S/S of infection	• Not to be given with TNF inhibitors • Not to be given with live vaccines	• Discontinue if serious infection occurs • Use with caution in patients with COPD • Subcut injection can be self-administered • Store subcut injection in refrigerator • Can be used alone or in combination with other non-biological DMARDs

Medications for Rheumatoid Arthritis *(cont'd)*

Generic • Brand • Dose/Dosage Forms	Contraindications	Primary Side Effects	Key Monitoring Parameters	Pertinent Drug Interactions	Med Pearls
Mechanism of action – inhibits Janus kinase thereby reducing cytokine signaling					
Tofacitinib • Xeljanz, Xeljanz XR • IR: 5 mg BID • ER: 11 mg daily • ER tabs, tabs	None	• Infection (especially latent TB reactivation, fungal infections and HBV reactivation) • Malignancy • GI perforation • Lymphocytopenia • Neutropenia • Anemia • ↑ LFTs • Dyslipidemia • Headache • Diarrhea	• PPD and HBV screening before initiating treatment • S/S of infection • CBC with differential • Lipid panel • LFTs	• CYP3A4 substrate • CYP3A4 inhibitors may ↑ effects/toxicity; dose when used with strong CYP3A4 inhibitors • CYP3A4 inducers may ↓ effects • Not to be given with TNF inhibitors • Not to be given with live vaccines	• Oral therapy offers advantage over many available biologics • Can be used alone or in combination with methotrexate or other non-biological DMARDs

OSTEOPOROSIS

Guidelines Summary

- Dietary and supplemental calcium and vitamin D are important prerequisites to pharmacological therapy. Without adequate calcium and vitamin D available, other therapies will be limited in their ability to improve bone architecture.

- Bisphosphonates are the first-line therapy for the prevention and treatment of osteoporosis in patients without contraindications.

- Oral bisphosphonates are approved for prevention and treatment of osteoporosis (including glucocorticoid-induced osteoporosis) in men and women.

- Efficacy of bisphosphonates beyond 5 years is limited, with rare but serious side effects such as osteonecrosis of the jaw (ONJ) and atypical femur fractures. It is reasonable to reassess fracture risk and consider therapy discontinuation after 3–5 years.

- Raloxifene is recommended as an alternative choice for the treatment of osteoporosis in patients with contraindications to bisphosphonates or in patients who are unable to comply with the appropriate bisphosphonate administration instructions.

- Calcitonin is reserved for third-line therapy because of a lack of compelling evidence indicating fracture reductions and lack of long-term data. Calcitonin is approved for the treatment of acute pain secondary to vertebral fractures and is well tolerated; therefore, this medication may have a specific role in certain situations.

- Teriparatide is approved for the treatment of osteoporosis and is indicated in patients with a history of fracture secondary to osteoporosis and in those with multiple risk factors for fracture who have not responded or are intolerant to bisphosphonate therapy, as well as for patients with glucocorticoid-induced osteoporosis.

- Denosumab is reserved for second-line therapy for the treatment of osteoporosis in postmenopausal females at high risk for fracture (i.e., previous osteoporotic fractures, multiple fracture risk factors, failed other therapies).

- Estrogens and tissue-selective estrogen complex (conjugated estrogens/bazedoxifene) are approved for the prevention of osteoporosis in postmenopausal women. Patients should consider potential risks (cardiovascular, breast cancer, venous thromboembolism) before initiating therapy with these agents. If the decision is made to initiate estrogen-based therapy for osteoporosis prevention, the lowest effective dose should be used for the shortest duration.

Osteoporosis Treatment Summary

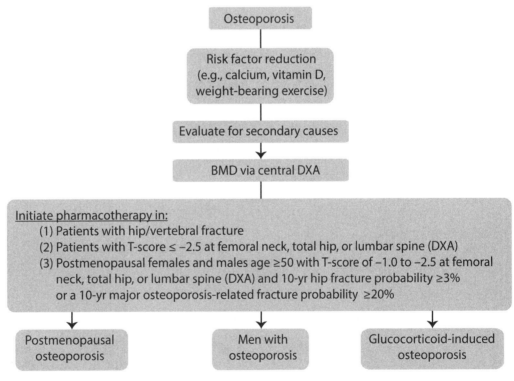

Abbreviations: BMD = bone mineral density

Management of Postmenopausal Osteoporosis

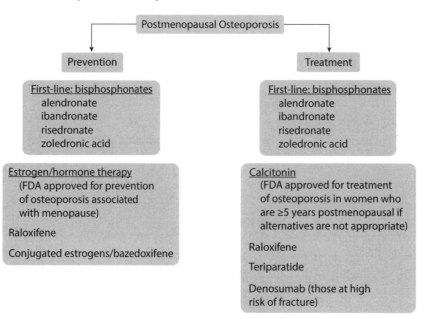

Management of Osteoporosis in Men

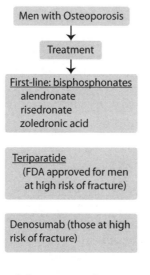

Management of Glucocorticoid-Induced Osteoporosis

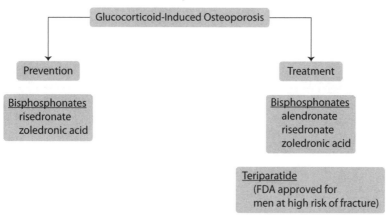

Medications for Osteoporosis

Generic • Brand • Dose/Dosage Forms	Contraindications	Primary Side Effects	Key Monitoring Parameters	Pertinent Drug Interactions	Med Pearls
Mechanism of action – bisphosphonates: adsorb to bone apatite and inhibit osteoclast activity					
Alendronate ☆ • Binosto, Fosamax • 10 mg daily or 70 mg weekly (treatment) • 5 mg daily or 35 mg weekly (prevention) • Effervescent tabs, solution, tabs Risedronate ☆ • Actonel, Atelvia • IR: 5 mg daily, 35 mg weekly, or 150 mg monthly • ER: 35 mg weekly • ER tabs, tabs Ibandronate ☆ • Boniva • PO: 150 mg monthly • IV: 3 mg every 3 mo • Injection, tabs	• Esophageal stricture • Hypersensitivity • Inability to sit upright or stand for ≥30 min • Creatinine clearance (CrCl) <35 mL/min • Hypocalcemia	• Nausea • Dyspepsia • Esophageal irritation • Ulceration • Myalgia/ arthralgia • ONJ • Atypical femur fractures	• BMD • Serum calcium concentrations • Serum 25(OH)D concentrations	• Absorption ↓ with antacids and products containing bi- or trivalent cations (e.g. iron, magnesium, aluminum, calcium, or zinc) (separate by ≥30 min) • NSAIDs may ↑ risk of GI symptoms	• Alendronate and risedronate IR tabs must be taken with 6–8 oz of water ≥30 minutes (60 min for ibandronate) prior to other medications/food • Alendronate oral solution should be followed by ≥2 oz of water; effervescent tabs should be dissolved in 4 oz of room-temperature water • Risedronate ER tabs must be taken with ≥4 oz of water immediately after breakfast • Patient should remain upright for ≥30 min (60 min for ibandronate) (for alendronate, must also remain upright until after first food of day)
Zoledronic acid • Reclast • 5 mg IV infusion yearly (every 2 yr for prevention) • Injection	• Hypersensitivity • CrCl <35 mL/min • Hypocalcemia	• Renal impairment • ONJ • Atypical femur fractures • Hypocalcemia • Myalgia/ arthralgia • Acute-phase reaction (fever, myalgia, flu-like symptoms)	• BMD • Renal function • Serum calcium concentrations • Serum 25(OH)D concentrations	• ↑ risk of hypocalcemia with loop diuretics • ↑ risk of nephrotoxicity with other nephrotoxic drugs (aminoglycosides, NSAIDs)	Acetaminophen may be given after drug is administered to minimize acute-phase reaction symptoms
Mechanism of action – selective estrogen receptor modulators: through selective binding to estrogen receptors, ↓ bone resorption and ↓ biochemical markers of bone turnover					
Raloxifene ☆ • Evista • 60 mg daily • Tabs	• History of pulmonary embolism, deep vein thrombosis, or retinal vein thrombosis • Pregnancy/ lactation	• Hot flashes • Leg cramps • Thromboembolism • Peripheral edema • ↑ sweating	• BMD • S/S of thromboembolism	Absorption ↓ by bile acid sequestrants (avoid concurrent use)	Lipid effects include ↓ low-density lipoprotein cholesterol (LDL-C) with no effect on high-density lipoprotein cholesterol (HDL-C)/triglycerides

Medications for Osteoporosis *(cont'd)*

Generic • Brand • Dose/Dosage Forms	Contraindications	Primary Side Effects	Key Monitoring Parameters	Pertinent Drug Interactions	Med Pearls
Miscellaneous Agents					
Mechanism of action – inhibits bone resorption through inhibition of osteoclast activity, to a small degree, stimulates bone formation through stimulation of osteoblast activity					
Calcitonin • Miacalcin • 1 spray (200 units) in 1 nostril daily intranasally • 100 units IM or subcut daily • Injection, nasal spray	Hypersensitivity	• Anaphylaxis • Hypocalcemia • Nasal irritation and dryness • Rhinitis • Malignancy	BMD	None	• Refrigerate injection and unopened nasal spray bottle; once opened, keep nasal spray at room temp while in use • Discard unused nasal spray after 30 days
Mechanism of action – acts as a parathyroid hormone (PTH) agonist; thereby ↑ bone formation by the stimulation of osteoblast activity and ↑ renal reabsorption of calcium					
Teriparatide • Forteo • 20 mcg subcut daily • Injection	Hypersensitivity	• Orthostatic hypotension • Dizziness • Nausea • Hypercalcemia • Hyperuricemia • Hypercalciuria	• BMD • BP • Urinary calcium • Serum calcium concentrations • Serum 25(OH)D concentrations	May predispose to digoxin toxicity	• ↓ risk of vertebral and nonvertebral fractures • Should not use for >2 yr • Black box warning: osteosarcoma • Store in refrigerator
Abaloparatide • Tymlos • 80 mcg subcut daily • Injection	None			None	
Mechanism of action – monoclonal antibody, bone-modifying agent					
Denosumab • Prolia • 60 mg subcut every 6 mo • Injection	• Hypersensitivity • Hypocalcemia • Pregnancy	• Anaphylaxis • Hypocalcemia • ONJ • Atypical femur fractures • Skin infections • Rash • Myalgia/arthralgia • Hyperlipidemia	• BMD • Serum calcium concentrations • Serum 25(OH)D concentrations • Serum phosphorus concentrations • Serum magnesium concentrations	None	Store in refrigerator

GOUT

Treatment of Acute Gouty Arthropathy

- Asymptomatic hyperuricemia does not require therapy.

- First-line treatment for gout includes the use of an NSAID. The majority of acute gout attacks will respond to an NSAID within 72 hours of therapy. Indomethacin is the most common NSAID used in the treatment of gout, but other NSAIDs are also appropriate. Please see the medication charts in the Pain Management chapter for more specific NSAID information.

- If patients have a contraindication to the use of an NSAID, evaluation of the time course of symptoms is necessary.

    - If gout symptoms have been present for <48 hours, colchicine is recommended for acute treatment.

    - If gout symptoms have been present for >48 hours, use of a corticosteroid is recommended.

- If the patient demonstrates an inadequate response to either NSAIDs or colchicine, corticosteroids should be considered.

- The use of oral (preferred) or parenteral corticosteroids is recommended for multi-joint involvement, while an intra-articular corticosteroid can be used to target one specific symptomatic joint.

- Allopurinol or febuxostat should never be used in the treatment of acute gout. These agents are reserved for chronic prophylactic therapy in patients with multiple gout exacerbations each year. If these agents are used in the treatment of an acute gout exacerbation, the symptoms may be worsened due to the mobilization of uric acid stores.

Prophylaxis of Gout

- Colchicine maintenance therapy is indicated for prophylaxis in patients with only slightly elevated serum uric acid levels.

- Allopurinol is indicated for prophylaxis of gout exacerbations in patients with a moderately elevated serum uric acid level and a history of nephrolithiasis, tophi, serum creatinine >2.0 mg/dL, or urinary uric acid excretion indicative of overproduction.

- Uricosuric drugs are indicated for prophylaxis of gout exacerbations in patients who are not candidates for allopurinol or febuxostat therapy and have a urinary uric acid excretion indicative of underexcretion.

- When initiating prophylactic therapy in a patient with gout, colchicine should be initiated with allopurinol, febuxostat, or a uricosuric and continued for the first 3–6 months of therapy to avoid causing an exacerbation.

- Pegloticase is indicated for refractory chronic gout in patients that do not respond to or have contraindications to traditional therapy.

Gout Treatment Summary

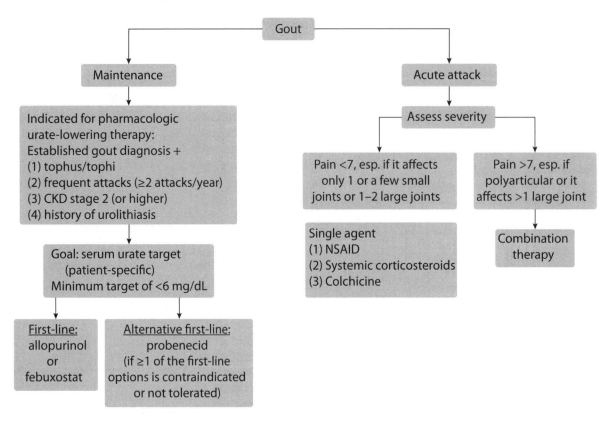

Drugs for Gout

Generic • Brand • Dose & Max	Contraindications	Primary Side Effects	Key Monitoring Parameters	Pertinent Drug Interactions	Med Pearls
Mechanism of action – inhibits lactic acid production, decreases uric acid deposition, reduces phagocytosis, and decreases inflammation					
Colchicine • Colcrys, Mitigare • 1.2 mg then 0.6 mg 1 hr later (max = 1.8 mg) • Caps, tabs	• Hypersensitivity • Serious GI, renal, hepatic or cardiac disorders	• N/V/D • Rare: bone marrow suppression, aplastic anemia, thrombocytopenia	• Serum uric acid • GI symptoms • Periodic CBC	• CYP3A4 and P-glycoprotein substrate • CYP3A4 inhibitors may ↑ effects/ toxicity • CYP3A4 inducers may ↓ effects	• Patients may be provided with a prescription to be filled on a PRN basis and used during an exacerbation • Used for treatment and prophylaxis
Mechanism of action – xanthine oxidase inhibitor: by inhibition of xanthine oxidase, impairs the conversion of xanthine to uric acid, thereby ↓ the production of uric acid					
Allopurinol☆ • Zyloprim • 100–800 mg daily • Tabs	Hypersensitivity	• Rash (Stevens-Johnson syndrome possible) • Leukopenia • GI upset	• Serum uric acid concentrations • Renal function	May ↑ levels/ risk of toxicity of mercaptopurine and azathioprine (↓ dose of mercaptopurine and azathioprine to 25% of usual dose)	Adjust dose in renal impairment
Febuxostat • Uloric • 40–80 mg daily • Tabs	Concurrent use with azathioprine or mercaptopurine	• ↑ LFTs • Arthralgia	• LFTs (2 and 4 months after initiation and periodically thereafter) • Serum uric acid concentrations	• May ↑ levels/ risk of toxicity of mercaptopurine and azathioprine (contraindicated) • May ↑ levels/ risk of toxicity of theophylline	• No renal dose adjustment necessary • Not to be used during acute gout flares
Mechanism of action – uricosuric agents: ↑ the renal clearance of uric acid by inhibiting tubular reabsorption					
Probenecid • Only available generically • 250–1,000 mg BID • Tabs	• Hypersensitivity • CrCl <50 mL/min • History of renal calculi • Overproducers of uric acid • Peptic ulcer disease	• GI upset • Rash • Nephrolithiasis	• Serum uric acid concentrations • Renal function	• May ↑ levels/ risk of toxicity of methotrexate • May ↑ levels of penicillins	May precipitate acute gouty attacks; avoid use during acute gouty arthritis

Drugs for Gout *(cont'd)*

Generic • Brand • Dose & Max	Contraindications	Primary Side Effects	Key Monitoring Parameters	Pertinent Drug Interactions	Med Pearls
Mechanism of action – catalyzes oxidation of uric acid to allantoin, thereby ↓ serum uric acid concentrations					
Pegloticase • Krystexxa • 8 mg IV infusion (over >2 hr) every 2 wk • Injection	• Glucose-6-phosphate-dehydrogenase deficiency • Risk of hemolysis • Methemoglobinemia	• Acute gout exacerbation • Infusion reactions • Anaphylaxis • HF exacerbation	• Serum uric acid concentrations • S/S of anaphylaxis/ infusion reactions 1 hr after infusion • S/S of HF exacerbation	None	• Indicated only for refractory cases • Patient should receive pre-treatment with antihistamine and corticosteroid • Gout flare prophylaxis with colchicine or NSAID 1 wk prior to administration is recommended
Mechanism of action – inhibits the transporter proteins involved in renal uric acid reabsorption, uric acid transporter 1 (URAT1), and organic anion transporter 4 (OAT4), which ↓ serum uric acid concentrations and ↑ renal clearance of uric acid					
Lesinurad • Zurampic • 200 mg daily • Tabs	• CrCl <45 mL/min • Kidney transplant recipients • Tumor lysis syndrome	• Headache • ↑ serum creatinine • Acute renal failure • Nephrolithiasis • Gastroesophageal reflux disease	• Serum uric acid concentrations • Renal function	• CYP2C9 substrate • CYP2C9 inhibitors may ↑ effects/ toxicity • CYP2C9 inducers may ↓ effects • May ↓ effects of hormonal contraceptives	Must be used in combination with xanthine oxidase inhibitor

PRACTICE QUESTIONS

1. Which of the following is NOT correctly matched with its trade name?

    (A) Methotrexate – Rheumatrex
    (B) Hydroxychloroquine – Azulfidine
    (C) Leflunomide – Arava
    (D) Etanercept – Enbrel
    (E) Infliximab – Remicade

2. A 60-year-old woman on etanercept 50 mg subcutaneously once weekly is requesting that her immunizations be updated. Which immunization would be contraindicated?

    (A) Varicella zoster
    (B) Seasonal influenza vaccine (intramuscular)
    (C) 23-valent pneumococcal vaccine
    (D) Tetanus, diphtheria, pertussis (Tdap)

3. A 64-year-old asymptomatic man with a medical history significant for hypertension and obesity takes bisoprolol 5 mg daily. His serum uric acid concentration is 7.3 mg/dL on routine laboratory examination. Which is the MOST appropriate therapeutic strategy?

    (A) Start allopurinol 100 mg/day.
    (B) Start febuxostat 40 mg/day.
    (C) Start probenecid 500 mg twice daily.
    (D) Therapy is not indicated because the patient has not yet experienced a gout attack.

4. A 52-year-old man with a medical history of hypertension, obesity, and gout (one episode, 6 months ago) takes enalapril 40 mg daily, amlodipine 10 mg daily, and aspirin 81 mg daily. He presents with symptoms, starting this morning, of gout in his left first metatarsophalangeal joint and left ankle. The metatarsophalangeal joint is swollen, inflamed, erythematous, and sensitive to light touch. Which is the BEST approach to therapy?

    (A) Colchicine 1.2 mg by mouth, then 0.6 mg 1 hour later
    (B) Colchicine 1.2 mg by mouth, then 0.6 mg 1 hour later; start allopurinol 300 mg once daily
    (C) Colchicine 1.2 mg by mouth, then 0.6 mg every hour as tolerated
    (D) Colchicine 1.2 mg by mouth, then 0.6 mg every hour as tolerated; start allopurinol 300 mg once daily

5. An 80-year-old woman is diagnosed with osteoarthritis of the right hand. Her medical history is significant for of peptic ulcer disease (PUD), hypertension, and hyperlipidemia. Which is the MOST appropriate therapy recommendation?

   (A) Glucosamine sulfate 500 mg by mouth three times daily
   (B) Naproxen 500 mg by mouth twice daily
   (C) Diclofenac 1% gel topically four times daily
   (D) Duloxetine 60 mg by mouth once daily

6. A 62-year-old man with hyperlipidemia, allergic rhinitis, and a history of PUD with an upper gastrointestinal bleed 2 years ago is diagnosed with osteoarthritis of the knee. He has tried maximum-dose, scheduled acetaminophen with insufficient pain relief. Current medications include atorvastatin and loratadine. Which is the BEST recommendation for the management of this patient's osteoarthritis of the knee?

   (A) Naproxen
   (B) Naproxen plus esomeprazole
   (C) Intraarticular corticosteroid
   (D) Diclofenac topical gel

7. A 44-year-old woman is newly diagnosed with rheumatoid arthritis (determined to be moderate–high disease activity) following more than 3 months of bilateral symptoms involving her metacarpophalangeal (MCP) and wrist joints. Laboratory results include AST 33 IU/L, ALT 36 IU/L, SCr 1.0 mg/dL, Hgb 13 g/dL, Hct 39%, (+) RF. Which is the MOST appropriate therapy selection?

   (A) Hydroxychloroquine
   (B) Methotrexate
   (C) Leflunomide
   (D) Adalimumab

8. A 56-year-old woman with rheumatoid arthritis complains of worsening joint pain in wrists and elbows over the past month. Upon physical exam, new rheumatoid nodules are noted on both elbows. Current medications include adalimumab, methotrexate, and folic acid. Prior medications include hydroxychloroquine (in combination with methotrexate), leflunomide, and etanercept. Which is the MOST appropriate therapy recommendation?

   (A) Replace adalimumab with abatacept
   (B) Replace methotrexate with sulfasalazine
   (C) Add sulfasalazine
   (D) Add minocycline

9. A 72-year-old woman with osteoporosis and a history of multiple vertebral fractures presents with intolerance to both alendronate and risedronate due to dyspepsia and esophageal irritation. She has followed administration instructions closely but continues to complain of bothersome side effects and indicates that she will no longer consider taking the medications. Her medical history is significant for chronic heart failure and history of venous thromboembolism (×2). Current medications include calcium, vitamin D, lisinopril, digoxin, furosemide, and rivaroxaban. Which of the following is the MOST appropriate therapy for her osteoporosis?

   (A) Ibandronate
   (B) Raloxifene
   (C) Denosumab
   (D) Teriparitide

ANSWERS AND EXPLANATIONS

1. **B**

Hydroxychloroquine is generic for Plaquenil. Azulfidine is the brand name for sulfasalazine. The other answer choices are correctly matched with their trade names. Methotrexate (A) is generic for Rheumatrex or Trexall.

2. **A**

Patients with RA receiving biologic DMARDs should not be administered live vaccines such as varicella zoster. Trivalent seasonal influenza vaccine (B) and 23-valent pneumococcal vaccine (C) are acceptable to give to all patients, according to the schedule recommended by the Centers for Disease Control and Prevention (CDC) and Advisory Committee on Immunization Practices (ACIP). The Tdap vaccine (D) may also be safely administered to patients who are considered (non-HIV) immune compromised or receiving immune system–compromising agents.

3. **D**

Patients should not receive treatment for asymptomatic hyperuricemia until they have experienced their first gouty attack. One to 2 weeks after the first attack, patients may begin uric acid–lowering therapy, and they should be treated to a serum uric acid concentration of <6 mg/dL.

4. **A**

Because this patient is suffering from an acute gouty attack, the use of allopurinol (B and D) is not appropriate. Allopurinol should be initiated only after the episode of acute gout has resolved. With respect to the colchicine dose, current recommendations support the lower cumulative dose due to equal efficacy and superior tolerability (fewer GI adverse events). The "as-tolerated" instructions for choices (C) and (D) put the patient at risk of overdosing and could potentially cause the patient GI adverse effects and even life-threatening hematologic effects.

5. **C**

First-line options for osteoarthritis of the hand include topical and oral NSAIDs, topical capsaicin, and tramadol. The ACR 2012 guidelines do not recommend glucosamine (A) for the treatment of OA of the hand. For patients over age 75, topical NSAIDs are preferred over oral NSAIDs, making choice (B) incorrect. Although duloxetine (D) is a second-line option in osteoarthritis of the knee and hip, this agent is not recommended prior to topical NSAIDs and is not preferred in OA of the hand.

6. **B**

Patients with a history of a GI bleed >1 year ago should receive an NSAID plus a proton pump inhibitor (B) or a COX2 selective NSAID. According to the ACR 2012 guidelines, oral NSAIDs such as naproxen (A) are the first-line option following inadequate response to maximum dose acetaminophen in patients with OA of the knee. Duloxetine, tramadol, and intraarticular injections (C) are reserved for patients with NSAID nonresponse or NSAID contraindications. Diclofenac topical gel (D) is also reserved for patients with NSAID contraindication or over the age of 75.

7. **B**

According to the 2015 ACR recommendations, treatment-naive patients with moderate–high disease activity should receive combination DMARD therapy with methotrexate unless contraindicated.

8. **A**

Based upon the 2015 ACR recommendations for rheumatoid arthritis treatment in patients with established disease, health care providers should replace adalimumab in patients with high disease activity (persistently worsening symptoms on escalating therapy); the options include an alternate anti-TNF agent, rituximab, or abatacept. Using an alternate nonbiologic DMARD such as sulfasalazine in place of (B) or in addition to methotrexate (C) would not likely alter the disease progression or symptoms at this stage. Minocycline (D) is reserved for patients with low disease activity and good prognostic features.

9. **C**

Denosumab is an appropriate agent for the treatment of osteoporosis in postmenopausal female patients at high risk of fracture (prior fractures) that have been intolerant to or failed alternate therapy options. Ibandronate (A) is a bisphosphonate; although this is the first-line class, the patient has not tolerated two agents in this class of medications. Raloxifene (B) is contraindicated due to the patient's history of venous thromboembolism. Teriparatide (D) would be an appropriate selection in a patient with osteoporosis and a history of fracture but would interact with this patient's digoxin, increasing the risk of digoxin toxicity.

Hematologic Disorders

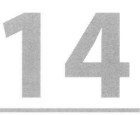

This chapter covers the following diseases:

- **Iron deficiency anemia**
- **Anemia of chronic kidney disease and dialysis**
- **Megaloblastic anemias**
- **Sickle cell disease**

IRON DEFICIENCY ANEMIA

Guidelines Summary

In children, adolescents, and women of reproductive age, a trial of iron is a reasonable approach if the review of symptoms, history, and physical examination are negative; however, the Hgb should be checked at one month. If there is not a 1 g/dL ↑ in the Hgb level in that time, possibilities include malabsorption of oral iron, lack of compliance, continued bleeding, or presence of an unknown lesion.

- Dose of elemental iron needed to treat IDA is 120 mg per for 3 months in adults and 3 mg/kg/day in children (max of 60 mg/day).
- An ↑ in the Hgb level of 1 g/dL after 1 month of treatment is an indicator of adequate response to iron therapy.
- Therapy should be continued for 3 months after correction of IDA to allow for replenishment of iron stores.
- Iron sulfate in a dose of 325 mg provides 65 mg of elemental iron, whereas 30 mg of iron gluconate provides 38 mg of elemental iron.
- GI absorption of elemental iron is enhanced in the presence of an acidic gastric environment, which can be accomplished through simultaneous intake of ascorbic acid (i.e., vitamin C).

- Patients should be counseled to take iron 2 hours before or 4 hours after antacids to minimize the potential for chelation and decreased absorption.

- Although iron absorption occurs more readily when taken on an empty stomach, this ↑ the likelihood of iron-induced stomach upset. The increased patient adherence that may result from taking the iron with food should be weighed against the inferior iron absorption that may occur.

- Laxatives, stool softeners, and adequate intake of liquids can alleviate the constipating effects of oral iron therapy.

- Indications for the use of intravenous (IV) iron include:

  - Intestinal malabsorption

  - Intolerance to oral iron, which often results in patient nonadherence

Medications for Iron Deficiency Anemia

Generic • Brand • Dose/Dosage Forms	Contraindications	Primary Side Effects	Key Monitoring	Pertinent Drug Interactions	Med Pearl
Mechanism of action – replaces iron found in Hgb, myoglobin; allows the transportation of oxygen via Hgb					
Ferrous sulfate, gluconate, fumarate • Sulfate: Fer-In-Sol, Fer-Iron, Slow-Fe • Gluconate: Ferate • Fumarate: Ferretts • Sulfate: 300 mg 2–4 × /day • Gluconate/fumarate: 60 mg 2–4 × /day • ER tabs, solution, tabs	• Hypersensitivity to iron salts • Hemochromatosis (GI tract absorbs excess iron) • Hemolytic anemia	• GI irritation • Epigastric pain • Nausea/vomiting (N/V) • Dark stools • Stomach cramping • Constipation	• Serum iron • TIBC • Serum ferritin • Reticulocyte count • Hgb/Hct	• ↓ absorption of tetracyclines, fluoroquinolones, levodopa, methyldopa, and penicillamine • Proton pump inhibitors (PPIs), H$_2$ blockers, and antacids can ↓ iron absorption	Administer with vitamin C or orange juice to ↑ absorption

Medications for Iron Deficiency Anemia *(cont'd)*

Generic • Brand • Dose/Dosage Forms	Contraindications	Primary Side Effects	Key Monitoring	Pertinent Drug Interactions	Med Pearl
Mechanism of action – iron complex taken up by reticuloendothelial system and then released for storage or for transport and incorporation into Hgb; eventually replenishes depleted iron stores in the bone marrow					
Iron dextran complex • Infed (IM or IV) • Dose (in mL) = 0.0442 (desired Hgb − observed Hgb) × lean body weight (LBW) + (0.26 × LBW) • Max dose = 100 mg/day	Hypersensitivity	• Anaphylaxis • Hypotension • Tightness in the chest • Wheezing • Flushing	• Anaphylactic reaction • Serum iron • TIBC • Serum ferritin • Transferrin saturation • Reticulocyte count • Hgb/Hct • Blood pressure • Heart rate	None	• Test dose is required • Anaphylaxis may still occur despite having an uneventful test dose • If flushing or hypotension occur, ↓ infusion rate
Sodium ferric gluconate • Ferrlecit • 125 mg via IV infusion (usually × 8 doses) • Injection	Hypersensitivity	• Anaphylaxis • Tachycardia • Hypotension • Chest pain • Dizziness		May ↓ absorption of oral iron	• A safer form of parenteral iron compared to iron dextran • No test dose required
Ferumoxytol • Feraheme • 510 mg via IV infusion followed by 510 mg via IV infusion 3–8 days later • Injection	• Hypersensitivity • History of allergic reaction to any IV iron product	• Anaphylaxis • Diarrhea • Constipation • Hypotension • Dizziness			• Patients with multiple drug allergies at ↑ risk for anaphylactic reaction • May interfere with MRI readings for up to 3 mo after use • No test dose required
Iron sucrose • Venofer • Hemodialysis-dependent: 100 mg IV 1–3 ×/wk during dialysis until cumulative dose of 1,000 mg achieved (10 doses) • Peritoneal dialysis-dependent: 300 mg IV, then 300 mg IV 14 days later, then 400 mg IV 14 days later • No dialysis: 200 mg IV administered on 5 separate occasions during a 14-day time period • Injection	Hypersensitivity	• Anaphylaxis • Hypotension • Headache • Chest pain • Dizziness			• Can be administered as a slow IV injection (2–5 min) or as an IV infusion (time is dose dependent) • No test dose required
Ferric carboxymaltose • Injectafer • <50 kg: 15 mg/kg IV, then 15 mg/kg IV ≥7 days later (max = 1500 mg/treatment course) • ≥50 kg: 750 mg IV, then 750 mg IV ≥7 days later • Injection	Hypersensitivity	• Anaphylaxis • Hypertension • Nausea • Flushing • Hypophosphatemia • Dizziness		Unknown	• Can be administered as a slow IV injection (100 mg/min) or as an IV infusion (over ≥15 min) • No test dose required

ANEMIA OF CHRONIC KIDNEY DISEASE AND DIALYSIS

Guidelines Summary

- Treatment guidelines are based on Hgb.
- ESAs should be used with caution in patients with malignancy if cure of malignancy is an option or if anemia can be managed via transfusion.
- The upper limit of Hgb should not exceed 11.5 g/dL in adults.
- In adults, ESAs should not be used to intentionally ↑ the Hgb > 13 g/dL.
- In pediatric patients, the range of Hgb should be 11–12 g/dL.
- Iron therapy may be used if transferrin saturation is < 30% and ferritin is < 500 ng/mL.

Medications for Anemia of Chronic Kidney Disease and Dialysis

Generic • Brand • Dose/Dosage Forms	Contraindications	Primary Side Effects	Key Monitoring	Pertinent Drug Interactions	Med Pearl
Erythropoietin Stimulating Agents					
Mechanism of action – induce erythropoiesis by stimulating the division and differentiation of committed erythroid progenitor cells; induce the release of reticulocytes from the bone marrow into the bloodstream					
Epoetin alfa • Procrit, Epogen • Initial: 50–100 units/kg IV or subcut 3 × /wk • Injection Darbepoetin alfa • Aranesp • CKD patients on dialysis: 0.45 mcg/kg IV or subcut weekly or 0.75 mcg/kg IV or subcut every 2 wk • CKD patients not on dialysis: 0.45 mcg/kg IV or subcut every 4 wk • Injection	• Hypersensitivity • Uncontrolled hypertension • Pure red cell aplasia	• Hypertension • ↑ mortality, myocardial infarction, stroke, or thromboembolism (if target Hgb >11 g/dL) • Seizures • Peripheral edema • Headache • Nausea • Arthralgia	• Hgb • Ferritin • Transferrin saturation • Iron stores • Blood pressure	None	• IV route preferred for patients on hemodialysis • In patients with CKD on dialysis, initiate treatment if Hgb <10 g/dL • Do not ↑ dose more frequently than every 4 wk • If Hgb ↑ by >1 g/dL in a 2-wk period, ↓ dose by ≥25% • If Hgb has not ↑ by >1 g/dL in 4-wk period, ↑ dose by 25% • For CKD patients on dialysis, if Hgb >11 g/dL, ↓ or interrupt dose • For CKD patients NOT on dialysis, if Hgb >10 g/dL, ↓ or interrupt dose

Medications for Anemia of Chronic Kidney Disease and Dialysis *(cont'd)*

Generic • Brand • Dose/Dosage Forms	Contraindications	Primary Side Effects	Key Monitoring	Pertinent Drug Interactions	Med Pearl
Dialysate Iron Replacement					
Mechanism of action – binds to transferrin for incorporation into hemoglobin					
Ferric pyrophosphate citrate • Triferic • 1 ampule: 2.5 gal. bicarbonate concentrate; 2 micromolar concentration	Hypersensitivity	• Peripheral edema • Urinary tract infection • Pain • Headache • Fatigue • Fistula thrombosis • Fistula hemorrhage	Predialysis iron status	None	Only used in dialysis patients

MEGALOBLASTIC ANEMIAS

Treatment Summary

- No major guidelines have been recently published on the treatment of pernicious anemia or folate deficiency.

- Treatment is directed toward replacing the deficient factor.

- Blood transfusions are rarely required.

- Treatment is often initiated with intramuscular injections before moving to oral formulations.

- With therapy, reticulocytosis should begin within 1 week, followed by an ↑ Hgb over 6–8 weeks.

- Coexisting iron deficiency is present in one-third of patients and is a common cause of incomplete response to therapy with vitamin B_{12} or folic acid.

Medications for Megaloblastic Anemias

Generic • Brand • Dose/Dosage Forms	Contraindications	Primary Side Effects	Key Monitoring	Pertinent Drug Interactions	Med Pearl
Mechanism of action – coenzyme for various metabolic functions, cell replication, and hematopoiesis					
Cyanocobalamin (vitamin B_{12}) • Nascobal • IM: Initial: 100– 1,000 mcg daily for 1 wk, then 100–1,000 mcg every 1–3 months • PO: 500–2,000 mcg daily, maintenance 1,000 mcg daily • Intranasal: 500 mcg in 1 nostril weekly	Hypersensitivity	• Anxiety • Itching • Diarrhea	• Serum vitamin B_{12} • Hgb/Hct • Reticulocyte count • Serum folate • Serum iron	• Metformin and PPIs may ↓ vitamin B_{12} absorption	Hydroxocobalamin is a longer-acting form of vitamin B_{12}
Mechanism of action – coenzyme in many metabolic systems, particularly for purine and pyrimidine synthesis					
Folic acid (folate) ☆ • Only available generically • 0.4–1 mg daily • Prevention of neural tube defects: 0.4–0.8 mg daily	Hypersensitivity	• Allergic reaction • Bronchospasm • Flushing • Malaise • Pruritus • Rash	• Serum folate • Hgb/Hct • Reticulocyte count • Serum iron	• May ↓ phenytoin and phenobarbital levels • Phenytoin and sulfasalazine may ↓ folate absorption	Products containing >0.8 mg of folic acid are Rx only

SICKLE CELL DISEASE

Guidelines Summary

Medication related considerations for patients with SCD:

- Prevent pneumococcal disease with the use of immunizations. Penicillin may also be used as a prophylactic agent up to age 5.

- Progestin-only hormonal contraceptives, levonorgestrel and intrauterine devices can be used in patients with SCD without concern.

- Rapidly assess and treat pain using nonopioid and opioid analgesics.

- May consider the use of hydroxyurea if an adult patient experiences three or more moderate-to-severe pain crises in a 12-month period.

PRACTICE QUESTIONS

1. Which of the following can be administered with ferrous sulfate to increase absorption?

    (A) Ascorbic acid
    (B) Calcium carbonate
    (C) Famotidine
    (D) Omeprazole

2. Which of the following is an adverse effect associated with epoetin alfa?

    (A) Bradycardia
    (B) Constipation
    (C) Hypertension
    (D) Thrombocytopenia

3. Absorption of which of the following medications may be impaired if given concurrently with oral ferrous sulfate? (Select ALL that apply.)

    (A) Amoxicillin
    (B) Ciprofloxacin
    (C) Tetracycline
    (D) Trimethoprim

4. JJ is a 28-year-old female who just confirmed that she is pregnant. Which of the following should be recommended for JJ to prevent neural tube defects?

    (A) Cyanocobalamin
    (B) Ferrous gluconate
    (C) Ferumoxytol
    (D) Folic acid

5. Which of the following is a precaution for using darbepoetin?

    (A) BP of 110/72
    (B) CKD
    (C) HgB of 13 g/dL
    (D) Palliative chemotherapy

6. Which of the following statements regarding cyanocobalamin is TRUE?

    (A) Injection solution is red to pink in color.
    (B) It is used for the treatment of folate deficiency.
    (C) It must be initiated with the nasal form.
    (D) Levels may be depleted by sulfonylureas.

ANSWERS AND EXPLANATIONS

1. **A**

Oral iron products need an acidic environment for absorption. Ascorbic acid (vitamin C) or a glass of orange juice can be administered with oral iron products to increase absorption. Calcium carbonate (B) is an antacid, famotidine (C) is an H_2 agonist, and omeprazole (D) is a proton pump inhibitor; all of these would decrease the acidification needed for iron absorption.

2. **C**

Hypertension is associated with the use of ESAs and should be monitored for while on therapy. If a patient has uncontrolled HTN before starting ESAs, it may preclude the use until the blood pressure is more optimally managed. Bradycardia (A), constipation (B), and thrombocytopenia (D) are not associated with ESAs.

3. **B, C**

Oral iron products can bind to both quinolone and tetracycline antibiotics, leading to a decreased serum concentration for the quinolone or tetracycline antibiotic if given concurrently. If iron needs to be given with either a quinolone or a tetracycline antibiotic, the antibiotic should be given 2–4 hours prior to or 2–8 hours after the oral iron product is administered.

4. **D**

Folic acid can be used to prevent neural tube defects. Cyanocobalamin (A) (vitamin B_{12}) is used to increase B_{12} levels and prevent pernicious anemia. Ferrous gluconate (B) and ferumoxytol (C) are used to increase iron levels.

5. **C**

ESA agents should not be used to maintain a Hgb > 13 g/dL, due to adverse cardiovascular events. ESAs may increase BP (A) but are only contraindicated in patients with uncontrolled HTN. CKD (B) is an indication for use of ESAs, but the upper limit of Hgb should not exceed 11.5 g/dL in adults. ESAs can be used in patients receiving palliative chemotherapy (D), but they should not be used in patients receiving curative chemotherapy.

6. **A**

The injection solution for cyanocobalamin is red to pink and is stable at room temperature. Cyanocobalamin is used to treat B_{12} deficiency, not folate deficiency (B). B_{12} therapy is often initiated with the IM formulation and is then transitioned to oral therapy; the nasal formulation (C) is rarely used. Levels of B_{12} may be depleted with metformin, not sulfonylureas (D).

Antidotes

16

The following chapter addresses drugs that are used as antagonist drugs:

- **General antidotes**

GENERAL ANTIDOTES

Activated Charcoal

Activated charcoal absorbs a wide range of toxins and is often given to reduce absorption within the GI tract. A single dose is generally effective, particularly if it is given within 1 hour of ingestion. Delayed use, however, may be beneficial for modified-release preparations or for drugs that slow GI transit time, such as those with antimuscarinic properties. Charcoal is generally well tolerated, although vomiting is common, and there is a risk of aspiration if the airway is not adequately protected. Repeated doses may be useful in eliminating some substances even after systemic absorption has occurred.

Active removal of poisons from the stomach by induction of emesis or gastric lavage has been widely used, but there is little evidence to support its role. Emesis should not be induced if the poison is corrosive or petroleum-based, or if the poison is removable by treatment with activated charcoal.

Gastric Lavage

Gastric lavage may occasionally be indicated for ingestion of noncaustic poisons that are not absorbed by activated charcoal, but only if less than 1 hour has elapsed since ingestion. Gastric lavage should not be attempted if the airway is not adequately protected.

Whole-bowel irrigation using a nonabsorbable osmotic agent such as a macrogol has also been used, particularly for substances that pass beyond the stomach before being absorbed (e.g., iron preparations or enteric-coated or modified-release formulations); however, its role is not established.

Antidotes

Toxic/Overdose Substance	Generic Name for Antidote • Brand Name/Dosage Form • Dose	Contraindications	Primary Side Effects	Key Monitoring	Med Pearl
Mechanism of action – pure opioid antagonist that competes and displaces narcotics at opioid receptor sites					
Opioids	Naloxone • Narcan, Evzio • 0.4–2 mg IV/IM/subcut every 2–3 min PRN; after reversal, repeat dose every 20–60 min PRN • Evzio: 0.4 mg IM/subcut every 2 min until emergency medical assistance is available • Narcan Nasal Spray: 1 spray (4 mg) every 2–3 min in alternating nostrils until emergency medical assistance is available • Injection, nasal spray	Hypersensitivity	• Tachycardia • Anxiety • Diaphoresis • Agitation • ↑ blood pressure (BP)	• Respiratory rate (RR) • Heart rate (HR) • BP	• Adverse effects can occur secondarily to reversal (withdrawal) • IV route is preferred due to quick effect • Nasal spray onset is longest (~8–13 min)
Mechanism of action – acts as a competitive antagonist at opioid receptor sites					
Opioids	Naltrexone • Vivitrol • PO: 25 mg initially, then 50 mg daily on weekdays with 100 mg on Saturdays **OR** 100 mg every other day; **OR** 150 mg every 3 days • IM: 380 mg every 4 wk • Injection, tabs	• Hypersensitivity • Acute opioid withdrawal • Failure to pass naloxone challenge • Positive urine drug screen for opioids	• Hepatotoxicity • Syncope • Headache • Sedation • Nausea/vomiting (N/V) • Depression • Suicidality • Injection site reactions • Muscle cramps	• Opioid withdrawal • Liver function tests (LFTs) • Mental status	• Do not give until patient is opioid-free for 7–10 days (to minimize risk of withdrawal) • Indicated for treatment of alcohol and opioid dependence • Highest affinity for mu receptors

Antidotes *(cont'd)*

Mechanism of action – competitively inhibits the activity at the benzodiazepine recognition site on the GABA/benzodiazepine complex

Toxic/Overdose Substance	Generic Name for Antidote • Brand Name/Dosage Form • Dose	Contraindications	Primary Side Effects	Key Monitoring	Med Pearl
Benzodiazepines	Flumazenil • Only available generically • 0.2 mg IV over 30 sec; if desired consciousness not achieved 30 sec after dose, repeat with 0.3 mg IV over 30 sec; if desired consciousness not achieved, can then repeat with 0.5 mg IV over 30 sec every minute • Injection	• Hypersensitivity • Receiving benzodiazepine for potentially life-threatening condition • Showing signs of serious cyclic antidepressant overdosage	• Palpitations • Blurred vision • Ataxia • Agitation • Dizziness • Seizures • ↑ sweating • Headache	• BP • HR • RR • Benzodiazepine reversal may result in seizures in some patients • May cause return of residual effects of benzodiazepines	• If patient has not responded 5 min after receiving a cumulative dose of 5 mg, the sedation is likely not due to benzodiazepines • Reversal may affect nonbenzodiazepines (eszopiclone, zaleplon, zolpidem)

Mechanism of action – competitively inhibits alcohol dehydrogenase, an enzyme that catalyzes the metabolism of ethanol, methanol, and ethylene glycol

• Methanol • Ethylene glycol	Fomepizole • Antizol • 15 mg/kg IV, then 10 mg/kg IV every 12 hr × 4 doses, then 15 mg/kg IV every 12 hr until ethylene glycol levels <20 mg/L and patient asymptomatic (with normal pH) • Injection	Hypersensitivity	• Headache • Nausea • Metallic taste • Drowsiness • Dizziness	• Plasma/urinary ethylene glycol or methanol concentrations • Plasma/urinary osmolality • Renal function • LFTs • Electrolytes • Arterial blood gas • Anion/osmolar gaps • S/S of methanol or ethylene glycol toxicity	• Therapy should be initiated immediately upon suspicion of methanol or ethylene glycol ingestion • Can be used alone or with hemodialysis

Mechanism of action – inhibits destruction of acetylcholine by acetylcholinesterase which prolongs effects of acetylcholine

Anticholinergic drugs	Physostigmine • Only available generically • 0.5–2 mg IM/IV to start; repeat every 10–30 min until response • Injection	• GI or genitourinary obstruction • Asthma • Gangrene • Severe cardiovascular disease • Concurrent use of depolarizing neuromuscular blocking agents	• Palpitation • Bradycardia • Restlessness • Seizure	• HR • RR • Electrocardiogram (ECG)	

Antidotes *(cont'd)*

Toxic/Overdose Substance	Generic Name for Antidote • Brand Name/Dosage Form • Dose	Contraindications	Primary Side Effects	Key Monitoring	Med Pearl
Mechanism of action – antigen-binding fragments (Fab) are specific for the treatment of digitalis intoxication					
Digoxin	Digoxin immune Fab • DigiFab • 40 mg will bind to 0.5 mg of digoxin • Injection	Hypersensitivity to sheep products	• Exacerbation of heart failure • Rapid ventricular response • Hypokalemia	• Serum potassium • BP • ECG • Renal function	Serum digoxin levels will greatly ↑ with digoxin immune Fab use and are not an accurate determination of body stores; do not monitor serum digoxin concentrations for several days to >1 wk
Mechanism of action – supplies a free thiol group which binds to and inactivates acrolein, the urotoxic metabolite of ifosfamide and cyclophosphamide					
• Cyclophospha-mide • Ifosfamide	Mesna • Mesnex • IV-only regimen: 20% of ifosfamide dose IV at time of ifosfamide dose, and then at 4 and 8 hr after ifosfamide dose • IV and PO regimen: 20% of ifosfamide dose IV at time of ifosfamide dose, then 40% of ifosfamide dose PO at 2 and 6 hr after ifosfamide dose • Injection, tabs	Hypersensitivity	• Anaphylaxis • Rash (including Stevens-Johnson syndrome) • N/V/D • Constipation • Leukopenia • Thrombocyto-penia • Anemia • Fatigue • Fever	• Urinalysis • Inputs/outputs	Only indicated for prevention of hemor-rhagic cystitis induced by ifosfamide; off-label use for prevention of hemor-rhagic cystits induced by cyclophosphamide
Mechanism of action – cardioprotective by converting intracellularly to a ring-opened chelating agent that interferes with iron-mediated oxygen free radical generation					
Doxorubicin	Dexrazoxane • Zinecard, Totect • 10:1 ratio of dexrazoxane: doxorubicin IV administered before doxorubicin • Injection	Hypersensitivity	• Myelosuppres-sion (additive to chemo-therapy) • Phlebitis	• Complete blood count with differential • LFTs • Renal function • Echocardiogram	• Only used if patients have received cumulative doxorubicin dose of 300 mg/m^2 and are continu-ing with doxorubicin therapy • Can also be used to treat anthracycline-induced extravasation (Totect)
Mechanism of action – free thiol metabolite is available to bind to and detoxify reactive metabolites of cisplatin					
Cisplatin	Amifostine • Ethyol • 910 mg/m^2 IV daily given 30 min prior to chemotherapy • Injection	Hypersensitivity	• Hypotension • N/V • Rash (includ-ing Stevens-Johnson syndrome) • Anaphylaxis • Hypocalcemia	• BP (every 5 min during the infusion) • Serum calcium	• Indicated to ↓ cumulative renal toxicity associated with repeated cisplatin administration (in ovarian cancer) • Antiemetic recommend prior to and in conjunction with amifostine • Hold antihypertensive medications for 24 hr before amifostine therapy

Antidotes *(cont'd)*

Toxic/Overdose Substance	Generic Name for Antidote • Brand Name/Dosage Form • Dose	Contraindications	Primary Side Effects	Key Monitoring	Med Pearl
Mechanism of action — combines with strongly acidic heparin to form a stable complex (salt) neutralizing the anticoagulant activity of both drugs					
Heparin	Protamine • Only available generically • 1 mg of protamine IV neutralizes ~100 units of heparin (max dose = 50 mg) • Injection	Hypersensitivity	• Hypersensitivity • Hypotension • Flushing • Dyspnea • Thromboembolism	• Activated partial thromboplastin time (aPTT) • BP • S/S of bleeding • S/S of thromboembolic events	Will also partially reverse anticoagulant effects of low-molecular weight heparins
Mechanism of action — promotes liver synthesis of clotting factors (II, VII, IX, X) which counteracts the mechanism of warfarin					
Warfarin	Vitamin K (phytonadione) • Mephyton • Depends on international normalized ratio (INR) and bleeding risk factors (i.e., INR >10: hold warfarin and give 2.5–5 mg vitamin K PO) • Injection, tabs	Hypersensitivity	• Anaphylaxis (especially with IV administration) • Thromboembolism	• Prothrombin time (PT) • INR • S/S of bleeding • S/S of thromboembolic events	• IM route should be avoided due to hematoma formation • Subcut is the preferred parenteral route • IV recommended only when major bleeding present at any INR • Expect INR to ↓ within 24–48 hr
Mechanism of action — monocolonal antibody fragment that binds to dabigatran and its metabolites					
Dabigatran	Idarucizumab • Praxbind • 5 g administered as 2 separate doses of 2.5 g IV ≤15 min apart • Injection	None	• Headache • Thromboembolism • Hypersensitivity	• aPTT • S/S of bleeding • S/S of thromboembolic events	Will not reverse effects of apixaban, edoxaban, or rivaroxaban
Mechanism of action — reduced form of folic acid: supplies the necessary cofactor blocked by methotrexate					
Methotrexate	Leucovorin • Only available generically • 15 mg PO/IM/IV every 6 hr × 10 doses until levels normalize • Injection, tabs	Vitamin B12-deficient megaloblastic anemias	• Anaphylaxis • Rash	Plasma methotrexate concentrations	Continue leucovorin until plasma methotrexate level <0.05 mmol/L
Mechanism of action — absorbs toxic substances or irritants, thus inhibiting GI absorption					
Numerous toxic substances	Activated charcoal • Actidose • 25–100 g/dose	• Unprotected airway • Non-intact GI tract • GI perforation • Intestinal obstruction	• Hypernatremia • Hypokalemia	• Constipation • Diarrhea	Sorbitol accelerates bowel evacuation

Antidotes *(cont'd)*

Toxic/Overdose Substance	Generic Name for Antidote • Brand Name/Dosage Form • Dose	Contraindications	Primary Side Effects	Key Monitoring	Med Pearl
Mechanism of action – exact mechanism of benefit in countering acetaminophen toxicity is unknown					
Acetaminophen	Acetylcysteine • Acetadote, Cetylev • PO: 140 mg/kg, then 70 mg/kg every 4 hr × 17 doses • IV: 150 mg/kg (max = 15 g) over 60 min, then 50 mg/kg (max = 5 g) over 4 hr, then 100 mg/kg (max = 10 g) over 16 hr • Effervecent tabs, injection	Hypersensitivity	• Anaphylaxis • N/V • Rash	• Serum acetaminophen concentrations • LFTs • Bilirubin • PT/INR • Hemoglobin/ hematocrit • Renal function	• Therapy should continue until acetaminophen levels are undetectable and there is no evidence of hepatotoxicity • Treatment should begin within 8 hr of acute ingestion
Mechanism of action – blocks the action of acetylcholine at parasympathetic sites in the smooth muscle, secretory glands, and the central nervous system					
Cholinergics	Atropine • AtroPen • 2 mg IM; may repeat with 2 additional doses every 10 min	None	• Anaphylaxis • N/V • Fatigue • Insomnia • Weakness • Tachycardia	• ECG • Respiratory status • HR • BP	Dose until symptoms subside
Mechanism of action – stimulates adrenergic receptors resulting in relaxation of smooth muscle of the bronchial tree, cardiac stimulation and dilation of skeletal muscle vasculature					
Hypersensitivity reactions	Epinephrine • Adrenalin, EpiPen, EpiPen Jr. • 0.2–0.5 mg IM or subcut every 5–15 min until improvement • EpiPen Jr.: 0.15 mg IM/subcut every 5–15 min until improvement	None	• Angina • Arrhythmias • Anxiety • Flushing • Dyspnea	• RR • HR • BP	IM administration in the anterolateral aspect of the middle third of the thigh is preferred
Mechanism of action – stimulates adenylate cyclase to produce increased cyclic AMP, which promotes hepatic glycogenolysis and gluconeogenesis					
Hypoglycemia	Glucagon • GlucaGen • 1 mg IV, IM, or subcut; may repeat in 15 min as needed	• Hypersensitivity • Insulinoma • Pheochromocy-toma	• Hypersensi-tivity • Hypotension • Nausea	• BP • Blood glucose • ECG • HR • Mental status	IV dextrose should be given as soon as available

PRACTICE QUESTIONS

1. Which drug is used to decrease toxicities associated with cisplatin?

   (A) Amifostine
   (B) Physostigmine
   (C) Nalmefene
   (D) Fomepizole
   (E) Leucovorin

2. How many doses of activated charcoal are typically effective?

   (A) 1
   (B) 2
   (C) 3
   (D) 4
   (E) 5

3. AS is a 22-year-old male that was found to have ingested at unknown amount of acetaminophen. He is brought to the hospital for management of his acetaminophen overdose. Which of the following should be monitored in a patient receiving acetylcysteine?

   (A) AST
   (B) Glucose
   (C) Methotrexate concentrations
   (D) Potassium

4. MJ is a 62-year-old females that presents to the ER complaining on uncontrollable nose bleeding. She alerts the physician that she is taking warfarin and is found to have an INR of 10.6. Which of the following agents could be given to MJ to correct her INR of 10.6?

   (A) Protamine
   (B) Vitamin K
   (C) Atropine
   (D) Glucagon

5. Atropine is used to treat which of the following?

   (A) Opioid toxicity
   (B) Hemorrhagic cystitis
   (C) Hypoglycemia
   (D) Cholinergic toxicity

6. A patient accidentally ingests antifreeze and has been diagnosed with ethylene glycol toxicity. Which of the following may be helpful in treating ethylene glycol poisoning?

   (A) Atropine
   (B) Flumazenil
   (C) Fomepizole
   (D) Nalmefene

7. A patient presents with an anaphylactic reaction secondary to nafcillin therapy that was administered despite a noted penicillin allergy. Which of the following may be used to treat the anaphylactic reaction?

   (A) Acetylcysteine
   (B) Activated charcoal
   (C) Leucovorin
   (D) Epinephrine

8. Which of the following should be monitored when glucagon is administered? (Select ALL that apply.)

   (A) Blood glucose
   (B) Hemoglobin A1c
   (C) ECG
   (D) Mental status

9. Which of the following is a contraindication to using physostigmine in the treatment of anticholinergic poisoning?

   (A) Asthma
   (B) Hyperglycemia
   (C) INR >4
   (D) Opioid withdrawal

10. Before starting naltrexone, which of the following should the patient achieve?

    (A) Normalization of blood pressure
    (B) Resolution of bradycardia
    (C) Negative urine drug screen
    (D) Normalization of platelet count

ANSWERS AND EXPLANATIONS

1. **A**

Amifostine is used to prevent cisplatin toxicities associated with renal toxicity. Physostigmine (B) is used primarily to reverse toxic CNS effects caused by anticholinergic drugs. Nalmefene (C) is used as a partial reversal of opioid drug effects. Fomepizole (D) is used for methanol and ethylene glycol poisoning, and leucovorin (E) is used as an antidote for folic acid antagonist.

2. **A**

Activated charcoal typically requires only a single dose to be effective, particularly if it is given within 1 hour of toxin ingestion.

3. **A**

Acetylcysteine is used in the treatment of acetaminophen overdose, which could produce liver toxicity and/or hepatic failure. AST, ALT, bilirubin, prothrombin time, and serum creatinine should be monitored in the presence of possible liver toxicity and acetylcysteine use.

4. **B**

An elevated INR is a result of an overdosage of warfarin. Vitamin K is the reversal agent and is recommend for use in patients with an INR >10 or significant bleeding. Protamine (A) can be used to reverse heparin; atropine (C) is used to reverse cholinergic toxicity; and glucagon (D) treats hypoglycemia.

5. **D**

Atropine is used to treat cholinergic toxicity. Nalaxone is used to treat opioid overdoses or respiratory depression associated with opioids (A). Hemorrhagic cystitis (B) secondary to ifosfamide is treated with mesna, and glucagon can be used to treat hypoglycemia (C).

6. **C**

Fomepizole is the antidote for ethylene glycol or methanol toxicity; it works by inhibiting alcohol dehydrogenase. Atropine is (A) used as an antidote for cholinergic toxicity. Flumazenil (B) is used to treat benzodiazepine toxicity. Nalmefene (D) is used to reverse opioid toxicity.

7. **D**

IV or subcutaneous epinephrine is used to treat anaphylactic reactions. Epinephrine stimulates adrenergic receptors to relax bronchial smooth muscle. Acetylcysteine (A) is used in the treatment of an acetaminophen overdose. Activated charcoal (B) is used to bind a wide-variety of toxins within in the GI tract. Leucovorin (C) is administered to treat methotrexate toxicity.

8. **A, C, D**

Blood glucose, ECG, and mental status are all correct monitoring parameters for glucagon. Blood glucose is monitored to evaluate the resolution of hypoglycemia. ECG and mental status are monitored to ensure patient stability in the presence of hypoglycemia. A1c levels (B) are not monitored, because A1c is a sign of glucose control over the previous 3 months; it would not be an indication of acute glucose control.

9. **A**

Asthma may be exacerbated by physostigmine and is a contraindication in the presence of anticholinergic toxicity. Hyperglycemia (B), an elevated INR (C), and opioid withdrawal (D) are not contraindications to use of physostigmine.

10. **C**

Before starting naltrexone, a patient should be in an opioid-free state. Naltrexone is used to maintain patients in an opioid-free state and should not be used in a patient who has taken opioids in the last 7–10 days.

Reproductive Health and Urologic Disorders

17

This chapter covers the following topics:

- **Contraception**
- **Hormone replacement therapy**
- **Erectile dysfunction**
- **Benign prostatic hyperplasia**
- **Urinary incontinence**

CONTRACEPTION

Therapy Selection

Available Prescription Therapies

- Combination estrogen and progestin
  - Monophasic
  - Multiphasic
- Progestin only
- Implantable
- Emergency contraception
  - Start within 72 hours of unprotected intercourse
  - Approved over-the-counter (OTC) (regardless of age)
  - Plan B (OTC)
    - » 2 tablets 0.75 mg levonorgestrel (taken every 12 hr × 2 doses)
  - Plan B One Step (OTC)
    - » 1 tablet by mouth, levonorgestrel 1.5 mg
  - Ella (Rx only)
    - » Ulipristal acetate 30 mg by mouth within 120 hr of unprotected intercourse

Advantages and Disadvantages of Contraception

Product Type	Advantages	Disadvantages
Combination products	Long history of superior efficacy; multiple formulations allow opportunity to try multiple-dose combination of estrogen/progestin components in different dosage forms (transdermal patch, oral, multiphasic, continuous); ↓ length of menses; ↓ incidence of cramping; ↓ risk of ectopic pregnancy	Drug interactions present; need for backup contraception with missed pills
Progestin only	Can be used safely in patients who are breastfeeding, are >35 years of age, and/or have systemic lupus erythematosus or intolerable estrogen-related side effects	Slightly less effective; require even stricter compliance than combinations; higher incidence of breakthrough bleeding; need for backup contraception with missed pills
Implantable	Longer-term efficacy	Not readily reversible; requires insertion at medical office

Adverse Effects Associated with Hormonal Imbalance

Estrogen Excess	Estrogen Deficiency	Progestin Excess	Progestin Deficiency
• Breast tenderness • Cyclic weight gain • Edema • Bloating • Hypertension • Melasma • Migraine • Nausea	• Vasomotor symptoms (hot flashes) • Spotting • Breakthrough bleeding (early) • ↓ libido • Dyspareunia	• ↓ libido • Depression • Fatigue • Weight gain • Acne • Hypomenorrhea • Vaginal candidiasis	• Heavy menstruation • Weight loss • Delayed menses • Spotting • Breakthrough bleeding (late)

Pharmacologic Contraceptives

Generic • Brand • Dose & Max	Contraindications	Primary Side Effects	Key Monitoring Parameters	Pertinent Drug Interactions	Med Pearls
Hormonal Contraceptives					
Oral monophasic/high-dose estrogen					
Ethinyl estradiol and norgestrel ☆ • Ogestrel • 50 mcg E. estradiol/0.5 mg norgestrel Ethinyl estradiol and ethynodiol diacetate • Zovia 1/50 • 50 mcg E. estradiol/1 mg E. diacetate Mestranol and norethindrone ☆ • Necon 1/50, Norinyl 1/50 • 50 mcg mestranol/1 mg norethindrone	• Pregnancy • Breast cancer • History of deep vein thrombosis (DVT) or pulmonary embolism (PE) • Lactation (<6 wk postpartum) • Smoker >35 years old	• Breast tenderness • ↑ breast size • Nausea • Edema • Bloating • Cyclic weight gain • DVT/PE • Headaches during active pills • Thrombo-phlebitis (rare) *Estrogen-excess side effects most common*	• Presence of side effects • Pregnancy	↓ effect of oral contraceptive: • Antibiotics (ampicillin, sulfonamides, tetracycline) • Anticon-vulsants (phenytoin, topiramate, barbiturates) • Protease inhibitors • Rifampin Need backup method of contraception during use and for ≥1 wk after; for chronic therapy with above medications use another form of contraception	Take 1 tablet daily at the same time of day for 21 days, followed by 7 days of inactive placebo pills

Pharmacologic Contraceptives *(cont'd)*

Generic • Brand • Dose & Max	Contraindications	Primary Side Effects	Key Monitoring Parameters	Pertinent Drug Interactions	Med Pearls
Oral monophasic/low-dose estrogen					
Ethinyl estradiol and levonorgestrel • Afirmelle, Aviane, Falmina, Lessina, Orsythia • 20 mcg E. estradiol/ 0.1 mg levonorgestrel • Altavera, Ayuna, Introvale, Kurvelo, Levora, Marlissa, Portia, Seasonale, Setlakin, Quasense • 30 mcg E. estradiol/0.15 mg levonorgestrel	• Pregnancy • Breast cancer • History of DVT or PE • Lactation (<6 wk postpartum) • Smoker >35 years old	• Nausea/vomiting (N/V) • Breakthrough bleeding • Spotting • Melasma • Headache • Weight change • Edema • DVT/PE • Side effects associated with hormonal imbalance (see preceding Adverse Effects table)	• Presence of side effects • Pregnancy	↓ effect of oral contraceptive: • Antibiotics (ampicillin, sulfonamides, tetracycline) • Anticonvulsants (phenytoin, topiramate, barbiturates) • Protease inhibitors • Rifampin Need backup method of contraception during use and for ≥1 wk after; for chronic therapy with above medications use another form of contraception	Seasonale is taken continuously for 84 days with 7 placebo pills; menses only every 3 mo
Ethinyl estradiol and drospirenone☆ • Beyaz (has added folate), Loryna, Melamisa, Nikki, Safyral (has added folate), Syeda, Yaela, Yasmin, Yaz • 20–30 mcg E. estradiol/3 mg drospirenone			• Serum potassium • Pregnancy		• ↓ duration of menses • Drospirenone is a structural analog to spironolactone
Ethinyl estradiol and norgestrel☆ • Cryselle, Elinest, Low-Ogestrel • 30 mcg E. estradiol/0.3 mg norgestrel			• Presence of side effects • Pregnancy		Take 1 tablet daily at the same time of day for 21 days, followed by 7 days of inactive placebo pills
Ethinyl estradiol and norethindrone acetate☆ • Aurovela 1/20, Aurovela 24 Fe, Aurovela Fe 1/20, Blisovi 24 Fe, Gildess 1/20, Gildess 24 Fe, Gildess Fe 1/20, Junel 1/20, Junel Fe 1/20, Larin 1/20, Larin 24 Fe, Larin Fe 1/20, Lo Loestrin Fe, Loestrin 21 1/20, Loestrin 24 Fe, Loestrin Fe 1/20, Microgestin 1/20, Microgestin Fe 1/20 • 10–20 mcg E. estradiol/1 mg norethindrone acetate					
Ethinyl estradiol and norethindrone☆ • Balziva, Briellyn, Femcon Fe, Gildagia, Nexesta Fe, Philith, Vyfemla, • 35 mcg E. estradiol/0.4 mg norethindrone • Brevicon☆, Cyclafem 0.5/35, Cyonanz, Modicon, Nortrel 0.5/35, Wera • 35 mcg E. estradiol/0.5 mg norethindrone • Alyacen 1/35, Cyclafem 1/35, Dasetta 1/35, Necon 1/35☆, Norinyl 1/35, Nortrel 1/35, Nylia 1/35, Ortho-Novum 1/35, Pirmella 1/35 • 35 mcg E. estradiol/1 mg norethindrone					
Ethinyl estradiol and desogestrel • Bekyree, Kariva, Kimidess, Pimtrea, Viorele, Volnea • 10–20 mcg E. estradiol/0.15 mg desogestrel • Desogen, Emoquette, Enskyce, Isibloom, Kalliga • 30 mcg E. estradiol, 0.15 mg desogestrel					

Pharmacologic Contraceptives *(cont'd)*

Generic • Brand • Dose & Max	Contraindications	Primary Side Effects	Key Monitoring Parameters	Pertinent Drug Interactions	Med Pearls
Oral monophasic/low-dose estrogen *(cont'd)*					
Ethinyl estradiol and levonorgestrel • Ashlyna, Daysee, Seasonique, Simpesse • 30 mcg E. estradiol/0.15 mg levonorgestrel/10 mcg E. estradiol	[Same as above]	[Same as above]	[Same as above]	[Same as above]	[Same as above]
Ethinyl estradiol and norgestimate ☆ • Estarylla, Mili, Mono-Linyah, Ortho-Cyclen, Previfem, Sprintec • 35 mcg E. estradiol/0.25 mg norgestimate					
Oral biphasic					
Ethinyl estradiol and norethindrone ☆ • Necon 10/11 • 35 mcg E. estradiol, 0.5–1 mg norethindrone	• Pregnancy • Breast cancer • History of DVT or PE • Lactation (<6 wk postpartum) • Smoker >35 years old	• N/V • Breakthrough bleeding • Spotting • Melasma • Headache • Weight change • Edema • DVT/PE • Side effects associated with hormonal imbalance (see Table 2)	• Presence of side effects • Pregnancy	↓ effect of oral contraceptive: • Antibiotics (ampicillin, sulfonamides, tetracycline) • Anticonvulsants (phenytoin, topiramate, barbiturates) • Protease inhibitors • Rifampin Need backup method of contraception during use and for ≥1 wk after; for chronic therapy with above medications use another form of contraception	• Created to ↓ overall hormone exposure • High incidence of breakthrough bleeding

Pharmacologic Contraceptives *(cont'd)*

Generic • Brand • Dose & Max	Contraindications	Primary Side Effects	Key Monitoring Parameters	Pertinent Drug Interactions	Med Pearls
Oral triphasic					
Ethinyl estradiol and norethindrone ☆ • Alyacen 7/7/7, Aranelle, Cyclafem 7/7/7, Dasetta 7/7/7, Necon 7/7/7, Nortrel 7/7/7, Nylia 7/7/7, Ortho-Novum 7/7/7, Pirmella 7/7/7, Tri-Norinyl • 35 mcg E. estradiol/0.5–1 mg norethindrone Ethinyl estradiol and desogestrel • Cyclessa, Velivet • 25 mcg E. estradiol/0.1–0.15 mg desogestrel Ethinyl estradiol and norgestimate ☆ • Ortho Tri-Cyclen, Tri-Estarylla, Tri-Linyah, Tri-Mili, Tri-Previfem, Tri-Sprintec • 35 mcg E. estradiol/0.18–0.25 mg norgestimate • Ortho-TriCyclen Lo, Tri-Lo-Estarylla, Tri-Lo-Sprintec • 25 mcg E. estradiol/0.18–25 mg norgestimate Ethinyl estradiol and levonorgestrel • Elifemme, Enpresse, Levonest, Myzilra, Trivora • 30–40 mcg E. estradiol/0.075–0.125 mg levonorgestrel	• Pregnancy • Breast cancer • History of DVT or PE • Lactation (<6 wk postpartum) • Smoker >35 years old	• N/V • Breakthrough bleeding • Spotting • Melasma • Headache • Weight change • Edema • DVT/PE • Side effects associated with hormonal imbalance (see Table 2)	• Presence of side effects • Pregnancy	Same as biphasic	• Many triphasics approved for treatment of acne as well • More difficult to deal with missed pills • ↓ overall hormone exposure
Oral four-phasic					
Estradiol valerate and dienogest • Natazia • Days 1–2: 3 mg estradiol valerate • Days 3–7: 2 mg estradiol valerate + 2 mg dienogest • Days 8–24: 2 mg estradiol valerate + 3 mg dienogest • Days 25–26: 1 mg estradiol valerate • Days 27–28: inactive	• Pregnancy • Lactation • Breast cancer • History of DVT or PE • Hepatic disease • Abnormal uterine bleeding • Vascular disease • Hypercoagulopathy	• N/V • Breakthrough bleeding • Spotting • Melasma • Headache • Weight change • Edema • DVT/PE • Side effects associated with hormonal imbalance (see preceding Adverse Effects table)	• Presence of side effects • Pregnancy	Same as triphasic	• Only 4-phasic option available • ↑ efficacy for heavy menstrual bleeding

Pharmacologic Contraceptives   *(cont'd)*

Generic • Brand • Dose & Max	Contraindications	Primary Side Effects	Key Monitoring Parameters	Pertinent Drug Interactions	Med Pearls
Transdermal					
Ethinyl estradiol and norelgestromin • Xulane • 35 mcg E. estradiol/0.15 mg norelgestromin	• Pregnancy • Breast cancer • History of DVT or PE • Lactation (<6 wk postpartum) • Smoker >35 years old	• N/V • Breakthrough bleeding • Spotting • Melasma • Headache • Weight change • Edema • DVT/PE • Side effects associated with hormonal imbalance (see preceding Adverse Effects table)	• Presence of side effects • Pregnancy	Same as oral contraceptives	• Safe with usual activities • Do not apply lotion to site of application • Improved compliance over oral • Apply weekly for 3 wk • Avoid if >90 kg
Other					
Ethinyl estradiol and etonogestrel ☆ • NuvaRing • 0.015 mg E. estradiol and 0.12 mg etonogestrel released daily • Inserted by patient intravaginally every 4 wk (active for 3 wk)	Negative pregnancy test needed for initiation	Same as oral contraceptives (systemic absorption occurs)	Same as oral contraceptives (systemic absorption occurs)	Same as oral contraceptives (systemic absorption occurs)	• May be removed before intercourse • Not to be used >4 mo after being dispensed
Oral progestin-only					
Norethindrone • Camila, Errin, Heather, Incassia, Jencycla, Micronor, Nor-QD • 0.35 mg daily Norgestrel • Ovrette • 0.075 mg daily	Negative pregnancy test prior to initiation	• ↓ libido depression • Fatigue • Weight gain • Acne • Hypomenorrhea	Presence of side effects	None	Can be used in breastfeeding women, those >35 yr who smoke, and those at risk of coronary heart disease
Parenteral progestin-only					
Medroxyprogesterone ☆ • Depo-Provera, Depo-Subq Provera 104 • 150 mg IM every 12 wk; or 104 mg subcut every 12 wk	• Must have negative pregnancy test to start therapy or to continue therapy if >14 wk since last injection • Breast cancer • Liver disease	• Weight gain • ↓ bone mineral density • Acne • Delayed return of fertility after discontinuation	Bone mineral density	None	• Supplement calcium and vitamin D due to potential bone loss • Do not use for >2 yr unless unable to use other forms of contraception

Pharmacologic Contraceptives   *(cont'd)*

Generic • Brand • Dose & Max	Contraindications	Primary Side Effects	Key Monitoring Parameters	Pertinent Drug Interactions	Med Pearls
Implantable/intrauterine					
Levonorgestrel ☆ • Mirena • 20 mcg released daily • Intrauterine • Kyleena • 17.5 mcg released daily • Intrauterine	• History or high risk of pelvic inflammatory disease (PID) or ectopic pregnancy • Breast cancer • Abnormal uterine bleeding • High risk for sexually transmitted infections (STIs) (multiple sexual partners) • Uterine or cervical cancer	• Spotting • Breakthrough bleeding • Amenorrhea • Mastalgia • Headache • Abdominal pain • PID	• Presence of side effects • Pregnancy	None	Remains in place for up to 5 yr
Levonorgestrel • Skyla • 6 mcg released daily • Intrauterine • Liletta • 15.6 mcg released daily • Intrauterine					Remains for 3 yr
Etonogestrel • Nexplanon • 68 mg subdermal implant in upper arm • Replace every 3 yr	History or high risk of PID or ectopic pregnancy	• Amenorrhea • Infrequent menses • Weight gain			Not studied in women >130% ideal body weight
Nonhormonal					
Copper–T380 • ParaGard • Intrauterine placement for up to 10 yrs	History or high risk of PID or ectopic pregnancy	• Heavy bleeding • Cramping	None	None	Can remain in place for up to 8–10 yr with efficacy

Doses Missed	Instructions for Patient
1	Take missed dose immediately and next dose at regular time
2 (during first 2 wk)	Take two doses daily for the next 2 days, then resume taking; use backup method for 7 days
2 (during third wk)	Sunday start: Take one dose daily until Sunday, dispose of current pack, then begin next pack without placebo pills. Backup method required for 7 days.
≥3	Other: Dispose of current pack and begin new pack. Backup method required for 7 days.

HORMONE REPLACEMENT THERAPY

Guidelines Summary

- All women should undergo careful evaluation prior to initiation of hormone replacement therapy (HRT), including comprehensive history and physical, mammography, and, potentially, bone densitometry.

- The benefit:risk ratio for HRT is highly individualized and based on a patient's symptoms, impact on quality of life, and degree of risk for adverse effects.

- The primary indication for HRT is vasomotor symptoms of hot flashes and night sweats.

- Local vaginal therapy is recommended when vaginal symptoms are the only complaint.

- Prevention of osteoporosis with HRT should be considered only for women with a very strong risk of osteoporosis and in whom other available therapies are not options.

- In women who are receiving HRT and who have an intact uterus, progestin is indicated as a means of decreasing the risk of endometrial hyperplasia and cancer that exists with unopposed estrogen use in these patients.

- Due to an unclear evidence-based benefit:risk ratio, HRT is not recommended for any of the following indications: cardiovascular disease, stroke prevention, hyperlipidemia, or dementia prevention.

- The Women's Health Initiative (WHI) indicated increased risks of venous thromboembolism, stroke, coronary disease, and breast cancer in women who receive HRT for an extended period of time. The risk was greatest in patients on estrogen-progestogen combination therapy and lower in estrogen only therapy.

- Combination therapy should be limited to 3–5 year or less whenever possible. Longer term use of estrogen only therapy may be considered.

- Nonhormonal options are available for the treatment of vasomotor symptoms in patients with contraindications to hormone therapy or preference to avoid hormone therapy. Evidence-based options include venlafaxine, paroxetine, fluoxetine, and gabapentin. (These agents are detailed in drug tables in the Neurological Disorders and Psychiatric Disorders chapters.) Brisdelle is a low-dose paroxetine product that is approved by the Food and Drug Administration solely for the treatment of vasomotor symptoms related to menopause.

Hormone Replacement Therapy

Generic • Brand • Dose/Dosage Form	Contraindications	Primary Side Effects	Key Monitoring Parameters	Med Pearls
Oral Preparations				
Estrogens				
Conjugated equine estrogens ☆ • Premarin • 0.3–2.5 mg daily	• Hypersensitivity • Abnormal bleeding • Breast cancer • History of DVT or PE • Pregnancy • Estrogen-dependent tumor • History of stroke or myocardial infarction (MI) • Hepatic impairment • Protein C, protein S, or antithrombin deficiency	• Nausea • Fluid retention • Bloating • Headaches • Mood changes • Breast tenderness • ↑ risk of DVT/PE, stroke, MI, and breast cancer • ↑ blood pressure (BP)	• Vaginal bleeding • S/S of DVT/PE • S/S of stroke • S/S of MI • BP • Pap smear • Breast exam • Mammogram	• Most studied • No generic equivalent • Should not be abruptly discontinued; taper
Micronized estradiol • Only available generically • 1–2 mg daily				• Long half-life • Most potent hepatic effects • Should not be abruptly discontinued; taper
Estropipate • Only available generically • 0.75–6 mg daily				
Esterified estrogens • Menest • 0.3–2.5 mg daily				Should not be abruptly discontinued; taper
Progestins				
Medroxyprogesterone ☆ • Provera • 2–10 mg daily	• Hypersensitivity • Abnormal bleeding • Breast cancer • History of DVT or PE • Pregnancy • Estrogen- or progesterone-dependent tumor • History of stroke or MI • Hepatic impairment	• ↓ libido • Cramping • Mood changes • Bloating • Nausea • Depression • Headache • ↑ risk of DVT/PE, stroke, MI, and breast cancer	• Vaginal bleeding • S/S of DVT/PE • S/S of stroke • S/S of MI • Pap smear • Breast exam • Mammogram	None
Micronized progestin • Prometrium • 200 mg daily				Primary use in patients with adverse effects associated with synthetic progestin
Selective Estrogen Receptor Modulator/Estrogen Agonist–Antagonist				
Ospemifene • Osphena • 60 mg daily	• Hypersensitivity • Abnormal bleeding • Breast cancer • History of DVT or PE • Pregnancy • Estrogen-dependent tumor • History of stroke or MI	• ↑ risk of DVT/PE, stroke, MI, and breast cancer • Vasomotor symptoms	• Vaginal bleeding • S/S of DVT/PE • S/S of stroke • S/S of MI • Pap smear • Breast exam • Mammogram	None

Hormone Replacement Therapy *(cont'd)*

Generic • Brand • Dose/Dosage Form	Contraindications	Primary Side Effects	Key Monitoring Parameters	Med Pearls
Combination Oral Preparations				
Conjugated equine estrogens and medroxyprogesterone ☆ • Prempro • 0.3–0.625 mg estrogen/ 1.5–2.5 mg progestin • Premphase • 0.625 mg/0 mg × 14 days then 0.625/5 mg × 14 days Estradiol and drospirenone • Angelique • 0.5–1 mg/0.25–0.5 mg daily Ethinyl estradiol and norethindrone acetate • FemHRT, Leribane, Fyavolv • 2.5–5 mcg/0.5–1 mg daily • Activella, Amabelz • 0.5–1 mg/0.1–0.5 mg daily	• Hypersensitivity • Abnormal bleeding • Breast cancer • History of DVT or PE • Pregnancy • Estrogen-dependent tumor • History of stroke or MI • Hepatic impairment • Protein C, protein S, or antithrombin deficiency	• Nausea • Fluid retention • Bloating • Headaches • Mood changes • Breast tenderness • ↑ risk of DVT/PE, stroke, MI, and breast cancer • ↑ BP	• Vaginal bleeding • S/S of DVT/PE • S/S of stroke • S/S of MI • BP • Pap smear • Breast exam • Mammogram	None
Transdermal and Topical Preparations				
17β Estradiol transdermal ☆ • Alora, Climara, Minivelle, Vivelle, Vivelle-Dot • 25–50 mcg/24 hours • Applied 1–2 × wk 17β Estradiol gel • Divigel, Elestrin, Estrogel • 0.25–1.25 g daily 17β Estradiol topical emulsion • Estrasorb • 2 packets (3.48 g) daily 17β Transdermal spray • Evamist • 1 spray (1.53 mg) daily; may ↑ to 2–3 sprays daily	• Hypersensitivity • Abnormal bleeding • Breast cancer • History of DVT or PE • Pregnancy • Estrogen-dependent tumor • History of stroke or MI • Hepatic impairment • Protein C, protein S, or antithrombin deficiency	• Skin irritation • Nausea • Fluid retention • Bloating • Headaches • Mood changes • Breast tenderness • ↑ risk of DVT/PE, stroke, MI, and breast cancer • ↑ BP	• Vaginal bleeding • S/S of DVT/PE • S/S of stroke • S/S of MI • BP • Pap smear • Breast exam • Mammogram	• Limited hepatic effects • Useful in patients with gastrointestinal disturbances • Side effects less common in general

Hormone Replacement Therapy *(cont'd)*

Generic • Brand • Dose/Dosage Form	Contraindications	Primary Side Effects	Key Monitoring Parameters	Med Pearls
Vaginal Preparations				
Conjugated estrogen cream • Premarin • 0.5 g 1–2 × /wk to daily intravaginally (for 21 days, 7 days off)	• Hypersensitivity • Abnormal bleeding • Breast cancer • History of DVT or PE • Pregnancy • Estrogen-dependent tumor • History of stroke or MI • Hepatic impairment • Protein C, protein S, or antithrombin deficiency	Systemic side effects possible but rare	• Presence of adverse effects • Efficacy	• Used in cases of vaginal symptoms only • Effective for stress incontinence
Estradiol ring • Estring • 2 mg intravaginally; should remain in place for 90 days • Femring • 0.05–0.1 mg intravaginally; should remain in place for 90 days				Long-term use associated with endometrial hyperplasia
17β Estradiol cream • Estrace • 2–4 g intravaginally daily × 1–2 wk, then 1–2 g daily × 1–2 wk, then 1 g/day 1–3 × /wk				• Used in cases of vaginal symptoms only • Effective for stress incontinence
Estradiol tablet • Vagifem • 1 tab (10 mcg) intravaginally daily × 2 wk, then 1 tab (10 mcg) twice weekly				Used in cases of vaginal symptoms only

Drug Interactions

	Interacting Drug(s)	Result
Estrogen	3A4 inducers: barbiturates, carbamazepine, phenytoin rifampin, St. John's wort	↓ effect of estrogen
	Levothyroxine, warfarin	↓ effect of interacting drug
	3A4 inhibitors: azole antifungals, macrolide antibiotics, ritonavir, grapefruit juice	↑ effect of estrogen
	Corticosteroids	↑ effect of interacting drug
Progestin	3A4 inducers: barbiturates, carbamazepine, phenytoin rifampin, St. John's wort	↓ effect of progestin

ERECTILE DYSFUNCTION

Guidelines Summary

- Initial treatment for most patients will consist of therapy with a phosphodiesterase-5 (PDE-5) inhibitor because these agents are known to be efficacious and are minimally invasive.

- PDE-5 inhibitors are contraindicated in patients who are currently taking nitrates, due to a risk of significant, dangerous hypotension when these agents are used concomitantly.

- If a patient does not respond to therapy with a PDE-5 inhibitor, alternate therapy options should be considered, including a different PDE-5 inhibitor, alprostadil intraurethral suppositories, intracavernous injection, vacuum constriction devices, and penile prostheses.

- Lifestyle modification and treatment of underlying cause/secondary cause should also be encouraged (hypertension, diabetes, hyperlipidemia).

Erectile Dysfunction Treatment Summary

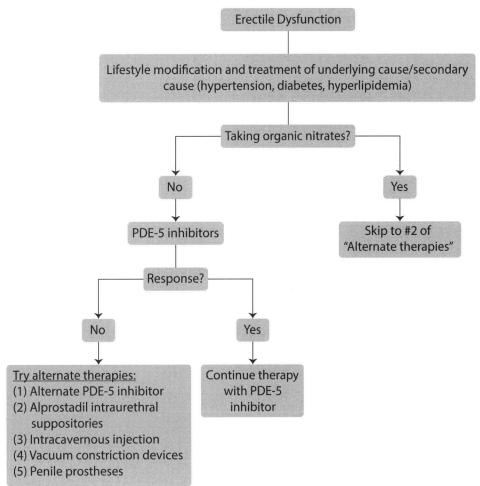

Medications for Erectile Dysfunction

Generic • Brand • Dose/Dosage Forms	Contraindications	Primary Side Effects	Key Monitoring Parameters	Pertinent Drug Interactions	Med Pearls
Oral					
Mechanism of action – PDE-5 inhibitors: enhance the activity of nitric oxide by inhibiting an enzyme (PDE-5) responsible for its degradation; enhanced nitric oxide allows relaxed smooth muscles and ↑ vasodilation and blood flow to the penis following stimulation					
Sildenafil☆ • Viagra • 25–100 mg PRN 0.5–4 hr prior to sexual activity (max = 1 dose daily) • Tabs Tadalafil☆ • Cialis • 5–20 mg PRN ≥30 min prior to sexual activity; or 2.5–5 mg daily • Tabs Vardenafil • Levitra, Staxyn • 5–20 mg (max = 10 mg for ODTs) PRN ~1 hr prior to sexual activity • ODTs, tabs Avanafil • Stendra • 50–200 mg PRN 15–30 min prior to sexual activity • Tabs	• Use with nitrates (continuous or intermittent) • Hypersensitivity • Concurrent use with riociguat	• Hypotension • Dizziness • Headache • Flushing • Dyspepsia • Priapism (not common) • Vision changes • Hearing changes	• Efficacy • Presence of side effects • BP	***Nitrates— Combination results in potentially fatal hypotension. Avoid concomitant use within 24 hours; 48 hours with tadalafil.*** • Concurrent use with alpha-blockers may ↑ risk of hypotension; avoid combination or use lowest dose of each agent used with close monitoring • 3A4 substrates • 3A4 inhibitors may ↑ effects/toxicity • 3A4 inducers may ↓ effects	Dose adjustments when used with strong 3A4 inhibitors: sildenafil (use initial dose of 25 mg); tadalafil (max dose = 10 mg every 72 hr; or 2.5 mg daily); vardenafil (max dose = 2.5–5 mg every 24–72 hr based on CYP3A4 inhibitor; do not use with ODTs); avanafil (avoid concurrent use)

Medications for Erectile Dysfunction   *(cont'd)*

Generic • Brand • Dose/Dosage Forms	Contraindications	Primary Side Effects	Key Monitoring Parameters	Pertinent Drug Interactions	Med Pearls
Topical					
Testosterone transdermal patch • Androderm • 2.5–6-mg patch daily • Transdermal patch Testosterone gel ☆ • AndroGel, Fortesta, Testim, Vogelxo • AndroGel 1%: 50–100 mg daily • AndroGel 1.62%: 40.5–81 mg daily • Fortesta: 40–70 mg daily • Testim: 50–100 mg daily • Vogelxo: 50–100 mg daily Testosterone intranasal gel • Natesto • 1 pump per nostril (total = 11 mg) TID Testosterone buccal • Striant • 30 mg BID (apply to gum, above incisor) Testosterone solution • Axiron • 60–120 mg daily (apply to axilla)	• Hypersensitivity • Breast or prostate cancer	• ↑ liver function tests (LFTs) • ↑ risk of DVT/PE, stroke, and MI • Edema • Hyperlipidemia • Depression • Aggression	• LFTs • Serum testosterone concentrations • Prostate-specific antigen • Lipid panel	May ↑ effects/toxicity of warfarin	• Only useful in ED due to hypogonadism • Schedule III controlled substance • Risk of abuse
Intramuscular					
Testosterone • Depo-Testosterone (cypionate), Generic (enanthate), Aveed (undecanoate) • Cypionate or enanthate: 50–400 mg IM every 2–4 wk • Undecanoate: 750 mg IM, then 750 mg IM 4 wk later, then 750 mg IM every 10 wk	• Hypersensitivity • Breast or prostate cancer • Serious cardiac, renal or hepatic disease	• ↑ LFTs • ↑ risk of DVT/PE, stroke, and MI • Edema • Hyperlipidemia • Depression • Aggression	• LFTs • Serum testosterone concentrations • PSA • Lipid panel	May ↑ effects/toxicity of warfarin	• Only useful in ED due to hypogonadism • Schedule III controlled substance

Medications for Erectile Dysfunction *(cont'd)*

Generic • Brand • Dose/Dosage Forms	Contraindications	Primary Side Effects	Key Monitoring Parameters	Pertinent Drug Interactions	Med Pearls
Intraurethral					
Alprostadil • Muse • 125–250 mcg pellets 5–10 min before intercourse	• Hypersensitivity • Urethral stricture • Chronic urethritis	• Urethral pain • Burning • Priapism • Hypotension	• Presence of side effects • Efficacy • BP	None	Duration of effect is 30–60 min
Intracavernosal					
Alprostadil • Caverject, Edex • 1–40 mcg 5–20 min before intercourse injected intracavernosal	• Hypersensitivity • Sickle-cell trait • Multiple myeloma • Leukemia	• Pain at injection site • Erythema • Priapism • Hypotension	• Presence of side effects • Efficacy • BP periodically	None	Self-injection training should be done in physician's office

BENIGN PROSTATIC HYPERPLASIA

Guidelines Summary

- Watchful waiting (no pharmacologic therapy) is appropriate for patients with mild symptoms (AUA-SI scores <8).

- In general, pharmacologic therapy is considered for patients with moderate–severe symptoms (AUA-SI scores ≥8).

- Alpha-antagonists are the treatment of choice for patients with LUTS and are used as monotherapy or in combination with 5-alpha reductase inhibitors or anticholinergics.

  - Nonselective alpha-antagonists such as terazosin and doxazosin are equally effective as the alpha 1A selective antagonists, tamsulosin, alfuzosin, and silodosin.

  - Nonselective alpha-antagonists require slow dose titration and lower BP; therefore, these agents should be used with caution in patients at risk for hypotension.

  - First-dose syncope and dizziness are common side effects, especially with the nonselective alpha-antagonists. Dosing at bedtime can minimize this side effect, but patients should be educated to stand up slowly to avoid falls.

  - Intraoperative floppy iris syndrome (IFIS) is a potential side effect of the alpha-antagonists that can significantly complicate cataract surgery. Patients with planned cataract surgery should not initiate new alpha-antagonist therapy until cataract surgery is complete.

- 5-alpha reductase inhibitors are appropriate as monotherapy or in combination with alpha-antagonists in patients with enlarged prostate glands. Concomitant therapy with alpha-antagonists will allow symptoms to improve during the initial 6 months of therapy when the 5-alpha reductase inhibitor is reaching maximal efficacy.

- Although earlier guidelines suggested use of 5-alpha reductase inhibitors in patients with prostate glands >50 mL (50 g), newer studies have demonstrated benefits in patients with prostate glands >30 mL (30 g).

■ Anticholinergic agents such as tolterodine may be considered in patient with LUTS (primarily irritative) and without an elevated postvoid residual (<250 mL). Please see the Urinary Incontinence section of this chapter for specifics related to anticholinergic medications.

PDE-5 inhibitors are now clinically indicated for daily use for the treatment of LUTS/BPH (tadalafil is approved by the Food and Drug Administration for this indication) but are generally reserved for patients who have not responded to more conventional therapies. Because PDE-5 inhibitors exhibit a significant drug interaction with nonselective alpha-antagonists, special care should be taken to monitor for and avoid this combination.

BPH Treatment Summary

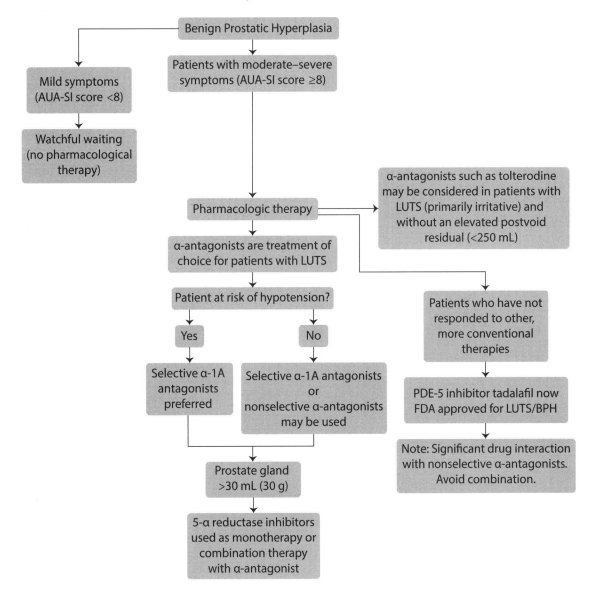

Medications for BPH

Generic • Brand • Dose/Dosage Forms	Contraindications	Primary Side Effects	Key Monitoring Parameters	Pertinent Drug Interactions	Med Pearls
Nonselective Alpha-1 Antagonists					
Doxazosin☆ • Cardura, Cardura XL • IR: 1–8 mg at bedtime • ER: 4–8 mg in A.M. • ER tabs, tabs	Hypersensitivity	• Orthostatic hypotension • Dizziness • Reflex tachycardia • Peripheral edema • Headache • Drowsiness • Priapism (rare)	• BP • Heart rate • LUTS	↑ risk of hypotension with PDE-5 inhibitors (avoid concurrent use)	• Dosed at bedtime (except for doxazosin ER which is dosed in A.M.) to prevent dizziness/falls during the day • ↑ risk of IFIS in patients undergoing cataract surgery
Terazosin☆ • Only available generically • 1–10 mg at bedtime • Caps					
Selective Alpha-1A Antagonists					
Tamsulosin☆ • Flomax • 0.4–0.8 mg daily	Hypersensitivity	• Orthostatic hypotension • Dizziness • Headache • Priapism (rare)	• BP • LUTS	• CYP2D6 and CYP3A4 substrate • CYP2D6 and CYP3A4 inhibitors may ↑ effects/toxicity; avoid use with strong CYP3A4 inhibitors • CYP3A4 inducers may ↓ effects • ↑ risk of hypotension with PDE-5 inhibitors • Cimetidine may ↑ levels	• Take ~30 min after a meal • Expensive relative to nonselective agents • ↑ risk of IFIS in patients undergoing cataract surgery
Alfuzosin • Uroxatral • 10 mg daily • ER tabs	• Hypersensitivity • Moderate to severe hepatic impairment • Concurrent use with strong 3A4 inhibitors			• CYP3A4 substrate • CYP3A4 inhibitors may ↑ effects/toxicity; concurrent use with strong CYP3A4 inhibitors contraindicated • CYP3A4 inducers may ↓ effects • ↑ risk of hypotension with PDE-5 inhibitors	• Take with food • Do not crush or chew • Expensive relative to nonselective agents • ↑ risk of IFIS in patients undergoing cataract surgery
Silodosin • Rapaflo • 8 mg daily • Caps	• Hypersensitivity • Severe renal or hepatic impairment • Concurrent use with strong 3A4 inhibitors	• Orthostatic hypotension • Dizziness • Headache • Diarrhea • Retrograde ejaculation • Priapism (rare)			• Adjust dose in renal impairment • Take with food • Expensive relative to nonselective agents • ↑ risk of IFIS in patients undergoing cataract surgery

Medications for BPH   *(cont'd)*

Generic • Brand • Dose/Dosage Forms	Contraindications	Primary Side Effects	Key Monitoring Parameters	Pertinent Drug Interactions	Med Pearls
5-Alpha Reductase Inhibitors					
Finasteride ☆ • Proscar • 5 mg daily • Tabs	• Hypersensitivity • Pregnant women or women of reproductive potential	• ↓ libido • ED • Gynecomastia	• PSA • LUTS	None	• Cause significant ↓ in PSA; should establish new PSA baseline ≥6 mo after initiation of therapy
Dutasteride ☆ • Avodart • 0.5 mg daily • Caps				• CYP3A4 substrate • CYP3A4 inhibitors may ↑ effects/toxicity • CYP3A4 inducers may ↓ effects	• Dutasteride caps and crushed/broken finasteride tabs should not be handled by pregnant women or women of childbearing potential (potentially teratogenic for male infants) • Men taking dutasteride should not donate blood for ≥6 mo after discontinuing therapy • Onset of effect can be up to 6 mo

Combination Products: See individual drug components for important points		
Brand	**Components**	**Dosing**
Jalyn	Dutasteride + Tamsulosin	1 cap (0.5 mg dutasteride/0.4 mg tamsulosin) daily (~30 min after a meal)

URINARY INCONTINENCE

Summary of Treatment Recommendations

- General
  - Nonpharmacological therapy is important as either monotherapy or an adjunct to pharmacotherapy. Options such as pelvic floor strengthening exercises and scheduled voiding are common.
- Stress incontinence
  - Options for treatment include topical estrogen, alpha agonists, and tricyclic antidepressants. Alpha agonists carry the risk of ↑ BP and heart rate, and should be used with extreme caution in patients with pre-existing hypertension or heart conditions.

- Urge incontinence
  - Options for treatment include antimuscarinic medications, mirabegron, and imipramine.
- Overflow incontinence
  - Treatment options are varied based upon the determined etiology. Since many cases of overflow incontinence are secondary to BPH, see the BPH section of this chapter for recommendations.

Medications for Urinary Incontinence

Generic • Brand • Dose/Dosage Forms	Contraindications	Primary Side Effects	Key Monitoring Parameters	Pertinent Drug Interactions	Med Pearls
Topical vaginal estrogen preparations: used in the treatment of stress incontinence (first-line) and urge incontinence (third-line); refer to the Hormone Replacement Therapy section of this chapter for more detailed information					
Tricyclic antidepressants: imipramine and desipramine are most commonly used in incontinence; used primarily in urge incontinence and stress incontinence; refer to the Psychiatric Disorders chapter for more detailed information					
Anticholinergic/Antimuscarinic Agents					
Oxybutynin ☆ • Ditropan XL • IR: 5 mg 2–4 × /day • ER: 5–30 mg daily • ER tabs, tabs • Oxytrol • Apply 1 patch (3.9 mg/day) twice weekly • Transdermal patch • Gelnique • 10%: Apply contents of 1 sachet (100 mg/g) daily • Transdermal gel	• Hypersensitivity • Urinary retention • Gastric retention • Narrow-angle glaucoma	• Dry mouth • Dry eyes • Constipation • Urinary retention • Dizziness • Somnolence • Hallucinations • Agitation • Confusion • Blurred vision • ↑ intraocular pressure • Angioedema	• S/S of incontinence • Presence of side effects	Additive effects with other anticholinergic medications	• Side effects less common with ER tabs and transdermal formulations • Transdermal patch available over-the-counter
Tolterodine ☆ • Detrol, Detrol LA • IR: 1–2 mg BID • ER: 2–4 mg daily • ER caps, tabs				• CYP2D6 and CYP3A4 substrate • CYP2D6 and CYP3A4 inhibitors may ↑ effects/toxicity • CYP3A4 inducers may ↓ effects • Additive effects with other anticholinergic medications	• Side effects less common with ER tabs • Adjust dose in renal or hepatic impairment

Medications for Urinary Incontinence *(cont'd)*

Generic • Brand • Dose/Dosage Forms	Contraindications	Primary Side Effects	Key Monitoring Parameters	Pertinent Drug Interactions	Med Pearls
Anticholinergic/Antimuscarinic Agents (cont'd)					
Darifenacin☆ • Enablex • 7.5–15 mg daily • ER tabs	[Same as above]	[Same as above]	[Same as above]	• CYP3A4 substrate • CYP3A4 inhibitors may ↑ effects/toxicity • CYP3A4 inducers may ↓ effects • Additive effects with other anticholinergic medications	• Adjust dose in renal or hepatic impairment • Max dose = 7.5 mg daily with strong CYP3A4 inhibitors
Solifenacin☆ • Vesicare • 5–10 mg daily • Tabs					• Adjust dose in hepatic impairment • Max dose = 5 mg daily with strong CYP3A4 inhibitors
Fesoterodine☆ • Toviaz • 4–8 mg daily • ER tabs					• Adjust dose in renal impairment • Max dose = 4 mg daily with strong CYP3A4 inhibitors
Trospium☆ • Only available generically • IR: 20 mg BID • ER: 60 mg daily • ER caps, tabs				• Metformin may ↓ levels • Additive effects with other anticholinergic medications	• Take 30 min before meals or on an empty stomach • Adjust dose in renal impairment and in patients ≥75 yr

Medications for Urinary Incontinence   *(cont'd)*

Generic • Brand • Dose/Dosage Forms	Contraindications	Primary Side Effects	Key Monitoring Parameters	Pertinent Drug Interactions	Med Pearls
Mechanism of action – beta-3 adrenergic receptor agonist					
Mirabegron • Myrbetriq • 25–50 mg daily • ER tabs	Hypersensitivity	• Hypertension • Angioedema • Headache	• BP • S/S of incontinence	• CYP2D6 inhibitor • May ↑ effects/toxicity of CYP2D6 substrates • May ↑ serum digoxin concentrations • May ↑ effects of warfarin • Additive effects with other anticholinergic medications	• Adjust dose in renal or hepatic impairment • Fewer anticholinergic side effects; may be a good option in elderly patients with anticholinergic side effects • Hypertension may limit use • Very expensive
Alpha Agonists					
Pseudoephedrine • Sudafed • 30–60 mg every 4–6 hr PRN (max = 240 mg/24 hrs) Phenylephrine • Many • 10–20 mg every 4 hr PRN	• Hypersensitivity • Concurrent use of monoamine oxidase inhibitors (MAOIs) • Uncontrolled hypertension	• ↑ BP • ↑ heart rate • ↑ blood sugar • Irritability • Insomnia	• BP • Heart rate • Fasting plasma glucose (if diabetes)	Concurrent use with MAOIs may ↑ risk of hypertensive crises	Use with caution in hypertension or pre-existing cardiac conditions

PRACTICE QUESTIONS

1. Which of the following is MOST accurate regarding the coadministration of sildenafil and nitroglycerin?

    (A) There is no drug interaction between the two medications.
    (B) There is a minor drug interaction between the two medications. The patient should be counseled to monitor for signs and symptoms of the interaction.
    (C) There is a major drug interaction between these two agents, but they can be safely coadministered as long as doses are separated by at least 1 hour.
    (D) There is a major drug interaction between sildenafil and some forms of nitroglycerin. The specific formulation of nitroglycerin should be determined before the medications are taken.
    (E) There is a major, potentially life-threatening drug interaction between the two agents. Coadministration should be avoided.

2. In which of the following clinical scenarios would hormone replacement therapy be contraindicated?

    (A) Breast cancer
    (B) Obesity
    (C) Stage 3 CKD
    (D) Diabetes mellitus
    (E) History of hysterectomy

3. Which of the following is the correct trade name for tadalafil?

    (A) Viagra
    (B) Levitra
    (C) Cialis
    (D) Caverject
    (E) Proscar

4. A 74-year-old man with benign prostatic hyperplasia (BPH) has taken terazosin for 6 months with some symptom improvement. He complains of persistent urinary urgency. His prostate size is 20 g and postvoid residual volume is 50 mL. Which medication is MOST appropriate in combination with his current treatment to address his symptoms?

    (A) Tolterodine
    (B) Dutasteride
    (C) Sildenafil
    (D) Saw palmetto

5. A 24-year-old woman on a monophasic oral contraceptive informs you that she missed the last 2 doses of her contraceptive tablets in the first 2 weeks of the pack. In addition to using a back up form of contraception for at least the next 7 days, which of the following is the MOST appropriate set of instructions to provide?

    (A) Take 1 extra dose today, the next dose at the regularly scheduled time, and resume 1 tablet daily.
    (B) Take 2 doses daily for next 2 days, then resume 1 tablet daily.
    (C) Take 1 tablet daily until Sunday, start a new pack without taking placebo pills.
    (D) Dispose of the current pack, wait until Sunday and restart a new pack on that day.

6. Which of the following contraceptives could be used safely in a 26-year-old woman who is 12 weeks postpartum and breastfeeding her baby?

    (A) Ortho Micronor
    (B) NuvaRing
    (C) Ovcon 35
    (D) Loestrin Fe

7. A 67-year-old man with BPH has an AUA-SI score of 10, prostate size of 15 g, and postvoid residual of 100 mL. He has a medical history of hypertension and cataracts and is scheduled to have cataract surgery in 2 weeks. Which of the following is the BEST recommendation?

    (A) Watchful waiting for 6 months.
    (B) Initiate alfuzosin today.
    (C) Initiate alfuzosin in 1 month.
    (D) Initiate dutasteride today.

ANSWERS AND EXPLANATIONS

1. **E**

There is a major, life-threatening drug interaction between these two medications. When coadministered, the two agents can result in a life-threatening drop in blood pressure. All forms of nitroglycerin carry this risk, and coadministration should be avoided within *at least* 24 hours.

2. **A**

Hormone replacement therapy is contraindicated in patients with breast cancer due to the potential to exacerbate tumor growth. Obesity, kidney disease, and diabetes are not contraindications to hormone replacement therapy. Patients with a history of hysterectomy may take unopposed estrogen but do not need progestin.

3. **C**

Cialis is the trade name for tadalafil. Viagra is the trade name for sildenafil, Levitra is the trade name for vardenafil, Caverject is the trade name for alprostadil, and Proscar is the trade name for finasteride.

4. **A**

Therapy with an anticholinergic drug such as tolterodine can be used in combination with alpha-blockers to treat symptoms of urinary urgency if the postvoid residual volume is below 250 mL. Dutasteride (B) is beneficial in combination with alpha-blockers in men with elevated prostate size (30–60 g or greater) and this patient's size is 20 g. Sildenafil (C) is appropriate for erectile dysfunction; however, phosphodiesterase inhibitors are reserved for patients that have not responded to conventional therapies, and tadalafil is the only currently FDA approved agent for LUTS associated with BPH. Saw palmetto (D) has limited evidence of benefit and would not be the best recommendation in this case.

5. **B**

Taking 2 doses daily for the next 2 days, then resuming 1 tablet daily is appropriate. An extra dose today, then resuming 1 tablet daily (A) would be correct if the patient had missed only 1 dose but it will not provide enough contraceptive medication if she missed 2 doses. Starting a new pack on Sunday (C and D) would be appropriate if the patient had missed 3 or more doses or if she had missed 2 or more doses in the third week of the pack.

6. **A**

Progestin-only contraceptives such as Ortho Micronor are safe options during breast-feeding. NuvaRing (B), Ovcon 35 (C), and LoestrinFe (D) are all estrogen-containing contraceptives and cannot be used during breastfeeding.

7. **B**

The patient's AUA-SI score (≥8) warrants pharmacological treatment, thus watchful waiting (A) is incorrect. Alpha antagonists including alfuzosin (C) would be the appropriate first-line therapy; however, it should not be started until after the patient's cataract surgery. Alfuzosin has the potential to cause intraoperative floppy iris syndrome (IFIS) in patients undergoing cataract surgery. And 5 alpha reductase inhibitors such as dutasteride (D) are reserved for patients with prostate glands >30 mL (30 g); this patient's prostate size is 15 g.

Preventive Medicine

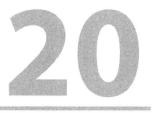

This chapter covers the following preventive health care measures:

- **Immunizations**
- **Weight loss**
- **Smoking cessation**

IMMUNIZATIONS

Immunizations

Vaccine • Brand Name • Route of Administration	Contraindications	Adverse Effects	Target Population	Medication Pearls
Live vaccines				
Herpes zoster (shingles) • Zostavax • Subcut	• History of anaphylaxis to gelatin or neomycin • Immunosuppression or immunodeficiency	• Injection site reactions • Headache • Flu-like symptoms • Fever	All patients ≥60 years of age	None
Live attenuated influenza • FluMist Quadrivalent • Intranasal	• Anaphylaxis to previous influenza vaccination • Hypersensitivity to egg protein • Children 2–17 years of age taking aspirin	• Runny nose • Nasal congestion • Fever • Sore throat • Headache • ↓ appetite • Weakness	All patients 2–49 years of age yearly	
Measles, mumps, rubella (MMR) • M-M-R II • Subcut	• Hypersensitivity to any vaccine component • Febrile illness • Immunosuppression or immunodeficiency • Pregnancy	• Injection site reactions • Arthralgia • Myalgia • Rash	Children ≥12 months	

Immunizations   *(cont'd)*

Vaccine • Brand Name • Route of Administration	Contraindications	Adverse Effects	Target Population	Medication Pearls
Live vaccines (cont'd)				
Rotavirus • Rotarix, RotaTeq • Oral	• Hypersensitivity • History of intussusception • Severe combined immunodeficiency disease	• Fever • Diarrhea • Vomiting • Otitis media • Nasopharyngitis	• Infants and children 6–24 weeks (Rotarix) • Infants and children 6–32 weeks (RotaTeq)	None
Varicella (chickenpox): • Varivax • Subcut	• Allergic reaction to vaccine, gelatin, or neomycin • Immunodeficiency or immunosuppression • Active, untreated tuberculosis • Pregnancy	• Injection site reactions • Rash • Fever • Malaise • Arthralgia	Children ≥12 months of age	
Inactivated vaccines				
Influenza • Afluria, Fluad, Fluarix Quadrivalent, Flucelvax, Flucelvax Quadrivalent, Flulaval Quadrivalent, Fluvirin, Fluzone High-Dose, Fluzone Intradermal Quadrivalent, Fluzone Quadrivalent • Intradermal (Fluzone Intradermal Quadrivalent) • IM (remainder)	• Allergy to previous influenza vaccination • Allergy to eggs (except for Flucelvax)	• Fever • Malaise • Myalgia • Injection site reactions	All patients ≥6 months of age	Yearly vaccination to account for antigenic drifts and ↓ antibody levels over time

Immunizations *(cont'd)*

Vaccine • Brand Name • Route of Administration	Contraindications	Adverse Effects	Target Population	Medication Pearls
Inactivated vaccines (cont'd)				
Diphtheria, tetanus, acelluar pertussis • DTaP: Daptacel, Infanrix • IM • Tdap: Adacel, Boostrix • IM • Td: Decavac, Tenivac • IM	**DTaP** • Serious allergic reaction to previous dose of diphtheria toxoid-, tetanus toxoid-, or pertussis-containing vaccine • Encephalopathy within 7 days of previous vaccination • Progressive neurologic disorders **Tdap** • Serious allergic reaction to diphtheria toxoid, tetanus toxoid and pertussis antigen-containing vaccine • Encephalopathy within 7 days of previous vaccination **Td** • Serious allergic reaction to tetanus toxoid or diphtheria toxoid containing vaccine	• Injection site reactions • Arthus reactions • Swelling • Fever	• DTaP: Children 6 week–6 years of age • Tdap: Single dose once >7 years of age or in third trimester of each pregnancy • Td: 1 dose every 10 years once ≥7 years of age	Tdap is needed only once per lifetime (except should be given during each pregnancy)
Human papillomavirus (HPV) • Cervarix (HPV2), Gardasil (HPV4), Gardasil 9 (HPV9) • IM	• Hypersensitivity • Allergy to yeast (Gardasil, Gardasil 9)	• Injection site reactions • Headache • Fever • Fatigue • Myalgia	• Cervarix: Females 9–25 years of age • Gardasil: Females and males 9–26 years of age • Gardasil 9: Females and males 9–26 years of age	• Cervarix protects against HPV types 16 and 18 • Gardasil protects against HPV types 6, 11, 16, and 18 • Gardasil 9 protects against HPV types 6, 11, 16, 18, 31, 33, 45, 52, and 58

Immunizations *(cont'd)*

Vaccine • Brand Name • Route of Administration	Contraindications	Adverse Effects	Target Population	Medication Pearls
Inactivated vaccines (cont'd)				
Streptococcus pneumoniae • Pneumovax 23 (PPSV23) • IM, subcut • Prevnar 13 (PCV13) • IM	• Severe allergic reaction to pneumococcal vaccine • Severe allergic reaction to any diphtheria toxoid-containing vaccine (PCV13)	• Injection site reactions • Fever • Myalgia	• PCV13: children 2–59 months of age; children 60–71 months of age with chronic heart disease, asthma, diabetes, asplenia, or immunosuppressive conditions; children ≥6 years of age, adolescents, and adults with asplenia or immunosuppressive conditions; and all patients ≥65 years of age • PPSV23: All patients ≥65 years of age; children, adolescents, and adults ≥2 years of age at ↑ risk for pneumococcal disease (asplena, sickle cell disease, heart failure, chronic obstructive pulmonary disease, asthma, diabetes, chronic liver disease, cigarette smokers, and immunosuppressed)	• PPSV23 not indicated for children <2 years of age • Second dose of PPSV23 recommended for patients ≥65 years of age with previous dose given ≥5 years ago
Meningococcal • MCV4: Menactra, Menveo • IM • MPSV4: Menomune • Subcut	• Hypersensitivity • Hypersensitivity to diphtheria toxoid (MCV4)	• Injection site reactions • Headache • Fever • Malaise	• MCV4: Adolescents 11–18 years of age with a booster dose after 5 years (if initial dose given before age 16); patients ≥2 months of age at ↑ risk of meningococcal disease (can be used up to age 55) • MPSV4: Unvaccinated adults >56 years of age who are at ↑ risk of meningococcal disease	MPSV4 should not be used in children <2 years of age

Immunizations *(cont'd)*

Vaccine • Brand Name • Route of Administration	Contraindications	Adverse Effects	Target Population	Medication Pearls
Inactivated vaccines (cont'd)				
Hepatitis A • Havrix, VAQTA • IM	• Hypersensitivity • Allergic reaction to vaccine or neomycin	• Injection site reactions • Fever	• All children ≥12 months of age • International travel other than Canada, Europe, Japan, New Zealand, or Australia • Men who have sex with men (MSM) • Illicit drug users • Laboratory workers • Patients with chronic liver disease or clotting disorders	None
Hepatitis B • Engerix-B, Recombivax HB • IM	• Hypersensitivity • Allergic reaction to previous hepatitis B vaccination or yeast	• Injection site reactions • Headache • Fatigue • Fever	• Infants at birth • All infants and children • Health care workers • International travel • Patients with multiple sexual partners • MSM • Injection drug users • Adults with diabetes mellitus • HIV • Chronic liver disease • End-stage renal disease	
Haemophilus influenza type B • ActHIB, Hiberix, PedvaxHIB • IM	• Hypersensitivity • Hypersensitivity to tetanus toxoid (ActHIB and Hiberix)	Injection site reactions	All infants and children through age 59 months	
Polio • IPOL • IM, subcut	Hypersensitivity		All infants and children >2 months of age	

WEIGHT LOSS

Guidelines Summary

Health care providers should evaluate a patient's BMI at each visit and create an individualized treatment plan. Weight loss plans need to include moderate caloric reduction, increased physical activity, and behavioral strategies that patients can use to sustain weight loss.

Medications for Weight Loss

Generic • Brand • Dose/Dosage Form	Contraindications	Primary Side Effects	Key Monitoring	Pertinent Drug Interactions	Med Pearls
Mechanism of action – inhibits gastric and pancreatic lipase to inhibit dietary fat					
Orlistat • Xenical, Alli (over-the-counter [OTC]) • Xenical: 120 mg TID with each meal • Alli: 60 mg TID with each meal • Caps	• Hypersensitivity • Chronic malabsorption syndrome • Pregnancy • Cholestasis	• Oily discharge/spotting • Fecal urgency • Hepatotoxicity • Nephrolithiasis • Cholelithiasis • Flatulence	• Weight • BMI • Serum glucose • Thyroid function • Liver function tests (LFTs) • Renal function	• May ↓ absorption of cyclosporine, warfarin, anticonvulsants, amiodarone, levothyroxine, and antiepileptic drugs levels • ↓ absorption of fat-soluble vitamins (A, D, E, K)	• Available OTC • Should supplement with multivitamin
Mechanism of action – stimulates hypothalamus to release norepinephrine (phentermine); suppresses appetite and ↑ satiety through inhibition of neuronal sodium channels and ↑ GABA activity (topiramate)					
Phentermine with topiramate • Qsymia • 3.75 mg/23 mg daily × 14 days, then 7.5 mg/46 mg daily × 12 wk; if 3% of baseline body weight has not been lost, discontinue therapy or ↑ dose to 11.25 mg/69 mg daily × 14 days, then 15 mg/92 mg daily • Caps	• Hypersensitivity to phentermine or sympathomimetics • Pregnancy • Hyperthyroidism • Glaucoma • Use of monoamine oxidase inhibitor (MAOI) within 2 wk	• Tachycardia • Headache • Insomnia • Xerostomia • Constipation • Paresthesia • Difficulty concentrating • Confusion • Memory issues • Speech problems • Depression • Dizziness • Kidney stones • Angle closure glaucoma • Visual field defects • ↓ sweating • Hyperthermia • Metabolic acidosis • ↑ SCr • Hypokalemia	• Weight • BMI • Heart rate (HR) • Blood pressure (BP) • Serum bicarbonate • Serum potassium • Serum glucose • Renal function • Suicidality • Intraocular pressure	• ↑ risk of hypertensive crisis with MAOIs • Other central nervous system (CNS) depressants, including alcohol, may ↑ CNS depressant effects • Concurrent use with loop or thiazide diuretics may ↑ risk of hypokalemia • Phenytoin or carbamazepine may ↓ topiramate levels • Concurrent use with valproic acid may ↑ risk of hyperammonemia or hypothermia • Concurrent use with zonisamide or acetazolamide may ↑ risk of metabolic acidosis or nephrolithiasis	• Schedule IV controlled substance • Adjust dose in renal or hepatic impairment • Teratogenic • Give in A.M. to minimize risk of insomnia • If patient has not lost 5% of baseline body weight by wk 12 of phentermine 15 mg/topiramate 92 mg daily, discontinue therapy

Medications for Weight Loss   (cont'd)

Generic • Brand • Dose/Dosage Form	Contraindications	Primary Side Effects	Key Monitoring	Pertinent Drug Interactions	Med Pearls
Mechanism of action – stimulates hypothalamus to release norepinephrine					
Phentermine • Adipex-P • 15–37.5 mg/day in 1–2 divided doses • Caps, tabs	• Hypersensitivity to phentermine or sympathomimetics • History of cardiovascular disease (e.g., coronary artery disease, stroke, arrhythmias, heart failure, uncontrolled hypertension) • Pregnancy • Breast feeding • Hyperthyroidism • Glaucoma • Use of MAOI within 2 wk • Agitation • History of drug abuse	• Hypertension • Tachycardia • Primary pulmonary hypertension • Valvular heart disease • Euphoria • Dizziness • Insomnia • Psychosis • Tremor	• Weight • BMI • BP • HR • S/S of valvular heart disease	↑ risk of hypertensive crisis with MAOIs	• Schedule IV controlled substance • Give before breakfast or 1–2 hr after breakfast
Mechanism of action – activates 5-HT2c receptors which stimulates pro-opiomelanocortin neurons that stimulate alpha-melanocortin-4 receptors which lead to ↑ satiety and ↓ appetite					
Lorcaserin • Belviq, Belviq XR • IR: 10 mg BID • ER: 20 mg daily • ER tabs, tabs	• Hypersensitivity • Pregnancy	• Headache • Dizziness • Nausea • Xerostomia • Constipation • Hypoglycemia • Difficulty concentrating • Memory issues • Priapism • Bradycardia • Leukopenia • Hyperprolactinemia • Serotonin syndrome	• Weight • BMI • Complete blood count • Serum glucose • Prolactin levels • S/S of valvular heart disease	• CYP2D6 inhibitor • May ↑ effects/toxicity of CYP2D6 substrates • ↑ risk of serotonin syndrome with MAOIs, selective serotonin reuptake inhibitors, serotonin-norepinephrine reuptake inhibitors, triptans, tricyclic antidepressants, fentanyl, lithium, dextromethorphan, meperidine, buspirone, linezolid, methylene blue, St. John's wort, and tramadol • Thioridazine • Antipsychotics • Ergot derivatives • Bupropion • Metoprolol • Tamoxifen • Serotonin modulators	• Schedule IV controlled substance • If patient has not lost ≥5% of baseline body weight by wk 12, discontinue therapy

Medications for Weight Loss   *(cont'd)*

Generic • Brand • Dose/Dosage Form	Contraindications	Primary Side Effects	Key Monitoring	Pertinent Drug Interactions	Med Pearls
Mechanism of action – not fully understood, weight loss thought to result from regulation of food intake via hypothalmus and mesolimbic influence.					
Naltrexone/ bupropion • Contrave • 8 mg/90 mg daily × 1 wk, then BID × 1 wk, then 16 mg/ 180 mg every A.M. and 8 mg/ 90 mg every P.M. × 1 wk, then 16 mg/180 mg BID • ER tabs	• Hypersensitivity to naltrexone or bupropion • Concurrent use of other products containing bupropion • Chronic opioid use • Uncontrolled hypertension • Seizure disorders • Bulimia • Anorexia nervosa • Abrupt discontinuation of alcohol, benzodiazepines, barbiturates, or antiepileptic drugs • Use of MAOI within 2 wk • Pregnancy	• Headache • Insomnia • Nausea/vomiting (N/V) • Constipation • Dizziness • Xerostomia • Seizures • Hypertension • Tachycardia • Anaphylaxis • Hepatotoxicity	• Weight • BMI • BP • HR • Renal function • LFTs • Suicidality	• CYP2B6 substrate • CYP2D6 inhibitor • CYP2B6 inhibitors may ↑ effects/toxicity • CYP2B6 inducers may ↓ effects • May ↑ effects/toxicity of CYP2D6 substrates • ↑ risk of hypertensive crisis with MAOIs	• Do not administer with a high-fat meal • Adjust dose in renal or hepatic impairment
Mechanism of action – GLP-1 analog which ↑ glucose-dependent insulin secretion, ↓ inappropriate glucagon secretion, slows gastric emptying, and ↓ food intake					
Liraglutide • Saxenda • 0.6 mg subcut daily × 1 wk, then ↑ by 0.6 mg daily at weekly intervals to target of 3 mg subcut daily • Injection	• Hypersensitivity • History of medullary thyroid carcinoma • Multiple endo-crine neoplasia syndrome type 2 • Pregnancy	• Tachycardia • Headache • Hypoglycemia • N/V/D • Constipation • Fatigue • Dyspepsia • Dizziness • ↓ appetite • Anaphylaxis • Cholelithiasis • Pancreatitis • Thyroid tumors	• Weight • BMI • HR • Serum glucose • Renal function • S/S of pancreatitis • S/S hypoglycemia • Thyroid tumors	• May delay absorption of other drugs due to ↑ gastric emptying time (administer other medications 1 hour prior) • Sulfonylureas and insulin ↑ risk of hypoglycemia	If patient has not lost ≥4% of baseline body weight by wk 16, discontinue therapy

SMOKING CESSATION

Guidelines Summary

- The model for treatment and intervention of tobacco use and dependence is summarized by the "5 A's":

  - **ASK.** Identify and document tobacco use status for every patient and every visit.

  - **ADVISE.** Urge every tobacco user to quit in a strong and personalized manner.

  - **ASSESS.** Evaluate if your patient is willing to make a quit attempt.

  - **ASSIST.** For patients willing to make a quit attempt, offer treatment options and additional counseling; for those not willing, use motivational strategies to promote quitting.

  - **ARRANGE.** Schedule follow-ups with those patients willing to make a quit attempt; for those not willing to make an attempt, address willingness to quit at the next visit.

- Tobacco dependence is a chronic disease that often requires repeated intervention and multiple attempts to quit. Effective treatments exist that can significantly increase rates of long-term abstinence.

- It is essential that health care providers consistently identify and document tobacco use status and treat every tobacco user seen in a health care setting.

- Tobacco dependence treatments are effective across a broad range of populations. Clinicians should encourage every patient willing to make a quit attempt to use the counseling treatments and medications recommended.

- Brief tobacco dependence treatment is effective. Clinicians should offer every patient who uses tobacco at least the brief treatments shown to be effective.

Medications for Smoking Cessation

Generic • Brand • Dose/Dosage Forms	Contraindications	Primary Side Effects	Key Monitoring	Pertinent Drug Interactions	Med Pearls
Mechanism of action – partial $\alpha_4\beta_2$ nicotinic receptor agonist; prevents nicotine stimulation of the mesolimbic dopamine system					
Varenicline ☆ • Chantix • 0.5 mg daily × 3 days, then 0.5 mg BID × 4 days, then 1 mg BID × 11 wk • Tabs	Hypersensitivity	• Somnolence • Abnormal dreams • N/V • Constipation • Suicidal/homicidal ideation • Irritability • Depression • Mania • Hostility • Agitation • Anxiety • Panic • Psychotic symptoms • Hallucinations • Paranoia • Delusions • Seizures • Hypersensitivity • Rash (including Stevens-Johnson syndrome)	• Nicotine consumption • Mood changes • Psychotic symptoms • Suicidal/homicidal ideation	• Concurrent use with nicotine replacement products may ↑ risk of N/V • ↑ effects of alcohol	• Start 1 wk prior to target stop day • Take after meal and with full glass of water
Mechanism of action – inhibits neuronal uptake of norepinephrine and dopamine					
Bupropion ☆ • Zyban • 150 mg daily × 3 days, then 150 mg BID × 7–12 wk • ER tabs	• Seizure disorders • Anorexia or bulimia • Abrupt discontinuation of alcohol, benzodiazepines, barbiturates, or antiepileptic drugs • Use of MAOI within 2 wk • Use of MAOI within 14 days • Hypersensitivity • Concurrent use of linezolid or methylene blue	• Insomnia • Xerostomia • Dizziness • Nausea • Constipation • Suicidal/homicidal ideation • Irritability • Depression • Mania • Hostility • Agitation • Anxiety • Panic • Psychotic symptoms • Hallucinations • Paranoia • Delusions • Seizures • Hypertension • Anaphylaxis	• Nicotine consumption • Mood changes • Psychotic symptoms • Suicidal/homicidal ideation • Seizure activity	• CYP2B6 substrate • CYP2D6 inhibitor • CYP2B6 inhibitors may ↑ effects/toxicity • CYP2B6 inducers may ↓ effects • May ↑ effects/toxicity of CYP2D6 substrates • ↑ risk of hypertensive crises with MAOIs	• Start 1 wk prior to target stop day • Can be coadministered with nicotine replacement patches

Medications for Smoking Cessation *(cont'd)*

Generic • Brand • Dose/Dosage Forms	Contraindications	Primary Side Effects	Key Monitoring	Pertinent Drug Interactions	Med Pearls
Mechanism of action – supplements nicotine, which exhibits primary effects via autonomic ganglia stimulation					
Nicotine • Nicoderm CQ, Nicorelief, Nicorette, Nicotrol, Thrive • Gum: 1 piece every 1–2 hr PRN during wk 1–6, then 1 piece every 2–4 hr PRN during wk 7–9, then 1 piece every 4–8 hr PRN during wk 10–12 as needed; max = 24 pieces/day) • Inhaler: 6–16 cartridges/day; duration of treatment = 3 mo • Transdermal patch: >10 cigarettes/day: 21 mg/day × 6 wk, then 14 mg/day × 2 wk, then 7 mg/day × 2 wk; ≤10 cigarettes/day: 14 mg/day × 6 wk, then 7 mg/day × 2 wk • Lozenge: 1 lozenge every 1–2 hr PRN during wk 1–6, then 1 lozenge every 2–4 hr PRN during wk 7–9, then 1 lozenge every 4–8 hr PRN during wk 10–12 as needed; max = 20 lozenges/day) • Nasal spray: 1 spray in each nostril 1–2 × /hr (max = 80 sprays/day); duration of treatment = 3 mo	• Smoking or chewing tobacco • Post-myocardial infarction • Life-threatening arrhythmias • Worsening angina	• Headache • Mouth or throat irritation • Dyspepsia • Cough	• Nicotine consumption • Nicotine toxicity (severe headache, dizziness, confusion)	None	• Can be coadministered with bupropion • Gum or lozenge: use 4-mg dose if smoke first cigarette within 30 min of waking; otherwise, use 2-mg dose • Do not eat or drink within 15 min of using gum or lozenge • Oral inhalation: patient should continuously puff for ~20 min

PRACTICE QUESTIONS

1. Which of the following is indicated to prevent HPV infections?

    (A) Gardasil
    (B) Menomune
    (C) Prevnar 13
    (D) Rotarix
    (E) Zostavax

2. Which of the following is a contraindication to using bupropion for smoking cessation?

    (A) Hepatic impairment
    (B) Obesity
    (C) Orthostatic hypotension
    (D) Active seizure disorder

3. Which of the following is contraindicated in a patient taking tacrolimus?

    (A) Hepatitis B vaccine
    (B) Pneumococcal vaccine
    (C) Tdap vaccine
    (D) Varicella vaccine
    (E) All of the above

4. Which of the following formulations are available for nicotine replacement? (Select ALL that apply.)

    (A) Lozenge
    (B) Tablet
    (C) Inhaler
    (D) Gum

5. Which of the following is indicated for weight loss?

    (A) Glargine
    (B) Glimepiride
    (C) Liraglutide
    (D) Pioglitazone

6. A patient needs to receive two live vaccines but is unable to receive both on the same day. How much time must elapse before the second vaccine may be given?

    (A) 1 day
    (B) 1 week
    (C) 2 weeks
    (D) 4 weeks

7. Which of the following should be monitored in a patient taking varenicline?

    (A) Behavioral changes
    (B) Bradycardia
    (C) Pulmonary function
    (D) Weight loss

8. Which of the following vaccines is indicated for all health care workers?

    (A) Haemophilus influenza type B vaccine
    (B) Hepatitis B vaccine
    (C) Human papillomavirus vaccine
    (D) Meningococcal vaccine

9. Which of the following is a counseling point for a patient taking orlistat?

    (A) No dietary modification is needed when taking orlistat.
    (B) Orlistat must be taken on an empty stomach.
    (C) Orlistat works best if taken at bedtime.
    (D) You may experience oily discharge or spotting.

10. Which of the following should be monitored in a patient taking Qsymia? (Select ALL that apply.)

    (A) Weight
    (B) Blood pressure
    (C) LFTs
    (D) Glucose

ANSWERS AND EXPLANATIONS

1. **A**

Gardasil is the vaccine that targets human papillomavirus types 6, 11, 16, and 18. Menomune (B) is the brand name of meningococcal vaccine. Prevnar (C) is the polysaccharide conjugate vaccine that targets pneumococcal disease. Rotarix (D) is the brand name for the rotavirus vaccine, and Zostavax (E) is the brand name for the herpes zoster vaccine.

2. **D**

Bupropion is contraindicated in patients with a seizure disorder because the medication causes CNS stimulation. Hepatic impairment (A) is not associated with bupropion, so the medication is not contraindicated in these patients. Weight loss may be seen with the use of bupropion, so the medication can be used in obese individuals (B). Bupropion may also cause blood pressure elevation, so orthostatic hypotension (C) is not a contraindication to use.

3. **D**

Live vaccines are contraindicated in a patient receiving immunosuppressive therapies. Varicella is a live, attenuated vaccine that, if given to an immunocompromised patient, may cause infection with chickenpox. Vaccines against hepatitis B (A), pneumococcal (B), and Tdap (C) infection are all inactivated vaccines.

4. **A, C, D**

Nicotine is available as a gum, lozenge, inhaler, patch, and nasal spray for the treatment of smoking cessation. It is not available as a tablet (B).

5. **C**

Liraglutide, a GLP-1 analog, is indicated to treat obesity under the brand name Saxenda. Liraglutide is also available under the brand name of Victoza, which is used to treat diabetes mellitus. Glargine (A), glimepiride (B), and pioglitazone (D) are not indicated for obesity management.

6. **D**

A four-week time period should separate doses of live vaccines if the live vaccines cannot all be given on the same day.

7. **A**

Behavioral changes such as depression, irritability, suicidal ideation, and agitation should be monitored for in patients taking varenicline for smoking cessation. Bradycardia (B), changes in pulmonary function (C), and weight loss (D) are not associated with the use of varenicline.

8. **B**

Health care workers should receive the hepatitis B vaccine due to potential exposure to blood or to blood-contaminated bodily fluids. OSHA requires the vaccine to be offered to those who have an occupational risk.

9. **D**

Orlistat may cause oily discharge or spotting, especially if dietary fat content is not limited. Patients taking orlistat for weight loss should limit dietary fat consumption and adhere to a low-calorie diet. Orlistat is taken three times per day with meals, not on an empty stomach (B) or at bedtime (C).

10. **A, B**

Qsymia is a combination of phentermine and topiramate. Due to the sympathomimetic activity of phentermine, blood pressure should be monitored; weight is also monitored to ensure the effectiveness of the drug. Qysmia is not associated with changes in liver function (C) or blood glucose levels (D), so those parameters do not need to be monitored.

Over-the-Counter Medications

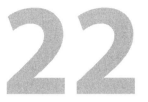

This chapter covers the following drug classes:

- **Vitamins**
- **Common herbals and supplements**
- **Decongestants**
- **Antihistamines**
- **Cough suppressants and expectorants**
- **Antidiarrheals**
- **Laxatives**
- **Antifungals**
- **Pediculocides**
- **Atopic dermatitis medications**
- **Poison ivy medications**
- **Sunscreens**

VITAMINS

Water-Soluble Vitamins

Vitamin	Function	Deficiency Manifestation	Recommended Daily Allowance (RDA)
B_1 (thiamine)	• Energy metabolism and production • Maintenance of nerve function	• Beriberi • Wernicke-Korsakoff syndrome	• Males: 1.2 mg • Females: 1.1 mg
B_2 (riboflavin)	• Energy metabolism and production • Maintenance of vision and skin	• Sore throat • Lesions of the lips and mucosa of the mouth • Glossitis • Normochromic, normocytic anemia	• Males: 1.3 mg • Females: 1.1 mg
B_3 (niacin)	• Energy metabolism and production • Maintenance of nervous and digestive systems and skin	Pellagra	• Males: 16 mg • Females: 14 mg
B_5 (pantothenic acid)	Energy metabolism and production	Paresthesia	5 mg
B_6 (pyridoxine)	• Production of red blood cells • Balance of sodium and potassium	Neuropathy	• Age 19–50 yr: 1.3 mg • Males >50 yr: 1.7 mg • Females >50 yr: 1.5 mg
B_7 (biotin)	• Fatty acid synthesis • Metabolism of amino acids	• Dermatitis • Enteritis • Hair loss	30 mcg
B_9 (folic acid)	• DNA synthesis • Production of red blood cells	• Neural tube defects • Megaloblastic anemia	400 mcg
B_{12} (cobalamins)	• Nerve function • Production of red blood cells • DNA synthesis	Megaloblastic anemia	2.4 mcg
C (ascorbic acid)	• Antioxidant • Enhances immune system	Scurvy	• Males: 90 mg • Females: 75 mg

Fat-Soluble Vitamins

Vitamin	Function	Deficiency Manifestation	RDA
A	Vision	• Night blindness • Xerophthalmia • Hyperkeratosis	• Males: 900 mcg (3,000 units) • Females: 700 mcg (2,330 units)
D	• Calcium and phosphorus regulation • Bone health	Rickets	• Age 19–70 yr: 15 mcg (600 units) • Age >70 yr: 20 mcg (800 units)
E	• Antioxidant • Smooth muscle and nerve function	Hemolytic anemia	15 mg
K	Blood clotting	Bleeding	• Males: 120 mcg • Females: 90 mcg

COMMON HERBALS AND SUPPLEMENTS

Common Usage

- Saw palmetto
  - Used in men to improve symptoms of benign prostatic hyperplasia (BPH)
- Glucosamine and chondroitin
  - Used widely for treating osteoarthritis and joint structure support
  - Glucosamine: important for maintaining elasticity, strength, and resiliency of the cartilage in articular (movable) joints
  - Chondroitin: promotes flexibility of cartilage
- Fish oils or omega-3 fatty acids
  - Used primarily for hypertriglyceridemia
  - Contain eicosapentaenoic acid (EPA) and docosahexaenoic acid (DHA), and are believed to be efficacious in many people
- St. John's wort
  - Used for mild to moderate depression
  - Used in Europe for centuries for mild to moderate depression and its efficacy is comparable with tricyclic antidepressants; one study suggests it is no more effective than a placebo or sertraline in moderate to severe depression; it should not be used with other selective serotonin reuptake inhibitors (SSRIs) or serotonin norepinephrine reuptake inhibitors (SNRIs)

- Coenzyme Q10
  - Used for cardiovascular diseases, including angina, heart failure, and hypertension, and may help with myalgias due to statin therapy
- Melatonin
  - Used for insomnia, particularly when adjusting to shift-work cycles or jet lag
  - Naturally secreted from the pineal gland and appears to be the sleep-regulating hormone of the body; adults experience about a 37% decrease in daily melatonin output between 20 and 70 years of age
- Echinacea
  - Used as an immune stimulant
  - Has been studied extensively in the area of flu and cold prevention/treatment
- Black cohosh
  - Used for women's health problems, especially postmenopausal symptom relief and painful menses
  - Should be avoided in pregnancy and lactation
- Ginger
  - Used primarily for motion sickness, dyspepsia, and nausea
  - Lacks sedative affects of other antinausea treatments
  - Has been studied in pregnant women at less than 17 weeks' gestation
- Ginkgo biloba
  - Used for vascular dementia, Alzheimer's, and ischemic stroke
  - The ginkgolides are potent platelet-activating factor antagonists
- Ginseng
  - Used to treat diabetes mellitus
  - May also help reduce mental and physical stress

Over-the-Counter Medications

Name • Alternate Name • Dose	Contraindications	Primary Side Effects	Key Monitoring Parameters	Pertinent Drug Interactions	Med Pearls
Mechanism of action – inhibits production of dihydrotestosterone (DHT), inhibits receptor binding, and accelerates the metabolism of DHT					
Serenoa repens • Saw palmetto • BPH: 160 mg BID	• Pregnancy or lactation • Age <12 yr	Nausea/vomiting (N/V)	BPH symptoms	• May ↑ toxicity of estrogens or estrogen-containing contraceptives • May ↑ risk of bleeding with warfarin	Data from meta-analysis do not support use
Mechanism of action – glucosamine is an amino-sugar that is naturally produced and is a key substrate in the synthesis of macromolecules for connective tissues; chondroitin absorbs water, adding to cartilage thickness, and is found in natural physiologic connective tissue; inhibits synovial enzymes that may contribute to cartilage destruction					
Glucosamine/ chondroitin • Glucosamine: 500 mg TID • Chondroitin: 400 mg TID	• Glucosamine: active bleeding • Chondroitin: none	• Flatulence • Abdominal cramps • ↑ blood glucose	Osteoarthritis pain	May ↑ risk of bleeding with antiplatelets or anticoagulants	
Mechanism of action – inhibit diacylglycerol transferase which leads to a ↓ in hepatic synthesis of triglycerides					
Omega-3 fatty acids • Fish oils • Hypertriglyceride-mia: 2–4 g/day	Active bleeding	Gastrointestinal upset	Lipid panel	May ↑ risk of bleeding with antiplatelets or anticoagulants	
Mechanism of action – ↑ concentrations of serotonin in the central nervous system (CNS) and may have some monoamine oxidase inhibitor (MAOI) effects					
Hypericum perforatum • St. John's wort • 300 mg TID	• Pregnancy or lactation • Concurrent use with CYP2C19, CYP3A4, or P-glycoprotein substrates	• Nausea • Xerostomia • Itching • Photosensitivity • Fatigue • Dizziness • Insomnia • Jitteriness • Headache	Depression symptoms	• CYP2C19 and CYP3A4 inducer • May ↓ effects of CYP2C19 or CYP3A4 substrates • ↑ risk of serotonin syndrome with MAOIs, SSRIs, SNRIs, triptans, tricyclic antidepressants (TCAs), fentanyl, lithium, dextromethorphan, meperidine, buspirone, linezolid, methylene blue, and tramadol	Minimum of 4–6 wk of therapy is recommended before results seen
Mechanism of action – involved in adenosine triphosphate generation and serves as a lipid-soluble antioxidant providing protection against free-radical damage within the mitochondria					
Ubiquinone • Coenzyme Q10 • 20–300 mg/day in 2–3 divided doses	None	• Abdominal discomfort • Headache • N/V	Heart failure symptoms	• May ↓ anticoagulant effects of warfarin • May ↑ risk of cardiotoxicity with anthracyclines	

Over-the-Counter Medications *(cont'd)*

Name • Alternate Name • Dose	Contraindications	Primary Side Effects	Key Monitoring Parameters	Pertinent Drug Interactions	Med Pearls
Mechanism of action – supplements the naturally deficient concentrations of melatonin					
N-acetyl-5-methoxytryp-tamine • Melatonin • 1–5 mg at bedtime	Autoimmune disease	• Morning sedation or drowsiness • Headache • Dizziness • Nausea	Sleep quality/quantity	• CYP1A2 inhibitor • May ↑ effects/toxicity of CYP1A2 substrates	Drugs that deplete vitamin B_6 may inhibit the ability of the body to synthesize melatonin
Mechanism of action – may stimulate white blood cell function, including cell-mediated immunity					
Echinacea purpurea/ angustifolia/ pallida • Echinacea • 50–1,000 mg TID on day 1, then 250 mg 4 × /day	• Hypersensitivty to plants in Asteraceae/ Compositae family (including ragweed, chrysanthemums, marigolds, daisies) • Immunosup-pressed patients • Rheumatoid arthritis • Systemic lupus erythematosus • Multiple sclerosis • Tuberculosis	• Itching • Rash • N/V	Cold symptoms	• CYP1A2 inhibitor • CYP3A4 inducer • May ↑ effects/toxicity of CYP1A2 substrates • May ↓ effects of CYP3A4 substrates • May ↓ effects of immunosuppressants	Should not use for >10 days in acute infection
Mechanism of action – contains phytoestrogens, which mimic estrogen					
Actaea racemosa or *Cimicifuga racemosa* • Black cohosh • 20–40 mg BID	• History of or at risk for breast cancer • Pregnancy or lactation • Aspirin sensitivity	• N/V • Rash • Hepatotoxicity	Menopausal symptoms	• CYP2D6 inhibitor • May ↑ effects/toxicity of CYP2D6 substrates	Contains salicylates
Mechanism of action – has local affects in the gastrointestinal (GI) tract and in the CNS					
Zingiber officinale • Ginger • 500–2500 mg/day in 2–4 divided doses	Active bleeding	Generally well tolerated	Degree of nausea	May ↑ risk of bleeding with antiplatelets or anticoagulants	Use during pregnancy for morning sickness remains controversial
Mechanism of action – the flavonoid component protects neurons and retinal tissue from oxidative stress and injury					
Ginkgo biloba • Ginkgo • 120–240 mg/day in 2–3 divided doses	• Pregnancy or lactation • Active bleeding	• Nausea • Constipation • Headache • Dizziness • Palpitations • Allergic skin reactions	Mini mental state exam	May ↑ risk of bleeding with antiplatelets or anticoagulants	None

Over-the-Counter Medications   *(cont'd)*

Name • Alternate Name • Dose	Contraindications	Primary Side Effects	Key Monitoring Parameters	Pertinent Drug Interactions	Med Pearls
Mechanism of action – ↓ postprandial glucose levels and stimulates the release of insulin					
Panax quinquefolius • Ginseng (American) • Usual: 100–400 mg daily • Diabetes: up to 3 g/day, 2 hr before a meal	Active bleeding	• Insomnia • Headache • Anorexia	Blood glucose	• May ↑ risk of bleeding with antiplatelets or anticoagulants • May ↑ effects of glucose-lowering drugs	Should not use for >3 mo

DECONGESTANTS

Guidelines Summary

- A pharmacist may appropriately recommend a decongestant once it is determined that the patient does not have any of the following:
    - Fever (temperature >101.5°F)
    - Chest pain
    - Shortness of breath
    - Uncontrolled hypertension
    - Cardiac arrhythmias
    - Insomnia
    - Anxiety
    - Worsening of symptoms or development of additional symptoms during self-treatment
    - Concurrent underlying chronic cardiopulmonary disease
    - Acquired immune deficiency syndrome or chronic immunosuppressant therapy
    - Frail patients of advanced age
    - Children <2 years of age
    - Current use of MAOIs
- Topical decongestants should not be recommended for longer than 3 days due to the risk of rhinitis medicamentosa, a condition of rebound nasal congestion brought on by overuse of intranasal vasoconstrictive medications.

Decongestants

Generic • Brand • Dose	Contraindications	Primary Side Effects	Key Monitoring Parameters	Pertinent Drug Interactions	Med Pearls
Oral Decongestants					
Mechanism of action – alpha-1 adrenergic stimulant					
Phenylephrine • Sudafed PE Maximum Strength • 10 mg every 4 hr PRN	• Uncontrolled hypertension • Ventricular tachycardia • Use of MAOI within 2 wk	• Restlessness • Hypertension • Tremor • Tachycardia • Insomnia	• Blood pressure • Heart rate • Anxiety	↑ risk of hypertensive crisis with MAOIs	Available OTC without restrictions
Pseudoephedrine • Sudafed • IR: 60 mg every 4–6 hr PRN • ER: 120 mg every 12 hr or 240 mg daily					• Available behind the counter • Must provide photo identification and sign log book to purchase • Amount purchased limited to ≤3.6 g/day or 9 g/mo
Topical Decongestants					
Oxymetazoline • Afrin • Intranasal: 2–3 sprays in each nostril BID	Hypersensitivity	• Dryness of nasal mucosa • Stinging • Rebound congestion	Rebound congestion	↑ risk of hypertensive crisis with MAOIs	Not recommended for longer than 3 days
Naphazoline • Clear Eyes • Ophthalmic: 1–2 drops every 6 hr PRN					
Phenylephrine • Neo-Synephrine • 1–2 sprays in each nostril every 4 hr					

ANTIHISTAMINES

Guidelines Summary

- Contact dermatitis
    - Identify the cause: chemicals, acids, solvent, fragrances, metals, poison ivy, etc.
    - Clean the area with mild soap and water.
    - Refer patient to physician if the rash causes edema or invades the eyelids, external genitalia, anus, or massive areas of the body.
    - Treatment includes topical treatment with hydrocortisone, bicarbonate pastes, and antihistamines.
- Allergic rhinitis and common cold
    - A pharmacist may appropriately recommend an antihistamine once it is determined that the patient does not have any of the following:
        » Symptoms of otitis media or sinusitis
        » Symptoms of lower respiratory tract infection
        » History of nonallergic rhinitis
- Insomnia
    - Transient or short-term insomnia with no underlying problems are appropriate for self-treatment.
    - Discuss good sleep hygiene practices—no caffeine after 5 P.M., no exercise in the evening.
    - If diphenhydramine is recommended, it should be taken at bedtime only as needed.
    - Patients who complain of continuing insomnia after 14 days of treatment should be referred to a physician.

Antihistamines

Generic • Brand • Dose/Dosage Forms	Contraindications	Primary Side Effects	Key Monitoring Parameters	Pertinent Drug Interactions	Med Pearls
First-Generation Histamine H₁ Antagonists					
Mechanism of action – competes with histamine for H₁ receptor sites on effector cells in the GI tract, blood vessels, and respiratory tract					
Clemastine • Tavist Allergy • 1.34 mg BID-TID (max = 8.04 mg/day) • Tabs	• Hypersensitivity • Concurrent use with MAOIs • Lactation • Asthma	• Sedation • Dry mouth • Constipation • Blurred vision • Urinary retention	Mental alertness	• Concurrent use with MAOIs may ↑ risk of anticholinergic effects • Additive effects with other anticholinergic medications	• Paradoxic reactions (including stimulatory effects) may be seen • Have more anticholinergic effects than second-generation H₁ antagonists • Diphenhydramine also available as injection • NOT for OTC use in children <2 yr
Chlorpheniramine • Chlor-Trimeton • IR: 4 mg every 4–6 hr PRN (max = 24 mg/day) • ER: 12 mg every 12 hr (max = 24 mg/day) • ER tabs, solution, tabs	• Hypersensitivity • Narrow angle glaucoma • BPH • Asthma			• CYP2D6 substrate • CYP2D6 inhibitors may ↑ effects/toxicity • Additive effects with other anticholinergic medications	
Brompheniramine • J-Tan PD • 1–2 mg every 4–6 hr PRN (max = 6 mg/day [2–5 yr]; 12 mg/day [6–11 yr]) • Solution, tabs	None			Additive effects with other anticholinergic medications	
Diphenhydramine • Benadryl, Sominex, Unisom, ZzzQuil • Allergy: 25–50 mg every 4–8 hr PRN (max = 300 mg/day) • Insomnia: 50 mg at bedtime PRN • Caps, chewable tabs, solution, strips, suspension, tabs	• Hypersensitivity • Lactation			Additive effects with other anticholinergic medications	
Doxylamine • Sleep Aid • 25 mg at bedtime PRN • Solution, tabs					

Antihistamines   *(cont'd)*

Generic • Brand • Dose/Dosage Forms	Contraindications	Primary Side Effects	Key Monitoring Parameters	Pertinent Drug Interactions	Med Pearls
Second-Generation Histamine H$_1$ Antagonists					
Mechanism of action – long-acting tricyclic antihistamines with selective peripheral H$_1$-receptor antagonistic properties; less blood-brain barrier penetration					
Loratadine • Alavert, Claritin • 10 mg daily • Caps, chewable tabs, ODTs, solution, tabs	Hypersensitivity	• Some sedation • Headache • Dizziness • Xerostomia	Relief of symptoms	Additive effects with other anticholinergic medications	• Available in combination with pseudoephedrine • Desloratadine (Clarinex) only available Rx • NOT for OTC use in children <2 yr
Cetirizine • Zyrtec • 5–10 mg daily • Caps, chewable tabs, ODTs, solution, tabs					• Available in combination with pseudoephedrine • Most sedating of the second-generation antihistamines • NOT for OTC use in children <2 yr
Fexofenadine • Allegra, Mucinex Allergy • 60 mg BID or 180 mg daily • ODTs, suspension, tabs		Headache			• Avoid taking with fruit juices • Available in combination with pseudoephedrine • Least sedating of the second-generation antihistamines • NOT for OTC use in children <2 yr

COUGH SUPPRESSANTS AND EXPECTORANTS

Guidelines Summary

- The primary goal of treating a cough is to reduce the number and severity of cough episodes.

- Cough suppressants (antitussives) should only be used to treat nonproductive coughs; should not be used for productive coughs.

- Codeine and dextromethorphan are the cough suppressants of choice for nonproductive cough.

- Antihistamines also have antitussive properties:
  - Diphenhydramine is a better choice for a cough associated with allergies but is highly sedating.
  - A second-generation antihistamine can also be considered since they are associated with less sedation.
- Expectorants include guaifenesin and water. Expectorants can be used to thin out the mucus or phlegm associated with a productive cough; they do NOT act as a cough suppressant.
- Patients should be excluded from self-treatment if they have any of the following:

Cough with thick yellow sputum or green phlegm	Unintended weight loss
Drenching nighttime sweats	History of asthma, COPD, or heart failure
Foreign-object aspiration	Cough duration >7 days
Fever (temperature >101.5°F)	Children <2 yr of age
Hemoptysis	Cough worsens during self-treatment

Cough Suppressants

Generic • Brand • Dose/Dosage Forms	Contraindications	Primary Side Effects	Key Monitoring Parameters	Pertinent Drug Interactions	Med Pearls
Mechanism of action – depresses the medullary cough center					
Dextromethorphan • Robitussin, Delsym • IR: 10–20 mg every 4 hr or 30 mg every 6–8 hr • ER: 60 mg BID • Max = 120 mg/day • Caps, ER suspension, gel, lozenges, solution, strips	Use of MAOI within 2 wk	• Confusion • Irritability	Relief of symptoms	• CYP2D6 substrate • CYP2D6 inhibitors may ↑ effects/ toxicity • ↑ risk of serotonin syndrome with MAOIs, SSRIs, SNRIs, triptans, TCAs, fentanyl, lithium, meperidine, buspirone, linezolid, methylene blue, St. John's wort, and tramadol	• Not for OTC use in children <2 yr • Chemically related to morphine; lacks narcotic properties except in overdose • May require Rx for use in children and adolescents in some states
Codeine • 7.5–15 mg every 4–6 hr (max = 120 mg/day)	• Hypersensitivity • Respiratory depression • Paralytic ileus • Severe or acute asthma • Gastrointestinal obstruction	• N/V • Constipation • Sedation	• CNS depression • Relief of symptoms	• CYP2D6 substrate • CYP2D6 inhibitors may ↑ effects/ toxicity • Other CNS depressants, including alcohol, may ↑ CNS depressant effects	10% of a codeine dose is demethylated in the liver to form morphine

Expectorant

Generic • Brand • Dose/Dosage Forms	Contraindications	Primary Side Effects	Key Monitoring Parameters	Pertinent Drug Interactions	Med Pearls
Mechanism of action – expectorant; irritates the gastric mucosa and stimulates respiratory tract secretions, thereby ↑ fluid volumes and ↓ mucous viscosity					
Guaifenesin • Mucinex • IR: 200–400 mg every 4 hr PRN • ER: 600–1,200 mg BID PRN • Max = 2,400 mg/day • ER tabs, oral packets, solution, tabs	Hypersensitivity	• Dizziness • Kidney stone formation	Relief of symptoms	None	More effective with water intake

ANTIDIARRHEALS

Guidelines Summary

■ Acute diarrhea can be managed with fluids, electrolyte replacement, dietary interventions, and nonprescription drug treatment.

■ Persistent and chronic diarrhea requires medical care, and patients are not candidates for self-treatment if either forms of diarrhea is present.

■ Patients should be excluded from self-treatment if any of the following apply:

  • <6 months of age

  • Severe dehydration

  • >6 months of age with persistent high fevers greater than 102.2°F

  • Blood, mucus, or pus in the stool

  • Protracted vomiting or severe abdominal pain

  • Pregnancy

  • Chronic or persistent diarrhea

Antidiarrheals

Generic • Brand • Dose/Dosage Forms	Contraindications	Primary Side Effects	Key Monitoring Parameters	Pertinent Drug Interactions	Med Pearls
Mechanism of action – acts directly on opioid receptors on intestinal muscles to inhibit peristalsis and prolong transit time					
Loperamide • Imodium A–D • 4 mg, followed by 2 mg after each loose stool, (max = 16 mg/day) • Caps, chewable tabs, solution, suspension, tabs	• Hypersensitivity • Abdominal pain without diarrhea • Children <2 yr • Primary tx for acute dysentery, acute ulcerative colitis, bacterial enterocolitis, and pseudomembranous colitis (*C. difficile*)	• Constipation • Abdominal cramping • Abdominal distention	• Bowel movement frequency • CNS depression • Paralytic ileus • S/S of dehydration	None	None
Mechanism of action – possesses both antisecretory and antimicrobial effects; may also provides some anti-inflammatory effects					
Bismuth subsalicylate • Pepto-Bismol • 524 mg every 30–60 min PRN for up to 2 days (max = 4,200 mg/day) • Chewable tabs, suspension	• Children or adolescents with influenza or chickenpox (due to risk of Reye's syndrome) • Hx of GI bleed • Pregnancy • Hypersensitivity to salicylates	• Discoloration of tongue and feces (grayish-black) • Hearing loss • Tinnitus	Bowel movement frequency	May ↓ absorption of tetracyclines and fluoroquino-lones (separate by 2 hr)	None
Mechanism of action – helps reestablish normal intestinal flora; suppresses the growth of potentially pathogenic microorganisms by producing lactic acid, which favors the establishment of an aciduric flora					
Lactobacillus • Culturelle, Lactinex • Culturelle: 1 caplet daily or BID • Lactinex: 4 tabs 3–4 × /day • Caps. chewable tabs, granules, powder, tabs, wafers	Hypersensitivity to milk protein	• Flatulence • Bloating	Bowel movement frequency	None	Lactinex must be stored in refrigerator
Lactase enzyme • Lactaid • 1–2 capsules taken with milk or meal	None	None	Bowel movement frequency	None	• Used in the treatment of lactose intolerance • Prevents osmotic diarrhea

LAXATIVES

Guidelines Summary

- Lifestyle modifications:
    - Educate patient about high fiber and increased hydration in diet.
    - Encourage patients to avoid postponing defecation.
    - Monitor bowel habits with a daily diary.
    - Encourage patients to maintain moderate exercise.
- Patients should be excluded from self-treatment if they have any of the following:
    - Marked abdominal pain or significant distention or cramping
    - Marked or unexplained flatulence
    - Fever
    - N/V
    - Paraplegia or quadriplegia
    - Daily laxative use
    - Unexplained changes in bowel habits and/or weight loss
    - Bowel symptoms that persist for 2 weeks
    - History of irritable bowel disease
- Pharmacologic therapy begins with bulk-forming agents and proceeds to osmotic laxatives.
- If these options are not helpful, stimulant laxatives should be considered.
- Enemas, suppositories, and lubricants are also available as options.

Medications for Constipation

Generic • Brand • Dose/Dosage Forms	Contraindications	Primary Side Effects	Key Monitoring Parameters	Pertinent Drug Interactions	Med Pearls
Mechanism of action – bulk-forming laxatives that work by absorbing water in the intestine to form a viscous liquid that promotes peristalsis					
Psyllium • Metamucil, Konsyl • 2.5–30 g/day in divided doses • Caps, packets, powder	• Fecal impaction • GI obstruction	• Abdominal cramps • Diarrhea	Bowel movement frequency	May ↓ absorption of other medications (space apart by 2 hr)	Take with full glass of water
Calcium polycarbophil • FiberCon • 2 tabs 1–4 × /day • Tabs					
Methylcellulose • Citrucel • 2 caps up to 6 × /day • 1 tbsp up to 3 × /day • Powder, tabs					

Medications for Constipation (cont'd)

Generic • Brand • Dose/Dosage Forms	Contraindications	Primary Side Effects	Key Monitoring Parameters	Pertinent Drug Interactions	Med Pearls
Mechanism of action – osmotic laxative that causes water retention in the stool					
Polyethylene glycol 3350 • GlycoLax, MiraLax • 17 g daily • Packets, powder	• GI obstruction • Hypersensitivity	• Abdominal cramps • Diarrhea • Bloating	Bowel movement frequency	None	Can reconstitute with 8 oz of water, juice, cola, or tea
Mechanism of action – stimulant laxatives that stimulates peristalsis by directly irritating the smooth muscle of the intestine					
Senna • Ex-Lax Maximum Strength, Senokot • 17.2 mg daily up to 34.4 mg BID • Chewable tabs, solution, tabs	• Fecal impaction • GI obstruction	• Abdominal cramps • Diarrhea	Bowel movement frequency	None	None
Bisacodyl • Dulcolax, Fleet Laxative • 5–15 mg PO daily • Rectal: 10 mg daily • Enema, suppository, tabs				Effect may be ↓ by milk, dairy products, or antacids (separate by 1 hr)	
Mechanism of action – stool softeners that ↓ surface tension of the oil-water interface of the stool, resulting in enhanced incorporation of water and fat which facilitates stool softening					
Docusate sodium • Colace • 100 mg PO BID • Rectal: 1 enema 1–3 × /day • Caps, enema, solution, tabs Docusate calcium • Kao-Tin • 240 mg daily	• Fecal impaction • GI obstruction	• Diarrhea • Cramping	Bowel movement frequency	None	Take with full glass of water
Mechanism of action – osmotic laxative that promotes bowel evacuation by causing osmotic retention of fluid which distends the colon with ↑ peristaltic activity					
Magnesium hydroxide • Phillips Milk of Magnesia • 1–2 tbsp daily or BID • Chewable tabs, suspension	Hypersensitivity	Diarrhea	Bowel movement frequency	May ↓ absorption of tetracyclines and fluoroquinolones (separate by 2 hr)	• Take with full glass of water • Use with caution in patients with renal impairment
Mechanism of action – lubricant laxative that eases passage of stool by ↓ water absorption and lubricating the intestines					
Mineral oil • Fleet Oil • 1–2 tbsp at bedtime • 1 enema × 1 • Enema, oil	• Children <6 yr • Pregnancy • Elderly • Difficulty swallowing	• Abdominal cramps • Diarrhea • Aspiration pneumonia	Bowel movement frequency	May ↓ absorption of fat-soluble vitamins (A, D, K, E)	Aspiration is possible, especially in elderly population

ANTIFUNGALS

Guidelines Summary

- Patients should be excluded from self-treatment if they have any of the following:
  - Causative factor unclear
  - Nails or scalp involved
  - Face, mucous membranes, or genitalia involved
  - Signs and symptoms of possible secondary bacterial infection
  - Excessive and continuous exudation, fever, malaise
- Apply a thin layer of medication to affected area for 2–4 weeks (product dependent), even after the signs and symptoms disappear.

Topical Antifungal Medications to Treat Tinea

Generic • Brand • Dose/Dosage Forms	Contraindications	Primary Side Effects	Key Monitoring Parameters	Pertinent Drug Interactions	Med Pearls
Mechanism of action – squalene epoxidase inhibitor results in deficiency of ergosterol within the fungal cell					
Butenafine • Lotrimin Ultra, Mentax • Apply daily × 2 wk (corporis/cruris) or 4 wk (pedis) • Cream	Hypersensitivity	• Burning • Contact dermatitis • Erythema • Irritation • Stinging	Clinical signs of improvement	None	Used to treat tinea pedis, tinea cruris, and tinea corporis
Terbinafine • Lamisil, Lamisil AT • Apply 1–2 × /day × ≥1 wk • Cream, gel					
Mechanism of action – binds to phospholipids in the fungal cell membrane, altering cell wall permeability and resulting in loss of intracellular elements					
Clotrimazole • Lotrimin AF • Apply BID	Hypersensitivity	• Burning • Contact dermatitis • Erythema • Itching	Clinical signs of improvement	None	Used to treat tinea pedis, tinea cruris, and tinea corporis
Miconazole • Desenex, Micatin • Apply BID × 2 wk (cruris) or 4 wk (corporis/pedis) • Cream, lotion, ointment, powder, powder spray, solution, spray					

Topical Antifungal Medications to Treat Tinea *(cont'd)*

Generic • Brand • Dose/Dosage Forms	Contraindications	Primary Side Effects	Key Monitoring Parameters	Pertinent Drug Interactions	Med Pearls
Mechanism of action – distorts the hyphae and stunts mycelial growth in susceptible fungi					
Tolnaftate • Tinactin • Apply BID × 2 wk (cruris) or 4 wk (corporis/pedis) • Cream, powder, powder spray, solution, spray	Hypersensitivity	• Burning • Contact dermatitis • Erythema • Itching	Clinical signs of improvement	None	Used to treat tinea pedis, tinea cruris, and tinea corporis
Mechanism of action – inhibits conversion of yeast to the hyphal form (active form) and interferes with fatty-acid biosynthesis					
Undecylenic acid • Fungi-Nail • Apply BID × 4 wk • Solution	Hypersensitivity	High alcohol concentrations may cause burning	Clinical signs of improvement	None	Used to treat tinea pedis and toe fungus

PEDICULOCIDES

Guidelines Summary

- All members of a household that contain a person with a lice infestation should be screened for lice and treated if they are infected.

- Treatment includes ovicidal agents. Retreatment is only needed for ovicidal agents if lice continue to be seen. Weakly ovicidal agents will require retreatment to make sure all nits have hatched and will be exposed to medication.

- Nonpharmacologic treatment includes washing all items such at hats, towels, and bedding that came into contact with the infected person within 48 hr of treatment in hot water and dried with hot air. If something cannot be washed in a washing machine, other options include dry cleaning or placing the items within a plastic bag for a two-week period.

- Patients should be excluded from self-treatment if they have any of the following:
  - Children <2 yr
  - Hypersensitivity to chrysanthemums
  - Secondary skin infection in lice-infested areas
  - Pregnancy
  - Lactation

Medications to Treat Pediculosis

Generic • Brand • Dose/Dosage Forms	Contraindications	Primary Side Effects	Key Monitoring Parameters	Med Pearls
Mechanism of action – inhibits respiration of lice by respiratory spiracle obstruction				
Benzyl alcohol • Ulesfia • 4–48 ounces based on length of hair • Lotion	None	• Pruritus • Erythema • Local irritation • Eye irritation	Eradication of lice and nits	• Rx only • Apply to *dry* hair, saturate scalp, leave on for 10 min, rinse, then repeat in 7 days
Mechanism of action – inhibits sodium influx into nerve cell membranes, causing repolarization and paralysis of the lice				
Permethrin • Elimite, Nix • Cream, lotion	Hypersensitivity	• Pruritus • Erythema • Scalp rash • Burning • Stinging • Scalp discomfort	Eradication of lice and nits	• Elimite is Rx only • Wash hair with conditioner-free shampoo, towel dry, apply sufficient amount of lotion or cream to saturate scalp and hair, leave on for no longer than 10 minutes, rinse with warm water, comb hair with nit comb; may repeat in 7 days, if needed • Do not use near eyes or inside the nose, ear, mouth, or vagina • Elimite can also be used for scabies
Mechanism of action – neurotoxicity caused by stimulation of nerve cells to produce repeated discharges and subsequent paralysis				
Pyrethrins and piperonyl butoxide • A–200, Licide, Pronto Plus, RID • Gel, oil, shampoo, solution	None	• Pruritus • Burning • Stinging • Skin irritation	Eradication of lice and nits	• Apply to *dry* hair, leave on for 10 minutes, wash and rinse, comb hair with nit comb, then repeat in 7–10 days • Do not use near eyes, in eyebrows or eyelashes, or inside nose, mouth, vagina • Solution should only be applied to bedding (not for human use)
Mechanism of action – ↑ permeabilty of cell membranes to chloride, resulting in hyperpolarization and death of lice				
Ivermectin • Sklice • Lotion	None	• Burning • Skin irritation	Eradication of lice and nits	• Rx only • Apply to *dry* scalp and hair, leave on for 10 minutes, rinse with warm water, comb hair with nit comb; do not repeat • Also available as cream (Soolantra) for rosacea
Mechanism of action – inhibits cholinesterase in lice, causing death				
Malathion • Ovide • Lotion	• Hypersensitivity • Neonates or infants	• Chemical burns • Local irritation • Stinging • Conjunctivitis	Eradication of lice and nits	• Rx only • Apply to *dry* hair and scalp, dry hair naturally (do not cover), shampoo off after 8–12 hr, comb hair with nit comb; may repeat in 7–9 days if needed

Medications to Treat Pediculosis   *(cont'd)*

Generic • Brand • Dose/Dosage Forms	Contraindications	Primary Side Effects	Key Monitoring Parameters	Med Pearls
Mechanism of action – CNS excitation and involuntary muscle contractions produce paralysis and death of lice				
Spinosad • Natroba • Suspension	None	• Erythema • Local irritation • Dry skin	Eradication of lice and nits	• Rx only • Apply to *dry* scalp and hair, leave on for 10 minutes, rinse with warm water, may then shampoo, comb hair with nit comb; may repeat in 7 days if needed
Mechanism of action – stimulates the nervous system of lice, causing seizures and death				
Lindane • Only available generically • Shampoo	• Hypersensitivity • Premature infants • Uncontrolled seizure disorders • Crusted skin conditions	• Ataxia • Dizziness • Burning • Neurotoxicity • Seizures • Dermatitis	• Eradication of lice and nits • Mental status • Seizures	• Rx only • Apply to *dry* hair and massage in for 4 min, add in water to form a lather, rinse hair thoroughly, comb hair with nit comb; do not repeat • Can also be used for pubic lice or scabies

ATOPIC DERMATITIS MEDICATIONS

Guidelines Summary

- Treatment of atopic dermatitis includes skin hydration, removal of known irritants, and topical steroid creams.
- Patients should be excluded from self-treatment any of the following apply
  - Age <2 years
  - Severe dermatitis or pruritus
  - Large body area involvement
  - Skin infection

Medications for Atopic Dermatitis

Generic • Brand • Dose/Dosage Forms	Contraindications	Primary Side Effects	Key Monitoring Parameters	Med Pearls
Mechanism of action – ↓ inflammatory mediators through the induction of phospholipase A2 inhibitory proteins and release of arachidonic acid				
Hydrocortisone • Cortaid • Applied up to 3–4 × /day • Cream	• Hypersensitivity • Diaper dermatitis	• Acneiform eruptions • Skin irritation • Dry skin • Hypopigmentation	Response to therapy	Avoid use on weeping lesions

POISON IVY MEDICATIONS

Guidelines Summary

- Remove clothing worn during exposure to urushiol. Wash exposed clothing separately to avoid contaminating other items.
- Wash skin with soap and water to remove urushiol.
- Treatment focuses on the relief of itching and may include the use of topical calamine or hydrocortisone.
- Avoid topical anesthetics, antihistamines, and antibiotics for mild symptoms to prevent sensitization of the skin and a drug-induced dermatitis.
- Nonpharmacologic treatment can include the use of colloidal oatmeal baths, tepid showers, and baking soda compressed.
- Patients should be excluded from self-treatment if they have any of the following:
  - Involvement of rash on the face, eyes, or genitalia
  - Difficulty breathing
  - Exposure to smoke from a burning poison ivy, poison oak, or poison sumac plant
  - Age <2 years
  - Widespread rash involving >25% of body surface area
  - Presence of infection
  - Presence of rash >2 weeks
  - Presence of numerous bullae

Medications for Poison Ivy

Generic • Dose/Dosage Forms	Contraindications	Primary Side Effects	Key Monitoring Parameters	Med Pearls
Mechanism of action – possesses astringent properties to dry weeping lesions; works as a skin protectant				
Calamine • Apply as often as necessary • Lotion	Hypersensitivity	Local irritation	Response to therapy	Do not use on open lesions

SUNSCREENS

Sunscreen

- The American Academy of Dermatology recommends that everyone wear sunscreen any day they will be outside and exposed to sunlight.
- Application of sunscreen should include agents that are:
  - Broad spectrum to cover exposure to both ultraviolet (UV) A and UVB rays
  - Water-resistant
  - Sun Protection Factor (SPF) of 30 or higher, which will block 97% of UVB rays
- Sunscreen terms:
  - SPF is measure of a suncreen's ability to block UVB rays. SPF is a factor that can estimate how much time one can spend in the sun without getting burned. If a burn would normally start in 10 minutes, using a product with an SPF of 30 will allow an exposure of approximately 300 minutes without a burn (30 times longer).
  - Water-resistant sunscreen is effective for up to 40 minutes in water.
  - Very water-resistant sunscreen is effective for up to 80 minutes in water.
- Guidelines for the application of sunscreen:
  - Sunscreen should not be applied to infants ≤6 mo.
  - Use enough sunscreen to coat the skin; may need ≥1 ounce to cover the body.
  - To protect lips, use a lip balm with at least an SPF of 30.
  - Apply 15 minutes before exposure to sun.
  - Reapply every 2 hours or after swimming.
  - Creams are best for application on dry skin and the face.
  - Sprays may be used, but ensure all areas have been covered.
  - Gels may be used for areas covered in hair.
  - Stick formulations are good for administration around the eyes.

PRACTICE QUESTIONS

1. Which of the following conditions might St. John's wort be used to treat?

    (A) BPH
    (B) Depression
    (C) Diabetes
    (D) Hypertriglyceridemia
    (E) Lactose intolerance

2. Which of the following vitamins is used to treat Wernicke-Korsakoff syndrome?

    (A) Thiamine
    (B) Folic acid
    (C) Pyridoxine
    (D) Riboflavin

3. Which of the following contain dextromethorphan?

    (A) Astepro
    (B) Delsym
    (C) Mucinex Allergy
    (D) ZzzQuil

4. Which of the following should be used for only 3 days to treat nasal congestion?

    (A) Diphenhydramine
    (B) Doxylamine
    (C) Loratadine
    (D) Naphazoline
    (E) Phenylephrine

5. A patient comes in complaining of bilateral knee pain caused by arthritis. He requests an herbal product. Which of the following herbal medications would help the patient's arthritis?

    (A) Echinancea
    (B) Melatonin
    (C) Osteo Bi-Flex
    (D) Saw palmetto

6. Which of the following is considered a second-generation or less sedating antihistamine?

   (A) Brompheniramine
   (B) Chlorpheniramine
   (C) Doxylamine
   (D) Fexofenadine
   (E) Pseudoephedrine

7. Which condition can terbinafine be used to treat?

   (A) Athlete's foot
   (B) Constipation
   (C) Diarrhea
   (D) Lactose intolerance
   (E) Seasonal allergies

8. Which of the following vitamins is/are fat soluble? (Select ALL that apply.)

   (A) Vitamin A
   (B) Vitamin B_6
   (C) Vitamin C
   (D) Vitamin D

9. Which of the following medications used to treat constipation should be used with caution in a patient with impaired renal function?

   (A) Ducolax
   (B) Konsyl
   (C) Milk of Magnesia
   (D) Miralax

10. Which of the following is a stool softener that can be used to treat constipation?

    (A) Colace
    (B) Fibercon
    (C) Metamucil
    (D) Miralax
    (E) Sennakot

ANSWERS AND EXPLANATIONS

1. **B**

St. John's wort is used to treat depression, as it increases the level of serotonin in the CNS. BPH (A) may be treated with saw palmetto, although meta-analysis data has not shown it to be useful. Diabetes (C) may be managed with the herbal supplement ginseng. Hypertriglyceridemia (D) may be treated with omega-3 fatty acids, and lactose intolerance (E) is treated with Lactaid.

2. **A**

Thiamine (vitamin B1) is used to treat Wernicke-Korsakoff syndrome. The syndrome occurs in severe thiamine deficiency.

3. **B**

Delsym contains dextromethorphan and is used a cough suppressant. Mucinex Allergy (A) is a brand name for fexofenadine. Astepro (C) is a nasal antihistamine that contains azelastine. ZzzQuil (diphenhydramine) (D) is an antihistamine used for the treatment of insomnia.

4. **D**

Nasal decongestants—oxymetazoline and naphazoline—should be used for only 3 days to prevent rebound nasal congestion. Diphenhydramine (A), doxylamine (B), and loratadine (C) are oral antihistamines that can be used for more than 3 days and treat postnasal drip or allergic reactions. Phenylephrine (E) is an oral decongestant that can be used for more than 3 days.

5. **C**

Osteo Bi-Flex (glucosamine and chondroitin) may be useful in treating arthritis pain by altering cartilage. Echinacea (A) may be used as an immune stimulant. Melatonin (B) may be useful for sleep disorders, and saw palmetto (D) may be used to treat benign prostatic hypertrophy.

6. **D**

Fexofenadine is a second-generation antihistamine and is less sedation that other first-generation antihistamines, including brompheniramine (A) and chlorpheniramine (B). Doxylamine (C) is a first-generation antihistamine used for the treatment of insomnia. Pseudoephedrine (E) is an oral decongestant.

7. **A**

Terbinafine is a topical antifungal used to treat athlete's foot. It should be applied to the affected area daily for at least 2 weeks, even after the condition appears to have cleared.

8. **A, D**

Vitamins A and D are fat soluble. Other fat-soluble vitamins include vitamin E and vitamin K. Fat-soluble vitamins may accumulate and cause toxicities if ingested in large quantities. B and C vitamins are water soluble and are excreted by the kidneys when the body has achieved adequate levels.

9. **C**

Milk of Magnesia should be used with caution in patients with renal impairment due to the potential of magnesium to accumulate in the body. Ducolax (bisacodyl) (A), Konsyl (psyllium) (B), and Miralax (PEG3350) (D), can all be used in patients with renal impairment.

10. **A**

Colace is a stool softener and is used to prevent and treat constipation. Fibercon (B) and Metamucil (C) are bulk-forming laxatives that should be taken with a full glass of water. Miralax (D) is an osmotic laxative, and Sennakot (E) is a stimulant laxative.

Part Three

Pharmaceutical Sciences, Calculations, Biostatistics, and Clinical Trial Design

Pharmaceutics

23

This chapter covers the following:

- **Physical pharmacy**
- **Pharmaceutical dosage forms**

Pharmaceutics encompasses a number of disciplines, including dosage form design, biopharmaceutics, and pharmacokinetics. This chapter focuses on dosage form design (drug dosage forms and the physical and chemical properties that allow these products to be manufactured).

PHYSICAL PHARMACY

Physical pharmacy is a branch of pharmaceutics that deals principally with the physical and chemical properties of drugs. It is a highly mathematical subject, but the NAPLEX is not concerned with these aspects except as they relate to chemical kinetics.

Preformulation

Preformulation is an important stage of drug development where the pharmaceutical company characterizes the following physicochemical properties of the drug.

Solubility and Lipophilicity

Every drug must be solubilized before it can be absorbed by the body. A drug must possess at least some aqueous solubility in order to be effective; poorly soluble compounds show incomplete and unpredictable absorption. However, at least some lipophilicity must also be present, as drugs must be able to pass through biological membranes in order to reach their sites of action which are often intracellular.

Dissolution rate is improved by ↓ particle size, which ↑ the surface area of the drug that comes into contact with the body fluids.

Ionization Behavior

Most drugs are administered as a salt and therefore carry a positive or negative charge in solution. That is, when such a drug goes into solution, a fraction of the molecules dissociate into ions (i.e., charged compounds). The proportion of ionized to unionized drug is very important because the two behave differently in the body:

- Ionized drug: More soluble, but cannot cross body membranes
- Unionized drug: Less soluble, but can cross body membranes

Remember: Until the drug is absorbed across the body membranes it cannot get to the site of action, but it needs to go into solution before that can happen. The equilibrium between the more soluble ionized form and the more absorbable unionized form of the drug is crucial.

The Henderson-Hasselbalch equation (see formula that follows) can be used to calculate exact ratios of ionized to unionized drug; however, the "Ionization Behavior of Weak Acids and Bases" table below will give you a rough estimate of the ionization behavior of weak acids and bases when comparing the pH of the absorption site to the pK_a. In most cases, you will be able to obtain a sufficiently accurate answer by using the table instead of the actual equation, saving valuable exam time.

$$pH = pK_a + \log \frac{[\text{Salt}]}{[\text{Acid}]} \text{ or } pH = pK_a + \log \frac{[\text{ionized}]}{[\text{unionized}]} \text{ if the drug is an acid}$$

$$pH = pK_a + \log \frac{[\text{Base}]}{[\text{Salt}]} \text{ or } pH = pK_a + \log \frac{[\text{unionized}]}{[\text{ionized}]} \text{ if the drug is a base}$$

Ionization Behavior of Weak Acids and Bases

	Acidic Drug	Basic Drug
$pH > pK_a$	More ionized	More unionized
$pH = pK_a$	Equal	Equal
$pH < pK_a$	More unionized	More ionized
Note that for pH more than 2 units away from pKa, expect almost complete ionization/unionization.		

The acid or base form is the unionized form and salt form is the ionized form of the corresponding acid or base. Accordingly, ionized and unionized can be substituted in the above equations in order to calculate the amount of ionization or unionization at a particular pH value. To identify which equation to use, you must first know if the drug in question is an acid or a base.

It is impossible to tell if a drug is an acid or a base by looking only at the pK_a. Some acids have a higher pK_a (phenytoin = 8.3) than do some bases (morphine = 8.0). You can tell if a drug is an acid or base, however, by what type of salt is used in its formulation. Weak acids form sodium, calcium, potassium, or other cationic salts; weak bases form hydrochloride or other anionic salts.

For example, warfarin is formulated as the sodium salt. Therefore, warfarin is an acid. The positively charged sodium ion is used to displace the proton (i.e., hydronium ion or positively charged hydrogen) from the proton-donating acid in its formulation. In solution, warfarin disassociates from sodium into a negatively charged molecule (i.e., ionized form). If the solution is acidic (e.g., gastric fluid), a proton is likely to be donated back to the negatively charged warfarin to produce the uncharged drug (unionized form). Of course, this is a dynamic state in which the drug is going back and forth between the ionized and unionized form based on the pH of the environment. Determining this ratio provides information about the drug's solubility and its ability to cross biological membranes in any given environment. This is the power of the Henderson-Hasselbalch equation and of the table presented.

Stability

Physical, chemical, and microbiological stability are all very important in preformulation studies. While physical instability does not generally result in ↓ drug concentrations, it can lead to problems with dose uniformity and pharmaceutical elegance (e.g., the mottled appearance that can develop in tablets over time, or the formation of a nonsuspendable sediment in a liquid dosage form).

Most drugs degrade by either zero- or first-order kinetics (see "Rate and Half-Life Equations" table). Drugs following zero-order degradation have a constant degradation rate that is independent of the drug concentration. First-order degradation, however, is concentration-dependent; therefore, the amount of drug degrading per unit of time is not constant.

Rate and Half-Life Equations

Order	Rate Equation		Half-Life Equation
Zero	$C = C_0 - k_0 t$		$t_{\frac{1}{2}} = 0.5 \dfrac{C_0}{k_0}$
First	$\log C = \log C_0 - \dfrac{k_0 t}{2.303}$	$C = C_0 e^{-kt}$	$t_{\frac{1}{2}} = \dfrac{\ln 2}{k_1} = \dfrac{0.693}{k_1}$

Where C is equal to concentration, C_0 is the initial concentration, K_0 is the zero-order degradation constant, t is time, $t_{1/2}$ is half-life, and K_1 is the first-order degradation constant.

With equations it is possible to calculate the concentration (or amount) of drug at any given time if its degradation rate constant is known. It is not, however, useful to memorize the first-order equation for the NAPLEX because the calculator provided does not include the exponential function (e). Therefore, the only way to calculate the concentration (or amount) of drug at any given time is to estimate the amount by understanding what the degradation constants represent.

The first thing to do is identify if the question is related to a zero-order or first-order process. If a graphical representation is presented for any problem, a zero-order process will be linear with a constant degradation over time. Therefore, the units for zero-order degradation constants are in terms of amount per unit time (e.g., mg/hr). First-order degradation will be a nonlinear decline that is asymptotic to the x-axis on a graph similar to a drug concentration-time curve seen in pharmacokinetics. The units of the first-order degradation constant are in terms of time^{-1} (e.g., yr^{-1}).

After identifying whether the degradation process is zero-order or first-order, the second step is to estimate how much drug is remaining (or degraded) over some amount of time. This is simple for zero-order processes because a constant amount is being lost over time. For example, if the starting amount of drug is 1,000 mg and 10 mg per year is degraded (i.e., $K_0 = 10$ mg/yr), after 10 years it will have lost 100 mg of drug and have 900 mg remaining. Many zero-order degradation problems can be rationalized without memorizing the equations in the table.

The estimation of amount of drug remaining following first-order degradation is not as straightforward and requires an in-depth understanding of the first-order degradation constant. The degradation constant is in terms of time^{-1}, as mentioned. This represents a percentage of drug lost per unit of time that is being presented. For example, a K_1 of 0.2 yr^{-1} indicates that 20% of the drug is lost every year. Thus, if the starting amount of drug is 1,000 mg of drug, 20% will be lost of that in the first year, or 200 mg, leaving 800 mg. The key in these estimations is to remember that in year 2, the starting amount is 800 mg because 200 mg was lost in year 1. To calculate the amount of drug lost after 2 years, subtract 20% of 800 mg (i.e., 160 mg) from 800 mg. Therefore, the amount of drug remaining after 2 years will be 800 mg minus 160 mg, for a total of 640 mg. This process must be repeated for year 3 and so on.

Solid-State Properties

Crystallization

Solids are present in crystalline or amorphous forms, or as a combination of the two. Crystalline forms show fixed geometric patterns, whereas the atoms in amorphous solids are randomly placed (as they would be in a liquid).

- Crystalline solids have definite melting points, whereas amorphous solids melt over a range of temperatures.
- Amorphous solids are more soluble than the corresponding crystalline forms.
- Solids tend to revert to the more stable crystalline form on storage.

Polymorphism

Polymorphs are one of several crystalline structures that have the same chemical formula but show different physical properties. The properties they exhibit can vary substantially, however, and this leads to pharmaceutical companies patenting different polymorphic forms based on variations in solubility, bioavailability, solid-state stability, or processing behavior (such as improved powder flow or tablet compaction).

A pharmacy-related example of polymorphism is ritonavir, a protease inhibitor used to treat human immunodeficiency virus. Initially, it was thought to exist in only one polymorphic form, with relatively poor aqueous solubility. It was marketed in a soft gelatin capsule, which contained an ethanol/water cosolvent system. After drug approval, several batches failed quality control tests. It was discovered that a second polymorphic form with even lower solubility had formed, causing the drug to precipitate out of the cosolvent system. The product had to be reformulated to include Kolliphor (polyethoxylated castor oil) as a solubilizing agent.

Rheology

Rheology is the science of flow properties, which is especially important when discussing liquid and semisolid dosage forms.

Viscosity and fluidity are two common terms associated with rheology. Viscosity refers to the resistance offered when part of the liquid flows past another part; fluidity is essentially the opposite. Viscous liquids are thick and slow-moving; fluid liquids are thin and flow more readily.

Testing

Numerous quality assurance tests exist for dosage forms. The four tests used for tablets and sometimes capsules are as follows: friability, hardness, disintegration, and dissolution testing.

Friability and hardness testing evaluate the ability of tablets to withstand manufacturing, packaging, and shipping. Hardness testing measures the force required to cause a tablet to break, and friability testing measures what percentage weight of a tablet is lost after it is tumbled for a specified amount of time in a friabilator.

Disintegration testing is performed by placing tablets into mesh-bottomed cylinders that are immersed in a solution and agitated at a specified rate.

PHARMACEUTICAL DOSAGE FORMS

Oral Delivery: Solids

Types of Immediate-Release Tablets

Type of Tablet	Key Features	Example
Compressed	All ingredients contained in a single layer; designed to be swallowed whole; may or may not be coated	Various
Multi-compressed	Contain separate layers of drug, for various reasons (incompatibility of drugs, immediate- plus extended-release in the same tablet, etc.)	Mucinex (guaifenesin)
Chewable	Disintegrate rapidly when chewed; usually mannitol-based (pleasant mouth feel, sweet taste)	Children's vitamins Dilantin Infatabs (phenytoin)
Buccal	Dissolve in cheek cavity; may be designed to erode slowly or quickly	Fentora (fentanyl)
Sublingual	Dissolve under the tongue; erode quickly and are absorbed rapidly	Nitrostat (nitroglycerin)
Effervescent	Contain drug that dissolves rapidly after adding to water; results in carbonated liquid that masks taste	Alka-Seltzer

Many immediate-release tablets are coated. This process can help mask unpleasant tastes and odors, as well as improve the appearance of the tablet, protect the drug from the atmosphere, and allow it to be swallowed more easily. The two types of coating used for immediate-release products are sugar and film coatings.

Types of Extended-Release Tablets

Type of Tablet	Key Features	Example
Enteric coating	Coating remains intact until drug reaches small intestine; can protect drug from stomach acid and enzymes, or can protect stomach from irritating drugs	Enteric-coated aspirin
Diffusion-controlled reservoir system	Beads or pellets are coated with polymer that releases drug at varying speeds; may involve several release rates	Drug-eluting stents
Diffusion-controlled matrix system	Drug is mixed into an inert plastic matrix; drug dissolves and leaves matrix	Glucotrol XL (glipizide)
Wax	Remains intact in GI tract and is eliminated in feces (inform patient that this is normal)	Desoxyn (methamphetamine)
Hydrophilic	Water causes matrix to swell; drug diffuses through gel layer, and may also be released as matrix erodes	Slo-Niacin (niacin)
Dissolution-controlled system	Rate of release affected by dissolution and tablet or bead erosion (some hydrophilic matrices fall into this category as well as diffusion-controlled)	Cardizem CD (diltiazem)
Ion-exchange resin	pH conditions of GI tract cause drug to be released from resin	Inderal (propanolol)
Osmotically controlled system	Tablet pulls water into system, then releases drug at controlled rate by osmotic pressure; tablet shell eliminated in feces (inform patient that this is normal)	Glucotrol XL (glipizide)
Complex formation	Drug is combined with other agents, forming a slowly soluble chemical complex	Rynatan allergy products

Types of Rapid-Release Solid Dosage Forms

Type of Product	Key Features	Example
Tablets	Product can contain large doses of drug	Claritin RediTabs (loratidine)
Strips	Dissolves before children can spit it out; cannot put large doses of drug into product	Zuplenz (ondansetron)
Lollipops	Absorbed through buccal mucosa	Actiq (fentanyl)

Oral Delivery: Liquids

Oral liquid dosage forms have the same advantages as other oral products, with the additional advantage of being easy to swallow for small children and others who cannot easily swallow solid dosage forms. Several disadvantages exist as well. Liquids are less portable and convenient than solids. Incorrect doses are much more likely, as patients or caregivers could measure using an inappropriate measuring device (i.e., not all spoons are standard size), and product may be spilled before being consumed. Also, taste can be a large issue, as more of the drug will reach a patient's taste buds than with the same drug in a tablet or capsule.

Solvents

Water is the most common solvent for pharmaceutical products; purified water prepared by distillation, reverse osmosis, or ion-exchange treatment is acceptable for oral use. Other commonly used solvents include ethyl alcohol, glycerin, sorbitol, propylene glycol, and some edible oils. Typically, solvents other than water are included to improve solubility and, in some cases, add sweetness to the final product (e.g., glycerin, sorbitol, and propylene glycol). Only small amounts of sorbitol and glycerin should be present in a given dose of liquid, as they may act as osmotic laxatives in higher quantities.

Types of Liquids

Single-phase liquid dosage forms are all variants of the solution. One or more soluble substances are dissolved in one or more solvents, including water. Therefore, the drug(s) must be water-soluble and stable in aqueous solution. The presence of other excipients in varying amounts results in the following designations:

Types of Single-Phase Liquid Dosage Forms

Type of Product	Key Features	Examples
Syrups	• Contain sugar or sugar substitutes • Contain little or no alcohol • Thickeners improve mouth feel and physically conceal the drug from taste buds • Taste pleasant; often used with children	Various cough/cold preparations
Elixirs	• By definition alcoholic, but some nonalcoholic commercial products are mislabeled as elixirs • Slightly sweet; artificial sweetener usually used since sucrose is not very soluble in alcohol • Less viscous than syrups	• Diphenhydramine • Phenobarbital • Digoxin

Types of Single-Phase Liquid Dosage Forms *(cont'd)*

Type of Product	Key Features	Examples
Tinctures	• 15–80% alcohol • Usually consist of drug extracted from plant material • Unpleasant taste; not commonly used today	• Opium tincture (1,000 mg morphine/100 mL) • Paregoric (camphorated opium tincture; 40 mg morphine/100 mL)
Spirits	• Alcoholic solutions of aromatic or volatile substances • High concentration of alcohol • Active ingredient may precipitate out when added to aqueous preparations	Flavoring agents
Aromatic waters	• Aqueous solutions of volatile oils • Very dilute	Flavoring and perfuming agents
Fluid extracts	• Similar to, but more potent than, tinctures • Used as drug source, not as dosage form	Herbal medications

Suspensions are multiphase products that contain finely divided solid particles distributed through the liquid phase. Some advantages exist over single-phase liquids. Drugs that have an unpleasant flavor are preferred as suspensions, since the drug does not interact with the taste buds as much when it is not dissolved. Also, drugs that have poor stability in water do not degrade as readily in suspension as they do in solution.

The primary concern with making suspensions is to have a particle size that is small enough to remain suspended in the dispersion medium of choice while not being so small that the particles start to attract each other and form clumps that will not resuspend. This can be achieved by two techniques, used separately or in combination: (1) use of structured vehicles and (2) controlled flocculation.

- Structured vehicles: ↑ viscosity and slow the sedimentation of suspended particles. These natural and synthetic polymer solutions are often used (cellulose gels, acacia, bentonite).

- Controlled flocculation: Add materials that promote loose aggregation of suspended particles, but keep their surfaces apart by charge or interaction of polymer chains. These particles will settle, but loosely, and resuspend easily.

Emulsions are dispersions that consist of nonmiscible liquids. These products are thermodynamically unstable and require an emulsifying agent to keep them combined properly.

Only oil-in-water (O/W) emulsions are used for oral dosage forms, as water needs to be in the external phase to be palatable to the patient; otherwise, all the patient would taste would be the oil in the outer portion of the product. Topical products can be either O/W or water in oil (W/O). Three types of emulsifiers are used, depending on the product being made:

- Surfactants: Contain hydrophilic and hydrophobic portions, which remain at the interface of the oil, and water phases to stabilize the product. Often used in combination.
- Hydrophilic colloids: Water-soluble polymers that form a film around oil droplets in O/W emulsions. Tend to ↑ viscosity of the product.
- Finely divided solids: Form a film of particles around the droplets of the dispersed phase, but allow interaction with the dispersion medium as well.

Topical Delivery

Topical products are used for three primary reasons: (1) to protect injured areas of the skin from the environment; (2) to hydrate the skin; and (3) to apply medication to the skin for local effect.

Powders and liquids are used as topical delivery systems, though not as frequently as semisolid preparations. Of the types of liquids mentioned in the oral delivery section, solutions, suspensions, and emulsions may all be used topically. Two external-use–only liquid products are:

- Liniments: Alcoholic solutions used to irritate the skin and relieve more deep-seated pain or discomfort (Heet, Absorbine Jr), or oleaginous emulsions used as emollients or protective agents. Liniments are applied by rubbing and are not suitable for application to bruised or broken skin.
- Collodions: Contain pyroxylin in an alcohol/ether base that evaporates, leaving an occlusive film on the skin; used to hold edges of incised wounds together.

Ointment Bases

Five types of ointment bases exist:

- Hydrocarbon/oleaginous: Greasy, petroleum-based products used for emollient effect (Vaseline, petrolatum)
- Anhydrous absorption: Greasy products that form W/O emulsions when aqueous solutions are added; can be used to incorporate solutions into an otherwise lipophilic base (hydrophilic petrolatum, anhydrous lanolin)
- W/O emulsion: Similar to anhydrous absorption bases, but already contain some water (hydrous lanolin, cold cream)
- O/W emulsion (water-removable): Creamy emulsions that are easily washed from the skin; may be diluted with water to form lotions (hydrophilic ointment, Lubriderm)
- Water-soluble: Greaseless, water-washable bases containing no oleaginous compounds; cannot add large amounts of water or will soften too much (PEG ointment)

Other topical product definitions are:

- **Creams:** Terminology often used to describe emulsion bases; soft, cosmetically acceptable topical products
- **Pastes:** Very thick semisolids containing at least 20% solids by weight
- **Gels:** Jelly-like dispersions that are water-soluble, water-washable, and greaseless

Rectal, Vaginal, and Urethral Delivery

Rectal, vaginal, and urethral dosage forms such as suppositories and enemas are less frequently prescribed than many other types of dosage form, but they do have an important place in certain types of therapy. They can be useful for local therapy in rectal or vaginal conditions, or when protecting susceptible drugs from GI tract degradation or first-pass metabolism.

Pulmonary Delivery

Metered-Dose Inhalers

Metered-dose inhalers (MDIs) are primarily used to deliver medications, including bronchodilators and corticosteroids, for the treatment of asthma and chronic obstructive pulmonary disease. While MDIs are portable and able to deliver precise quantities of potent drugs, many patients have difficulty using them properly.

Dry-Powder Inhalers

Dry-powder inhalers (DPIs) avoid some of the difficulties with MDIs. They are generally easier for patients to use correctly, since the device can be primed before use and the patient does not have to coordinate their breaths with device actuation. Ease of use, however, depends significantly on the particular type of device.

The Diskus device is a classic example of the discrete-dose style of DPI. Individual doses are contained in foil packets, protecting them from humidity and allowing for dose consistency if the device is dropped. Some discrete-dose devices are single-dose units, and the drug is added when the device is ready to be actuated (Rotahaler, Aerosilizer, Handihaler); this is often a necessity if a drug is heat-sensitive and must be kept refrigerated until use, such as Spiriva (tiotropium bromide). The Twisthaler, on the other hand, is an example of a reservoir device. All of the doses are contained in a central compartment; and if the device is dropped or exposed to humidity, all doses are affected. Of currently marketed products, only the Twisthaler and Flexhaler are reservoir devices.

Nebulizers

Nebulizers allow the drug to be delivered directly to the lung in high concentration and without the use of propellant. Two types exist: (1) jet and (2) ultrasonic. Jet nebulizers can be used with either solutions or suspensions, and operate by the Bernoulli principle, whereby compressed air from the machine flows at high speed over the medicated liquid, atomizing it and carrying it to the patient. Ultrasonic nebulizers can only be used with solutions. Ultrasonic nebulizers use the vibrations of high-frequency sound waves to move liquid from the machine through the face mask. Vibrations are timed to coincide with inhalation; therefore, less medication is lost with the ultrasonic than with the jet nebulizers.

Nasal Delivery

Nasal delivery shares many of the advantages of pulmonary delivery. Drugs that are inactivated by the GI tract or that undergo first-pass metabolism are protected, and large-molecule drugs can be absorbed across the nasal mucosa. The nose has a dense vasculature, which aids in absorption. Viscosity enhancers and mucoadhesives are often included in the formulations to ↑ residence time, as nasal drainage can be a problem. In addition to the many drugs available via nasal delivery (e.g., desmopressin, calcitonin, butorphanol, corticosteroids), the route shows promise for vaccine delivery, with FluMist being the first approved example.

The most commonly used nasal products are saline solutions for dry nasal mucosa, nasal decongestants, and intranasal corticosteroids.

Parenteral Delivery

Injectable products have many advantages over other dosage forms but also have more potential complications. No drug is lost to first-pass metabolism or acid- or enzyme-mediated degradation in the GI tract, which makes injection a particularly useful route for protein drug delivery. Additionally, the products must be sterile (see following table for various sterilization methods used), free from undesired particulate matter, and pyrogen-free.

Sterilization Methods Used in Industry

Method	How Does It Work?	Advantages	Disadvantages	Products Sterilized by This Method
Steam sterilization	Heat coagulates and kills microorganisms	• Method of choice when applicable • Lower heat than dry heat sterilization	• Cannot use with heat- or moisture-sensitive drugs • Autoclave can have cools spots	• Aqueous solutions in closed containers • Surgical instruments • Glassware
Dry heat sterilization	Heat coagulates and kills microorganisms	Useful for moisture-sensitive material	• Cannot use with heat-sensitive drugs • Autoclave can have cool spots	• Glassware • Surgical equipment • Oleaginous materials • Powders • Moisture-sensitive material
Filtration	Bacteria and particulate matter are physically removed by membrane filters	Inexpensive	• Technique failure • Membrane defects • Drug can absorb to membrane	• Small volumes of thin liquid • Heat-sensitive liquid formulations
Ionizing radiation	Gamma radiation mutates and kills bacteria	Effective for most microorgranisms	Expensive setup	Sterilizing plastic medical devices
Gas sterilization	Ethylene and propylene oxide gases alkylate microbial protein	Good for heat- and moisture-sensitive materials	• Possibility of toxic residue • Explosion hazard • Expensive setup • Cannot penetrate glass to sterilize material in sealed containers	• Heat-sensitive material • Moisture-sensitive material • Medical and surgical equipment wrapped in plastic

Multiple-dose injectable products must contain a preservative in order to ensure that the product remains sterile after the initial use.

Ocular and Otic Delivery

Drug delivery to the eye is complicated by two factors: (1) drug loss due to blinking and lacrimal drainage and (2) poor drug penetration through the corneal membrane. Polymers are typically used as viscosity enhancers to prolong the retention time and ↓ lacrimal drainage; some polymers, such as hyaluronic acid, have mild adhesive properties that prolong the retention time even further.

Most ocular products are solutions; however, suspensions, ointments, and gels may also be used. These dosage forms prolong drug contact with the eye and may be preferable in some situations.

Ocular products must be sterile when dispensed, and all multidose products must contain preservative. This helps prevent serious ocular infections, which can lead to corneal ulcers and blindness.

Otic products are generally solutions or suspensions, which frequently contain glycerin or propylene glycol to ↑ the viscosity and maximize contact between the product and the ear canal. The hygroscopic nature of these solvents also helps them draw moisture out of the tissues, which can ↓ inflammation and the amount of moisture available for any microorganisms to grow. Most otic products fall into one of the following categories:

- Anti-infective and anti-inflammatory products: May contain analgesics and local anesthetics to ↓ pain associated with otitis externa or otitis media
- Ear-wax removal agents: Contain surfactants (which emulsify ear wax) or peroxides (which release oxygen and disrupt the integrity of the ear wax), which facilitate removal of the ear wax

Transdermal Delivery

Transdermal delivery differs from topical delivery in that the drug is intended for systemic use. The drug molecules must therefore be small enough to penetrate the stratum corneum and reach the general circulation. Some transdermal ointments (nitroglycerin ointment) exist, but most products are available as transdermal delivery systems (patches).

Patches

Transdermal patches attach to the skin with adhesive and contain the drug either in a polymer matrix or in a drug reservoir covered by a rate-controlling membrane. An excess amount of drug is typically present to ensure that a concentration gradient exists, causing the drug to exit the patch and enter the skin passively. Patches provide more uniform blood concentrations than conventional release products and can improve patient compliance since, depending on the drug, they can be worn for 1 to 7 days. GI absorption problems and first-pass metabolism also are avoided with transdermal delivery.

PRACTICE QUESTIONS

1. Which of the following dosage forms must be sterile?

    (A) Ophthalmic suspension
    (B) Oral suspension
    (C) Topical suspension
    (D) Suspension for rectal administration
    (E) Otic suspension

2. A 15-year-old patient with ADHD who had been stable on a dose of 10 mg BID of Focalin is transitioning to Focalin XR 20 mg QD. After 2 weeks, he returns to the doctor complaining of distractedness during school and a jittery feeling in the morning an hour or two after taking his medication. When asked how he is taking his medication, he states that due to difficulty swallowing he has been opening the capsules of Focalin XR and mixing them with chunky applesauce, which he chews before swallowing. How do you explain the patient's current symptoms?

    (A) The new dose of Focalin XR is too high and should be reduced.
    (B) The patient is experiencing dose-dumping because he is opening the capsules.
    (C) The patient is experiencing dose-dumping because he is chewing the capsule contents with the applesauce.
    (D) The severity of the patient's ADHD has increased and he is suffering from a new-onset anxiety disorder.
    (E) The patient is experiencing dose-dumping because the capsule contents are interacting with the applesauce.

3. What environmental advantage do HFA inhalers have over CFC inhalers?

    (A) They contain less packaging.
    (B) They are less likely to lead to ozone depletion.
    (C) They do not contain mercury.
    (D) They are a pump spray instead of an aerosol spray.
    (E) They do not use petroleum-based mineral oil as an emulsifier.

4. An insulin injection decomposes at a rate of 0.15 yr^{-1}. How many units of an initial 100-unit solution remain after 3 years?

    (A) 70 units
    (B) 67 units
    (C) 65 units
    (D) 63 units
    (E) 61 units

5. Using the graph below, indicate which of the following statements is TRUE.

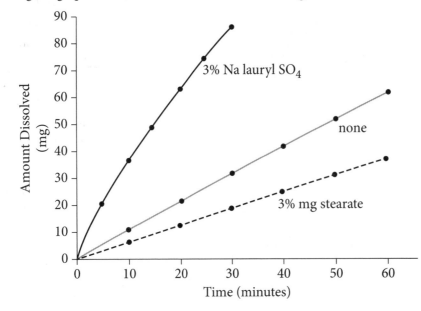

Figure 1. Effect of lubricant on dissolution rate of salicylic acid contained in the compressed tablets.

(A) Sodium lauryl sulfate appears to decrease the rate of dissolution.
(B) At 10 minutes, approximately 10 mg of salicylic acid have dissolved when formulated with sodium lauryl sulfate.
(C) The rate of dissolution of tablets containing magnesium stearate is greater than the control.
(D) The dissolution rate for tablets with 3% magnesium stearate follows zero-order kinetics.
(E) None of the above statements is true.

6. What approximate percentage of phenytoin sodium (pK$_a$ = 8.3) is unionized at a physiological pH of 7.3?

(A) 99%
(B) 90%
(C) 45%
(D) 10%
(E) 1%

ANSWERS AND EXPLANATIONS

1. **A**

All ophthalmic dosage forms must be sterile, and either packaged in single-dose containers or formulated to contain a preservative. Sterility is not required for any of the other routes, as the drug is being applied either to an epithelial surface (topical, otic) or to the GI mucosa (oral, rectal). These surfaces are not sterile in their natural state, and dosage forms applied to them need not be sterile.

2. **C**

Focalin XR derives its extended-release properties from a coating on the beads contained within the capsule. It is therefore appropriate to open the capsule and consume the contents with food or in liquid; applesauce is specifically mentioned in the manufacturer instructions as appropriate. However, crushing or chewing the beads destroys the coating, causing dose-dumping. The patient's jitteriness in the morning and inattention later in the day are symptomatic of too high a dose being absorbed in the morning, and too little medication remaining in his system later in the day.

3. **B**

HFA inhalers were designed to replace CFC inhalers, which are being phased out due to the Montreal Protocol and the effect of CFCs on ozone depletion. HFA inhalers are similar in size to CFC inhalers. Neither type of product contains the other excipients mentioned in the question.

4. **E**

The first step toward answering this problem is to determine if this is a zero-order or first-order degradation process. The units of the degradation rate constant are in time^{-1}, which indicates a nonlinear process and, therefore, a first-order degradation. The rate constant is given as 0.15 yr^{-1}, indicating that 15% of the insulin injection is lost every year. In year 1, 15% of the initial 100 units are lost, leaving 85 units. In year 2, 15% of the remaining 85 units are lost; that is, 12.75 units (85 × 0.15) are lost, and 85 − 12.75 = 72.25 units remain after year 2. In year 3, 15% of the 72.25 units are lost, or 10.84 units (72.25 × 0.15), and 72.25 − 10.84 = 61.41 units remain after year 3. This result is rounded to the answer 61 units.

5. **D**

The rate of dissolution follows zero-order kinetics. This can be observed on the graph because there is a linear relationship between the amount dissolved (*y*-axis) and time (*x*-axis). Because this graph is on a linear scale (i.e., it is NOT a log or natural log scale) and the relationship is linear, it is a zero-order process. Choice (A) is incorrect because the rate of dissolution (or any rate) is directly related to the slope of a line. A steeper slope indicates a faster rate. Because sodium lauryl sulfate had a steeper slope than control, it indicates that those tablets dissolved faster. The same concept applies to choice (C), which is incorrect. Choice (B) is also incorrect: Drawing a straight line up from 10 minutes on the *x*-axis to the line indicating sodium lauryl sulfate demonstrates that approximately 40 mg of the salicylic acid has dissolved, not 10 mg.

6. **B**

The first step to answer this question is to determine if phenytoin is an acidic or basic drug. Phenytoin is formulated with sodium; this indicates that phenytoin is a weak acid. The sodium ion replaces a proton on the phenytoin molecule in its salt formulation and disassociates in solution. Once phenytoin is identified as an acid, it is clear that the following equation applies:

$$pH = pK_a + \log \frac{[\text{Salt}]}{[\text{Acid}]}$$

The salt in the numerator is the ionized form of the drug; the denominator indicates the drug itself, which is unionized. The next step is to fill in the pH and pK_a given in the equation and change the ratio to be ionized over unionized as follows:

$$7.3 = 8.3 + \log \frac{\text{ionized}}{\text{unionized}}$$

To solve this equation, first, move all numeric values to one side of the equation:

$$-1 = \log \frac{\text{ionized}}{\text{unionized}}$$

Second, get rid of the log function by taking each side of the equation to the power of 10:

$$10^{-1} = 10 \; ^\wedge \log \frac{\text{ionized}}{\text{unionized}}$$

The 10 to a log power on the right side of the equation cancels out, and converting from scientific notation gives the following:

$$0.1 = \frac{\text{ionized}}{\text{unionized}}$$

Note that this is a good time to review general principles of using logarithmic functions and scientific notation. These functions will not be available on the NAPLEX calculator; understanding the simple principles is needed to calculate these problems.

Any number on either side of an equation can be divided by 1 without altering the math, thus the 0.1 on the left side of the equation can be divided by 1 to give ratios on both side of the equation:

$$\frac{0.1}{1} = \frac{\text{ionized}}{\text{unionized}}$$

Add the 0.1 to the 1 (total drug parts = 1.1). This shows that 0.1 of a total of 1.1 is ionized and 1 of 1.1 is unionized. The question asks for the percentage unionized, so divide 1 by 1.1. The result is a value of 90.9%, which is approximately 90%.

Pharmacokinetics

26

This chapter covers the following:

- **Plasma drug concentration profiles**
- **Theoretical compartments**
- **Basic pharmacokinetic parameters**
- **Multiple dosing**
- **Nonlinear pharmacokinetics**

PLASMA DRUG CONCENTRATION PROFILES

Plasma drug concentration versus time curve graphs are used extensively in pharmacokinetics. A known dose of drug is given to a patient, and blood samples are taken at various time intervals following drug administration. The concentration of drug in plasma following IV and oral administration is measured and plotted in the following figure. The shape of the curve depends on the relative rates of absorption (oral drug), distribution, and elimination of the drug.

Plasma Concentration versus Time Curves for Intravenous and Oral Drug Administration

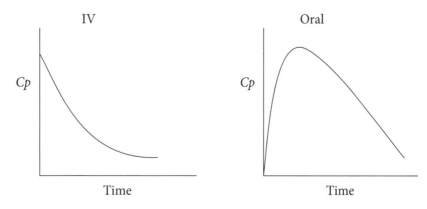

The preceding graphs represent drug plasma concentration (Cp) versus time profiles following an IV bolus and oral administration of a mock drug. Following IV administration, the drug will reach its maximum plasma concentration (C_{max}) at time 0 (leftmost point on the X-axis). Therefore, the time to maximum plasma concentration (T_{max}) is at time 0 following an IV bolus.

Following the lag time for absorption, a rise in drug plasma concentration is seen until it reaches a plateau, which represents the C_{max} on the oral curve. The time of this plateau (i.e., C_{max}) is the T_{max}. At T_{max}, there is a brief time period where this is no net change in drug plasma concentration. This represents the time when the rate of drug absorption is equal to that of elimination. Beyond the C_{max}, elimination will be greater than absorption and is represented by a decline in the drug plasma concentration.

THEORETICAL COMPARTMENTS

From a pharmacokinetic perspective, the body is considered to consist of compartments, inside each of which the drug can be considered evenly distributed.

- One-compartment model:
  - Central compartment includes plasma and well-perfused tissue with rapid distribution (e.g., liver, kidneys).
  - Drug distributes rapidly and uniformly to this compartment.
- Two-compartment model:
  - Central compartment is still present, and includes plasma and well-perfused organs (e.g., liver, kidneys).
  - There is a slow distribution of drug into a peripheral compartment that consists of poorly perfused tissue (e.g., muscles, connective tissue).

One-Compartment Model

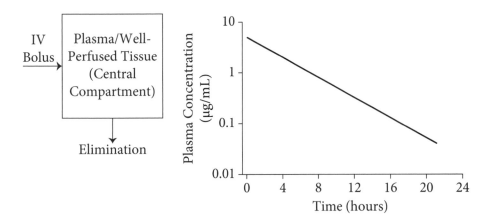

The basic structure of a one-compartment drug is displayed on the left, with a corresponding plasma concentration-time curve on the right. Note that the Y-axis is on a logarithmic scale, which linearizes the relationship. At time 0, the drug is administered into the central compartment. This can be observed on the concentration-time curve by the C_{max} at time 0. The central compartment represents plasma and tissue to which the drug rapidly distributes. The slope of the concentration time curve on a log or natural log scale is directly proportional to the first-order elimination rate constant and therefore the drug half-life. The elimination rate constant can be calculated by taking the difference of the natural log of two concentrations and dividing by the difference of the two corresponding times.

Two-Compartment Model

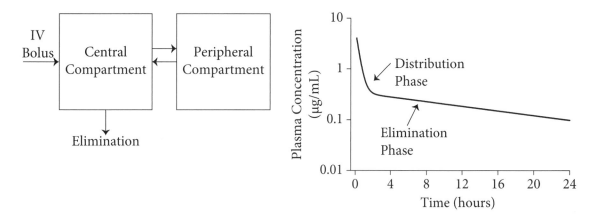

The general structure of a two-compartment model is displayed on the left of the figure. The right side of the figure represents the log concentration-time profile following an IV bolus of a two-compartment drug. As displayed on the concentration-time curve, there are two distinct slopes labeled as the distribution phase and the elimination phase. The *Cmax* following an IV bolus in a two-compartment model is still at time 0. However, the slope of the line at time 0 is representative of both the elimination from the central compartment and slow distribution into peripheral tissue. This phase, commonly called the *distribution phase* of the drug, is not directly representative of elimination. There-fore, it is inappropriate to calculate an elimination rate constant or half-life while a drug is in the distribution phase. Once drug accumulates in the peripheral tissue to a point of equilibrium (i.e., drug diffuses from peripheral tissue back into the central compart-ment), the change in the concentration-time curve is solely due to the elimination of the drug. The half-life of the drug can be calculated only in the elimination phase.

BASIC PHARMACOKINETIC PARAMETERS

Bioavailable Fraction

The bioavailable fraction (F) is the portion of dose administered that reaches the systemic circulation. For IV administration, $F = 1$. A drug given by any other route can have an F ranging from 0 to 1; the F will never be >1. Two factors can $\downarrow$ the F of a drug:

- Incomplete absorption
- First-pass metabolism

Elimination Rate Constant

The first-order elimination rate constant, k, represents the fraction of drug eliminated per unit time, and thus has units of reciprocal time (i.e., hr^{-1}). It can be obtained graphically (see the figure that follows) or from the drug $t_{1/2}$:

$$k = \frac{\ln 2}{t_{1/2}} = \frac{0.693}{t_{1/2}}$$

Graphical Calculation of Elimination Rate Constant

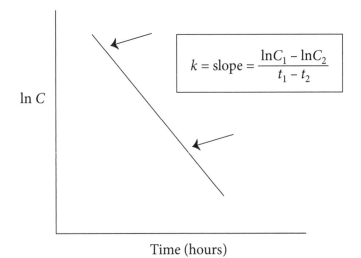

$$k = \text{slope} = \frac{\ln C_1 - \ln C_2}{t_1 - t_2}$$

ln C

Time (hours)

Half-Life

The elimination $t_{1/2}$ of a drug is the time required for its serum concentration to $\downarrow$ by half. It can be obtained mathematically or graphically:

$$t_{1/2} = \frac{\ln 2}{k} = \frac{0.693}{k}$$

The $t_{1/2}$ can also be calculated from clearance (CL) and volume of distribution (V_d). While these parameters do not influence or depend on one another, half-life depends on both of them:

$$t_{1/2} = 0.693 \times \left(\frac{Vd}{CL}\right)$$

Clearance

CL refers to the efficiency of the body in removing drug from the blood. The liver and kidney are the primary organs involved, and body CL refers to the sum of the hepatic (CL_h) and renal clearances (CL_r), plus any CL from other organs, usually negligible:

$$CL = CL_h + CL_r$$

Knowledge of drug CL can help determine when dosage adjustments are needed in patients with hepatic or renal impairment.

Volume of Distribution

Apparent V_d describes the volume of body fluids required to account for all drugs in the body. Several equations can be used to calculate apparent V_d, depending on the information you have available:

$$V_d = \frac{\text{Dose}}{C_{peak}} = \frac{F \times \text{Dose}}{AUC \times k} = \frac{CL \times t_{1/2}}{0.693}$$

V_d has the following effect on $t_{1/2}$:

- Small V_d:
  - Drug mostly located in blood
  - Liver and kidneys only clear drug in blood
  - Fewer passes needed to rid body of drug
  - Shorter $t_{1/2}$
- Large V_d:
  - Drug is extensively distributed into extravascular tissues
  - Liver and kidneys only clear drug in blood
  - More passes are required to clear drug from body
  - Longer $t_{1/2}$

Area under the Curve

Area under the curve (AUC) is a measure of the extent of drug exposure. It is defined as the area under the drug plasma level – time curve from $t = 0$ to infinity. It can be calculated by the trapezoidal rule, or by the other listed equations, and has units of concentration/time. S is the salt factor for a given drug formulation and refers to the percentage of administered product that is the active moiety (the acid or base, not the salt).

Trapezoidal rule:

$$AUC = \frac{C_{n-1} + C_n}{2}(tn - t_{n-1})$$

where n refers to the concentration and time associated with it and $n-1$ is the previous concentration and associated times.

Other equations:

$$AUC = \frac{F \times S \times D_0}{CL} = \frac{F \times D_0}{k \times V_D}$$

AUC is often directly proportional to dose, such that $\uparrow$ the dose of a drug from 500 mg to 1,000 mg will lead to a twofold $\uparrow$ in AUC.

MULTIPLE DOSING

Two things affect how much drug accumulates between the first dose and a dose at steady state:

- Elimination constant or half-life
- Dosing interval

We cannot control the half-life; it is dependent on the drug in question. However, the dosing interval can be adjusted to increase or decrease the drug accumulation factor. A simple estimation of this can be described by:

- Dosing interval < drug half-life → C_{SS} will be much higher than the concentration after the first dose.
- Dosing interval = drug half-life → C_{SS} will be twice as high as the concentration after the first dose.
- Dosing interval > drug half-life → C_{SS} will be similar to the concentration after the first dose (because the drug is almost completely washing out before the next dose is given).

Peak-to-Trough Ratio

Multiple intermittent dosing results in peak and trough drug concentrations. As will be discussed, a dose and dosing interval (τ) are calculated to achieve a desired steady-state plasma concentration average ($C_{SS,\ avg}$). The $C_{SS,\ avg}$ represents the average concentration between the peak and trough. Shorter dosing intervals for a particular dose will lead to a decreased $P{:}T$ ratio, meaning that less fluctuation in peak-to-trough is occurring.

Loading Doses

Loading doses are often used to achieve target plasma drug concentrations as quickly as possible. These large initial doses (which may be given as either a single dose or divided doses over a specified period of time) are especially important in life-threatening conditions such as myocardial infarction, status asthmaticus, and status epilepticus. Loading doses should not be used when there is not an urgent need to achieve target blood concentrations immediately or the patient cannot be supervised for possible toxicity. Loading doses for narrow-therapeutic-index drugs should ideally occur within a clinical setting.

$$F \times \text{Loading dose} = C_{ss(target)} \times V_d$$

Loading doses are commonly given by the IV route, so the F will be equal to 1 in these cases. If an oral loading dose is being administered, the bioavailability of the drug MUST be taken into consideration.

If the patient already has drug in his or her system, this needs to be taken into consideration. Simply take the desired concentration ($C_{ss(target)}$) and subtract out the concentration already in the system. Just be sure the units are identical when performing this calculation.

Constant IV Infusion

Constant-rate infusions do not generate fluctuations in plasma concentrations. Determining the rate for such infusions is relatively simple:

1. Determine the target steady-state plasma concentration (C_{SS}).
2. Find the appropriate population CL.
3. Look up S (if drug is a salt).
4. Calculate infusion rate (R). (The infusion rate is in the units of amount per time [e.g., mg/min].)

$$R = \frac{C_{ss} \times CL}{S}$$

In most instances, S will be equal to 1 and can be ignored. Clearance adjustment factors may be available for some drugs.

Intermittent Oral Dosing

Dose rate in intermittent oral dosing is calculated in a similar fashion to IV infusions. Remember to take F into account with oral dosing, however, since bioavailability may not be equal to IV products. The equation to calculate a dosing rate (dose divided by dosing interval, τ) for an intermittent infusion or oral dosing to a desired steady-state plasma concentration is displayed:

$$\frac{F \times \text{Dose}}{\tau} = C_{ss}, avg \times CL$$

where F is the bioavailability (equal to 1 for IV infusion), dose is the amount administered, τ is the dosing interval, Css, avg is the average steady-state plasma concentration, and CL is the clearance. This is an important equation that can be used to calculate maintenance dosing of drugs to desired steady-state concentrations.

NONLINEAR PHARMACOKINETICS

So far, this chapter has referred to general pharmacokinetic principles. These principles are applicable to most drugs without significant modification, and they result in linear mathematical models. Several assumptions are made when different or multiple doses are given:

- Drug clearance remains constant.
- Doubling the dose results in a doubling of the concentration and AUC.

These assumptions are not always accurate. With some drugs, giving a single low dose of the drug leads to the expected linear pharmacokinetics. However, when higher doses are given, or when the medication is taken chronically, the drug no longer fits the linear pharmacokinetic profile.

Pharmacokinetic Relationships: Linear versus Nonlinear

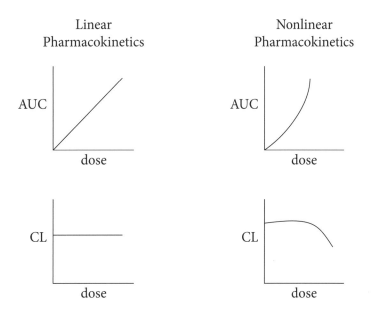

Nonlinear pharmacokinetics generally occur when one or more enzyme- or carrier-mediated systems are saturated. These systems are often referred to as capacity-limited.

Most elimination processes can be saturated if enough drug is given. Certain drugs (phenytoin in particular) show nonlinear behavior even at normal drug doses.

For drugs exhibiting nonlinear behavior, dose increases lead to half-life increases, and AUC is not proportional to the amount of bioavailable drug. The behavior is described by the Michaelis-Menten equation:

$$\frac{dC}{dt} = \frac{V_{max} - C_{SS}}{K_M + C_{SS}}$$

V_{max} (the maximum elimination rate) and K_M (the Michaelis constant, equal to one-half the concentration at V_{max}) are dependent on both the drug and the enzyme system.

PRACTICE QUESTIONS

1. A patient is being started on IV digoxin. What plasma concentration of digoxin would you expect after a loading dose of 0.75 mg? Patient weight $= 65$ kg $\times V_d = 6$ L/kg

    (A) 167 mcg/L
    (B) 2.6 mcg/L
    (C) 125 mcg/L
    (D) 1.95 mcg/L
    (E) 11.5 mcg/L

2. What is the half-life of procainamide in a patient whose total clearance is estimated to be 18 L/h and the volume of distribution is 140 L?

    (A) 10.8 hours
    (B) 7.4 hours
    (C) 5.4 hours
    (D) 4.6 hours
    (E) 2.7 hours

3. An investigational drug was intravenously injected into a patient, and serum samples were obtained at specific time intervals, displayed in the table below. What is the half-life of this drug?

Time Following IV Administration (min)	Serum Drug Concentrations (mg/dL)
10	8.6
20	7.5
30	6.5
60	4.2
80	3.2
100	2.4
120	1.8

    (A) 58 minutes
    (B) 48 minutes
    (C) 38 minutes
    (D) 28 minutes
    (E) 18 minutes

4. Which of the following statements is TRUE regarding the administration of theophylline depicted in the following graph?

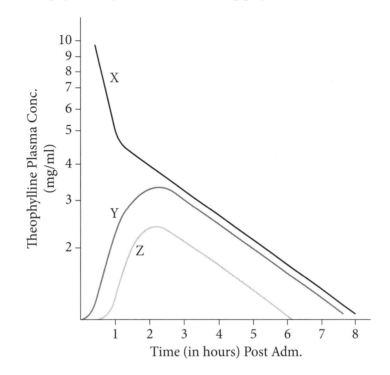

This graph illustrates the time course of the mean plasma theophylline (administered as the ethylenediamine salt) concentrations when 0.5 g is administered (X) intravenously, (Y) as a retention enema, and (Z) as an oral tablet.

(A) The elimination half-life of theophylline is 3.5 hours.
(B) Theophylline is eliminated from the body by zero-order kinetics.
(C) The bioavailability of theophylline is not affected the route of administration.
(D) The retention enema and oral tablet are bioequivalent to each other.
(E) None of the above statements is true.

5. A patient taking 40 mg of propranolol PO enters the hospital and is switched to propranolol IV. What would be an appropriate dose in milligrams, considering the drug undergoes approximately 90% first-pass effect?

(A)   4
(B) 20
(C) 40
(D) 80
(E) 120

6. The apparent V_d of gentamicin in a patient is 8 L. What dose of the antibiotic should be given to a patient with a current plasma concentration of 2 mg/L when a 6 mg/L concentration is desired?

   (A) 48 mg
   (B) 40 mg
   (C) 32 mg
   (D) 12 mg
   (E) 6 mg

7. 250 mg of an antibiotic with a half-life of 9 hours is given every 6 hours to a patient with a clearance rate of 1.54 L/hr. What is the steady-state concentration of this drug assuming 80% is absorbed?

   (A) 64.2 mg/L
   (B) 51.3 mg/L
   (C) 33.3 mg/L
   (D) 21.6 mg/L
   (E) 3.7 mg/L

ANSWERS AND EXPLANATIONS

1. **D**

$$\text{Use } C = \frac{\text{Dose}}{V_d} = \frac{0.75\,\text{mg}}{\dfrac{6\text{L}}{\text{kg}} \times 65\,\text{kg}} = \frac{1,000\,\text{mcg}}{1\,\text{mg}} = \frac{1.95\,\text{mcg}}{\text{L}}$$

2. **C**

$$t_{1/2} = 0.693 \times \frac{V_d}{CL}$$

$$t_{1/2} = 0.693 \times \frac{140}{18} = 5.4 \text{ hours}$$

3. **B**

The elimination rate constant can be directly calculated by first calculating the slope of the line on a natural log scale. The slope is equal to the negative value of the elimination rate constant. Theoretically any two time points and concentrations in the table can be used, but in practice it is important that you avoid choosing points in a distribution phase. It advisable to choose the later time points, as shown here.

$$-k = \text{slope} = \frac{\ln C_1 - \ln C_2}{t_1 - t_2}$$

$$-k = \text{slope} = \frac{\ln 3.2 - \ln 1.8}{80 - 120}$$

$$k = 0.0144$$

$$t_{1/2} = \frac{0.693}{k} \approx 48 \text{ minutes}$$

This answer can also be estimated by simply looking at the time it takes for any given concentration to decrease by half. For example, it took 40 minutes (difference between 120 and 80) for the concentration to go from 3.2 to 1.8. This is just a little less than half, so you know that the half-life of the drug must be slightly >40 minutes. Indeed, the calculated half-life was 48 minutes. This is a good method to check your calculations.

4. **A**

The half-life can be estimated from any of the three administration routes because the elimination phases are parallel to each other and have similar slopes. This indicates that they have identical elimination rate constants and half-lives. The key is to identify two concentrations (one that is half the value of the other) in the elimination phase of any of the routes. The half-life of theophylline can be estimated from the IV curve (X in the graph) because concentration 4 mg/mL and 2 mg/mL are in the elimination phase in the curve. To estimate the half-life, use a straight edge to extrapolate from 4 mg/mL on the y-axis to the IV curve (X on the graph) and then down from that point to the time (x-axis value) that theophylline was at 4 mg/mL. This time is approximately 2 hours following IV administration. Do the same extrapolation for the 2 mg/mL concentration. The time of the 2 mg/mL concentration is approximately 5.5 hours. Therefore, between 2 and 5.5 hours (or 3.5 hours) after IV administration, the concentration of theophylline decreased by half its value from 4 mg/mL to 2 mg/mL. Therefore, choice (A) is a true statement. Choice (B) is false because the elimination of theophylline is linear on the log-axis, indicating a first-order process. Choice (C) is false because the bioavailability is clearly altered by the route of administration. This can be seen by the vastly different AUCs given the same total dosages of each route. Choice (D) is false because the C_{max} and AUCs are different between the retention enema and the oral dose. These, along with T_{max}, must be similar to demonstrate bioequivalence.

5. **A**

If 90% of the oral drug is lost to a first-pass effect, then the bioavailability (F) cannot be greater than 10%. Therefore, one would administer 10% of the oral dose by the IV route; 10% of 40 mg is 4 mg.

6. **C**

$$F \times \text{Loading dose} = C_{SS\,(target)} \times V_d$$

In this case, an IV drug is being administered, so F is equal to 1. Additionally, there is drug onboard at 2 mg/L with a target of 6 mg/L. These concentrations can be subtracted from each other to get the concentration for the $C_{SS(target)}$ value.

6 mg/L (desired C_{SS}) − 2 mg/L (onboard C) = 4 mg/L

$F \times \text{Loading dose} = 4 \times 8 = 32$ mg

7. **D**

$$\frac{F \times \text{Dose}}{\tau} = C_{SS,avg} \times CL$$

$$\frac{0.8 \times 250\,\text{mg}}{6\,\text{hours}} = C_{SS,avg} \times 1.54\,\text{L/hr}$$

$$C_{SS,avg} = 21.6\text{ mg/L}$$

Calculations

27

This chapter covers the following:

- **Problem-solving techniques**
- **Fundamentals of units and measurement**
- **Density, specific gravity, and specific volume**
- **Percentage, ratio strengths, and parts per million**
- **Dilution, concentration, and alligation**
- **Electrolyte solutions**
- **Compounding calculations**

PROBLEM-SOLVING TECHNIQUES

Ratio-Proportion and Dimensional Analysis

Ratio-proportion is a one-step calculation technique that is probably the easiest to use for simple (one- or two-step) calculations. In this process, you set up a likeness between a fraction involving known quantities and one that includes your unknown, and solve the equation by cross-multiplying. An example is given here, illustrating how to convert 3 fluid ounces to milliliters:

$$\frac{30\,\text{mL}}{1\,\text{fl oz}} = \frac{x\,\text{mL}}{3\,\text{fl oz}}$$

$$(30\,\text{mL})(3\,\text{fl oz}) = (x\,\text{mL})(1\,\text{fl oz})$$

$$\frac{(30\,\text{mL})(3\,\text{fl oz})}{(1\,\text{fl oz})} = x\,\text{mL}$$

$$x = 90\,\text{mL}$$

To avoid rounding errors, keep as many decimal points as possible until the last step in the calculation. If the question is fill-in-the-blank style, it will instruct you regarding how many decimals points to include in the final answer.

Dimensional analysis is a technique, often used in chemistry and other sciences, which allows you to set up long calculations in a single step. Using the short example given earlier, the problem would be solved:

$$3 \text{ fl oz} \times \frac{(30 \text{ mL})}{(1 \text{ fl oz})} = 90 \text{ mL}$$

As you can see, the fluid ounces cancel out and leave you with the correct units of milliliters. This serves as an internal error-check and may be helpful in longer, more complex problems.

FUNDAMENTALS OF UNITS AND MEASUREMENT

- Avoirdupois refers to solid measures only (pounds and ounces).
  - 1 pound = 16 ounces
- Common or household liquid measurements start with the teaspoon:
  - 1 teaspoon (tsp) = 5 mL
  - 3 tsp = 1 tablespoon (T) = 15 mL
  - 2 T = 1 fluid ounce (fl oz) = 30 mL = 1/8 cup
  - 1 cup = 8 fl oz
  - 1 pint = 16 fl oz (or 2 cups)
  - 1 quart = 32 fl oz (or 4 cups)
  - 1 gallon = 128 fl oz (or 16 cups)

Avoirdupois System	Metric System
1 lb	454 g
2.2 lb	1 kg
1 oz	28.4 g
1 grain	64.8 mg

Apothecary System	Metric System
1 tsp	5 mL
1 T	15 mL
1 fl oz	29.6 mL (30 mL is an acceptable estimate)
1 cup	240 mL
1 pint	473 mL
1 quart	946 mL
1 gallon	3,785 mL

Prefix	Conversion Factor	Example
Kilo (k)	1,000 or 10^3	1 kilograms (kg) = 1,000 grams (g)
Deci (d)	0.1 or 10^{-1}	1 deciliter (dL) = 0.1 liters (L)
Centi (c)	0.01 or 10^{-2}	1 centimeter (cm) = 0.01 meters (m)
Milli (m)	0.001 or 10^{-3}	1 milligram (mg) = 0.001 grams (g)
Micro (μ)	0.000001 or 10^{-6}	1 microliter (μL) = 0.000001 liters (L)
Nano (n)	0.000000001 or 10^{-9}	1 nanogram (ng) = 0.000000001 grams (g)

DENSITY, SPECIFIC GRAVITY, AND SPECIFIC VOLUME

Density should be treated like a conversion factor, since you are converting between mass and volume.

Example: 450 mL of phenol weighs 482.56 g. What is its density? Express your answer in g/mL.

$$\frac{482.56 \text{ g phenol}}{450 \text{ mL}} = 1.07 \text{ g/mL}$$

Specific gravity (SG) is the density of a substance relative to a reference substance (usually water). It is a unitless number, because it is equal to density divided by density—the units cancel out. Since water has a density of 1 g/mL, the SG will be numerically identical to the density of the substance expressed in g/mL.

Example: 150 mL of formaldehyde weighs 121.82 g. What is its specific gravity?

$$\frac{\dfrac{121.82 \text{ g formaldehyde}}{150 \text{ ml}}}{\dfrac{1 \text{ g water}}{1 \text{ mL}}} = 0.81$$

Thus, formaldehyde has a SG of 0.81, which is the same as the density if presented in g/mL.

PERCENTAGE, RATIO STRENGTHS, AND PARTS PER MILLION

Since drugs are administered as dosage forms that contain more than just the active ingredient, the amount of the active ingredient needs to be expressed.

Percent describes the number of parts of active drug relative to 100 parts of the total. In pharmacy, simply stating % is incomplete; you must attach the appropriate descriptor from the following list:

- % w/w: g of active drug per 100 g of product
- % w/v: g of active drug per 100 mL of product
- % v/v: mL of active drug per 100 mL of product

Examples:

    (1)   10% w/v = 10 g of drug in every 100 mL of the total

    (2)   10% w/w = 10 g of drug in every 100 g of the total

Ratio strength is another way of expressing concentration, in terms of parts of active drug related to any number of parts of the whole. Ratio strength is usually expressed in terms of 1 part of active drug relative to the total number of parts of the product, as opposed to percent, which is any number of parts of active drug relative to 100 parts of product.

Example: Express 1 g of epinephrine in 1 L of solution as a percent strength and as a ratio strength.

First convert the units to g and mL:

    1 L = 1,000 mL

To convert to **percentage strength**, set the denominator on the right side of the ratio-proportion equation to 100 and calculate for the numerator.

$$\frac{1\,\text{g epinephrine}}{1{,}000\,\text{mL}} = \frac{\text{g active}}{100\,\text{mL product}} = 0.1\%\,\text{w/v}$$

To convert to **ratio strength**, set the numerator on the right side of the ratio-proportion equation to 1 and calculate for the denominator.

$$\frac{1\,\text{g epinephrine}}{1{,}000\,\text{mL}} = \frac{1\,\text{active}}{x\,\text{mL product}} = 1{:}1{,}000\,\text{w/v}$$

Parts per million (ppm) is a special case of ratio strength. Instead of fixing the numerator as 1, in this case you fix the denominator constant as 1,000,000. Parts per billion (ppb) and trillion (ppt) are handled in an analogous fashion.

DILUTION, CONCENTRATION, AND ALLIGATION

In some cases, you may receive a prescription in which you need to either dilute a product you have on hand or make a product more concentrated. These problems can generally be solved by:

1. Using the equation: (quantity) × (concentration) = (quantity) × (concentration)
2. Determining the quantity of active ingredient needed and then calculating the quantity of the available solution (usually a concentrated stock solution) that will provide the needed amount of active ingredient

Example:

If 250 mL of a 15% v/v solution of methyl salicylate in alcohol are diluted to 1,500 mL, what will be the percentage strength of this diluted solution?

$$250 \text{ mL} \times 15\% = 1{,}500 \text{ mL} \times x\%$$

$$x = 2.5\% \text{ v/v}$$

Alligation

Alligation is a method of solving problems that involves mixing multiple products that have different percentage strengths.

Alligation Alternate

This method allows calculation of the number of parts of two or more components of a given strength when they are mixed to prepare a mixture of a desired strength. Crosswise subtraction is used to determine the amounts needed of each component. This method can be used regardless of how concentration is expressed (mg/mL, ratio, parts, %).

Example:

In what proportion should a 20% benzocaine ointment be mixed with an ointment base to produce a 2.5% w/w benzocaine ointment?

Since there is no active drug in the ointment base, its strength can be expressed as 0%. To complete this problem, set up a table with the high concentration (i.e., 20%) in the upper left corner and the low concentration (i.e., 0%) in the lower left corner. The desired concentration (i.e., 2.5%) is placed in the center column between the low and high concentrations. Subtract diagonally to calculate the parts of the low and high concentration solutions to be mixed. See the following table for the appropriate setup of this problem.

Strengths to Be Mixed	Desired	Difference in Strength Mixed (crosswise subtraction of absolute values)
20%		2.5 parts (2.5−0) of 20% ointment
	2.5%	
0%		17.5 parts (20 − 2.5) of ointment base

Therefore, 2.5 parts of the 20% w/w ointment should be added to 17.5 parts of the ointment base. For example, if 12 g were to be dispensed in the preceding problem, you would use the following parts.

Parts of high concentration: 2.5 parts

Parts of low concentration: 17.5 parts

Total parts (i.e., high plus low concentration): 20 parts

To calculate the amount of the *high* concentration to be mixed:

$$\frac{2.5\,\text{parts}}{20\,\text{parts}} = \frac{x\,\text{g}}{12\,\text{g}}$$
$$x = 1.5\,\text{g}$$

To calculate the amount of the *low* concentration to be mixed:

$$\frac{17.5\,\text{parts}}{20\,\text{parts}} = \frac{x\,\text{g}}{12\,\text{g}}$$
$$x = 10.5\,\text{g}$$

ELECTROLYTE SOLUTIONS

Millimoles and Milliequivalents

A review of several chemistry concepts will be useful before beginning milliequivalent calculations.

- Moles (mol): Measurement of the amount of a substance; Avogadro's number of particles (6.023×10^{23})
- Atomic weight: Found on the periodic table; 1 mol of that atom weighs that many grams (also, 1 mmol of that atom weighs that many mg)
- Molecular weight (MW): The sum of all the atomic weights for all of the atoms in the molecule. 1 **mole** of the molecule will weigh the value of the molecular weight in **grams**. However, in electrolyte solutions and osmolarity calculations, it is necessary to convert to millimoles. This can be visualized in the following important equations:

$$\text{moles} = \frac{\text{Amount (grams)}}{\text{Molecular weight}}$$

$$\text{millimoles} = \frac{\text{Amount (milligrams)}}{\text{Molecular weight}}$$

- Molar solution: The molarity of a solution is the moles of solute in every 1 L of solution. This is an important concept on the NAPLEX, as questions can ask for the answer in terms of molarity; therefore, on the last step of the problem, you would then need to calculate how many moles there are in 1 L for the solutes in the problem.

The following table displays the valence of the most common ions. This information will likely not be provided on the NAPLEX.

Valence	Ions
+1	Sodium, potassium, lithium
+2	Barium, calcium, magnesium, zinc
+3	Aluminum
+1 or +2	Copper
+2 or +3	Iron, manganese
−1	Acetate, chloride, bicarbonate
−2	Sulfate, carbonate
−1, −2, or −3	Phosphate, citrate

In the magnesium chloride example, Mg^{+2} is divalent; it takes two Cl^- to make as much negative charge as one Mg^{+2}. Therefore, the correct formula is $MgCl_2$, not $MgCl$. $NaCl$, however, is made up of two monovalent ions, so the charges are equal.

The concept of equivalents is important in pharmacy when dispensing electrolytes or small drug molecules as salts. For example, a prescription that is written for 40 mg of potassium chloride does not contain the same amount of elemental potassium as a prescription written for 40 mg potassium acetate. The reason is that the 40 mg in each prescription is the total weight of potassium and the salt form (i.e., chloride or acetate).

To overcome this problem for electrolytes, the prescriptions will be written in terms of milliequivalents (mEq). For example, a prescription that calls for 40 mEq of potassium chloride will contain the same amount of elemental potassium as a prescription that calls for 40 mEq of potassium acetate.

Use the following equation to calculate mEq:

$$\text{milliequivalents (mEq)} = \frac{\text{Amount (milligrams)}}{\text{Molecular weight}} \times \text{valence}$$

Example:

How many milligrams of potassium citrate powder (MW = 324.41) should be weighed to compound 1 dose of the following prescription?

Rx   *Potassium citrate 20 mEq PO TID*

Recall that potassium has a valence of +1 and citrate has a −3, so the formula must have 3 potassium ions for every citrate or $K_3(C_6H_5O_7)$.

$$20\,mEq = \frac{x\,mg}{324.1} \times 3$$
$$x = 2{,}160\,mg$$

Therefore, 20 mEq of potassium citrate provides 20 mEq of potassium and 20 mEq of citrate. This means that a quantity of 2,160 mg of potassium citrate would provide 20 mEq of potassium and 20 mEq of citrate.

Osmolarity and Isotonicity

Osmotic pressure is the pressure that exists across a semipermeable membrane due to the free movement of solvent but not solute. Because cell membranes are semipermeable, this concept is important in patients. When administering parenteral drugs, you must balance the osmolarity of your medication with the osmolarity of the body. If not, tissue damage, pain, and possibly death can result due to cells swelling or shrinking with the movement of solvent.

Solutions are considered isotonic when each one has the same osmotic pressure; in pharmacy and medicine, the reference solution is the plasma (280–300 mOsm/L). Hypertonic solutions have higher osmotic pressure than this; hypotonic solutions have lower osmotic pressure. Some other facts you should remember about osmotic pressure are:

- It is a colligative property, based on the number of particles in solution.
- It can be calculated directly, using dissociation constants.
  - NaCl dissociates into sodium and chloride 80% in aqueous solution.
  - For every 100 particles, 80 will have dissociated (making 160 particles) and 20 will not → 180 particles (20 + 160).

  $$\frac{180\,particles\,after\,dissociation}{100\,particles\,before\,dissociation} = 1.8 = i$$

- To calculate the milliosmoles (mOsm) in a given solution, multiply the millimoles by the theoretical number of particles that the compound would dissociate into in solution.

$$mOsm = \frac{Amount\,(mg)}{Molecular\ weight} \times Theoretical\ number\ of\ particles$$
$$(or\ disassociation\ constant)$$

- The NAPLEX may ask for answers to be written in terms of milliosmolarity. To calculate milliosmolarity you need to calculate the amount of milliosmoles in the quantity of solution in the problem and convert to 1 L at the end.

Example:

Calculate the osmolarity of NS in mOsm/L. MW NS = 58.5 and $i = 1.8$.

NS = normal saline = 0.9% w/v NaCl in water

$$\frac{0.9\,g}{100\,mL} = \frac{x\,g}{1,000\,mL}$$

$x = 9\,g$ or 9,000 mg of NaCl per liter

$$x\,mOsm = \frac{9,000\,mg}{58.5} \times 1.8$$

$$x = 276.9\,mOsm/L$$

COMPOUNDING CALCULATIONS

Use of Prefabricated Dosage Forms in Compounding

Example:

Rx	Aspirin	300 *mg*
	Lactose	qs
	M.ft. cap DTD #60	

Using 325-mg aspirin tablets (weighing 430 mg each) as the source drug, how many tablets are needed to compound this prescription? How many grams of the crushed powder should be weighed out?

$$\frac{300\,mg\,ASA}{capsule} \times 60\,capsules \times \frac{tablet}{325\,mg\,ASA} = 55.38\,tablets \rightarrow 56\,tablets$$

$$55.38\,tablets \times 430\,mg\ total\ tablet\ weight = 23,813\,mg = 23.813\,g$$

Reconstitution Calculations

Example:

Cefadroxil powder for oral suspension comes in a strength of 250 mg/5 mL. The reconstitution instructions are to add 70 mL of purified water to yield a final solution volume of 100 mL. How many grams of cefadroxil powder are in the bottle?

$$\frac{250 \text{ mg cefadroxil}}{5 \text{ mL suspension}} \times 100 \text{ mL} = 5{,}000 \text{ mg} = 5 \text{ g}$$

Drip Rate Calculations

IV medications are regulated by one of the following methods:

- Drip chambers
  - Deliver drops of defined volume
  - Flow is adjusted by the nurse to a set number of *whole* drops per minute
  - Standard sets are 10 gtt/mL or 15 gtt/mL
  - Pediatric and critical care drugs may use microdrop infusion sets: 60 gtt/mL
- Infusion pumps
  - Deliver a rate of mL/hr
  - Round to the nearest 0.1 mL

Example:

17 mL of concentrated vancomycin solution is added to a 100-mL piggyback bag of NS. This solution is to be infused over 1 hour. What is the infusion rate?

$$\frac{17 \text{ mL vancomycin} + 100 \text{ mL NS}}{60 \text{ min}} = 117 \text{ mL}/60 \text{ min} = 117 \text{ mL/hr}$$

What is the infusion rate in drops/min if the drug is administered using an infusion set that delivers 10 gtt/mL?

$$\frac{117 \text{ mL}}{60 \text{ min}} \times \frac{10 \text{ gtt}}{\text{mL}} = 19.5 \text{ gtt/min} = 20 \text{ gtt/min}$$

Parenteral Nutrition

Calculations Involving Calories

The usual term is Calorie (with a capital C), which is equal to 1 kilocalorie. Therefore, Calories and kilocalories are synonymous.

To calculate the caloric requirements for a hospitalized patient, first calculate that patient's basal energy requirement. The calculated basal energy expenditure is then multiplied by a stress factor (usually between 1 and 2) to obtain a total energy expenditure (TEE).

The normal adult requires 25–35 Cal/kg/day. The Calories provided by a TPN can be estimated as follows:

Dextrose in the hydrated form (D_5W, $D_{70}W$, etc.)	3.4 Cal/g
Carbohydrates	4 Cal/g
Fats	9 Cal/g
Protein	4 Cal/g

Dextrose in water is the hydrated form and is used in TPN. Although dextrose is a carbohydrate, water molecules are attached to the dextrose to make it more soluble. Therefore, when calculating caloric content of a TPN, 3.4 Cal/g should be used for the dextrose content.

To prevent essential fatty acid deficiency, particularly a deficiency of linoleic acid, fats are incorporated into TPNs usually two to three times weekly. Fats are provided through infusion of oil emulsions. Fatty oil emulsions are approximately isotonic, have a milky appearance, and can be infused into peripheral blood vessels. Every milliliter of 10% fat emulsion has 1.1 Calories, whereas every milliliter of 20% fat emulsion has 2 calories.

Calculations Involving Amino Acids

The average adult requires approximately 1 g/kg/day of amino acids. Amino acids are included in TPN primarily to provide protein and nitrogen supplementation. On average, 16% of an amino acid solution is nitrogen content.

Example:

How many milliliters of an 8.5% amino acid solution are required to provide 20 g of nitrogen?

$$\frac{16\,\text{g nitrogen}}{100\,\text{g amino acids}} = \frac{20\,\text{g nitrogen}}{x\,\text{g amino acids}}$$

$$x = 125\,\text{g amino acids}$$

$$\frac{8.5\,\text{g amino acids}}{100\,\text{mL}} = \frac{125\,\text{g amino acids}}{x\,\text{mL}}$$

$$x = 1{,}470\,\text{mL}$$

Of importance is the Cal/g nitrogen ratio. The desired ratio is 125/1 up to 150/1. That is, a formula should provide at least 125 Calories for each gram of nitrogen being infused.

Compounding Considerations for TPNs

Both calcium and phosphate are essential components of TPN formulas. Sources of calcium include the chloride and gluconate salts. Phosphorus is supplied as combinations of mono- and disodium phosphates or mono- and dipotassium phosphates. The exact ratio depends on the pH of the solution.

Depending upon the relative concentrations of the soluble calcium salts and the phosphate salts, a chemical reaction may occur forming the very **insoluble dibasic calcium phosphate** ($CaPO_4$). This fine, white precipitate may form slowly and be difficult to visualize, especially if a milky fatty oil emulsion is also included in the TPN.

Methods for lessening the incompatibility problem:

1. Keep Ca and PO_4 concentrations below certain limits (solubility curves are available for various mixtures).
2. Agitate the mixture after each ingredient addition.
3. Add Na or K phosphates first and calcium salt last.
4. Add the Na or K phosphates to the amino acid solution, and the calcium salt to the dextrose solution; then, mix by shaking.
5. Use a 0.2 micron filter for nonfat emulsion formulas; a 1.2 micron filter is needed for fatty oil emulsions.

PRACTICE QUESTIONS

1. How many milliliters of water should be mixed with 240 mL of syrup containing 85% w/v sucrose to make a syrup containing 60% w/v sucrose?

    (A) 80 mL
    (B) 100 mL
    (C) 160 mL
    (D) 240 mL
    (E) 340 mL

2. If 10 mL of a solution are to contain 3 mEq of sodium ion, how many 1-g sodium chloride (MW 58.5) tablets would be required to compound 250 mL of solution?

    (A) 2
    (B) 3
    (C) 4
    (D) 5
    (E) 6

3. You have been asked to prepare 500 mL of a benzalkonium chloride solution. The concentration of the solution you prepare must be such that if 20 mL of your solution are diluted to a liter, a 1:1,470 solution is formed. How many milliliters of a 17% w/v benzalkonium chloride solution will you need to compound the solution?

    (A) 17 mL
    (B) 20 mL
    (C) 100 mL
    (D) 147 mL
    (E) 500 mL

4. A pharmacist has 75 grams of 3% w/w zinc oxide paste in stock, to which she adds 5 g of pure zinc oxide. What is the percent concentration of zinc oxide in the final product?

    (A) 2.4% w/w
    (B) 3% w/w
    (C) 7.25% w/w
    (D) 9.06% w/w
    (E) 9.67% w/w

5. How many milligrams of boric acid are needed to compound the following prescription? (The E values are as follows: zinc chloride 0.62, phenacaine HCl 0.17, and boric acid 0.52.)

Rx	Zinc chloride	0.2% w/v
	Phenacaine HCl	1% w/v
	Boric acid	qs
	Purified water qs	60 mL

(A) 92 mg
(B) 189 mg
(C) 339 mg
(D) 364 mg
(E) 699 mg

6. How many milligrams of sodium chloride are needed to compound the following prescription? (The E value of phenylephrine HCl is 0.32.)

Rx	Phenylephrine HCl	0.5% w/v
	Sodium chloride	qs
	Purified water qs	30 mL

(A) 48 mg
(B) 86 mg
(C) 150 mg
(D) 222 mg
(E) 270 mg

7. How many milliliters of a 1% (w/v) stock solution of epinephrine HCl are needed for the following prescription?

Rx	Epinephrine HCl sol. 1:500 w/v	60 mL

(A) 0.012 mL
(B) 0.12 mL
(C) 1.2 mL
(D) 12 mL
(E) 120 mL

8. Calculate the percentage (v/v) of witch hazel in the following prescription.

   Rx   Sulfur ppt   15 g

             Witch hazel   45 mL
             Alcohol
             Calamine lotion qs   120 mL

   (A) 12.5%
   (B) 25%
   (C) 27.3%
   (D) 37.5%
   (E) 45%

9. The following prescription is written for penicillin suspension to be administered: 1.5 teaspoonfuls PO TID for 12 days. How many milliliters of the suspension should be dispensed?

   (A) 23 mL
   (B) 54 mL
   (C) 90 mL
   (D) 270 mL
   (E) 810 mL

10. A 40-pound child is to receive Dilantin 2.5 mg/kg PO BID. How many milliliters of Dilantin suspension (125 mg/5 mL) should be dispensed for a 30-day supply?

    (A) 55 mL
    (B) 109 mL
    (C) 240 mL
    (D) 265 mL
    (E) 528 mL

11. A patient who weighs 167 pounds is receiving phenylephrine at a dose of 2 mcg/kg/min. How many milligrams of phenylephrine does the patient receive over 2 hours?

    (A) 0.30 mg
    (B) 9.1 mg
    (C) 18.2 mg
    (D) 40 mg
    (E) 5,060 mg

12. A formula for 2,000 levothyroxine tablets contains 274 mg of levothyroxine. How many micrograms of levothyroxine are in each tablet?

    (A) 0.137 mcg
    (B) 1.37 mcg
    (C) 13.7 mcg
    (D) 137 mcg
    (E) 1,370 mcg

13. The formula for an analgesic ointment is 10 g menthol, 95 g benzocaine, 5 g camphor, 40 g mineral oil, and 850 g petrolatum. How many grams of benzocaine are needed to prepare 5 lbs. of this product?

    (A) 0.22 g
    (B) 215.7 g
    (C) 238.3 g
    (D) 253.7 g
    (E) 1,045 g

14. A solution of iodine in chloroform has a strength of 1.4% (w/v). How many milliliters of chloroform must be evaporated from the original 180 mL to adjust the iodine concentration to 2.4% (w/v)?

    (A) 50 mL
    (B) 75 mL
    (C) 105 mL
    (D) 125 mL
    (E) 155 mL

15. How many grams of zinc oxide should be mixed with 8% (w/w) zinc oxide ointment to make 250 g of a 12% (w/w) zinc oxide ointment? Round your answer to one decimal place.

    (A) 10.9 g
    (B) 18.5 g
    (C) 37.9 g
    (D) 100 g
    (E) 239.1 g

16. A patient is to receive 2 mEq of sodium chloride per kilogram of body weight. If the patient weighs 186 lbs., how many milliliters of a 0.9% solution of sodium chloride (MW = 58.5) should be administered?

    (A) 11 mL
    (B) 321 mL
    (C) 550 mL
    (D) 1,099 mL
    (E) 5,320 mL

17. How many milliosmoles of calcium chloride (MW = 147) are represented in 200 mL of a 10% (w/v) calcium chloride solution?

    (A) 8.8 mOsm
    (B) 136 mOsm
    (C) 272 mOsm
    (D) 408 mOsm
    (E) 816 mOsm

18. If an ointment contains 60% (w/w) of polyethylene glycol 400 (specific gravity = 1.13), how many milliliters of polyethylene glycol are needed to prepare 1 kg of ointment?

    (A) 53 mL
    (B) 68 mL
    (C) 354 mL
    (D) 531 mL
    (E) 678 mL

19. How many milliliters of water should be added to 50 mL of zephiran chloride 1:750 solution to obtain a 1:10,000 strength solution?

    (A) 100 mL
    (B) 200 mL
    (C) 250 mL
    (D) 617 mL
    (E) 667 mL

20. You receive a prescription for fluticasone HFA 440 mcg BID with instructions to dispense a 90-day supply. Fluticasone HFA is available commercially as 220 mcg/metered dose with 120 doses per inhaler. How many inhalers should be dispensed for a 90-day supply?

    (A) 1 inhaler
    (B) 2 inhalers
    (C) 3 inhalers
    (D) 4 inhalers
    (E) 6 inhalers

21. You receive a prescription for insulin glargine 65 units subcut once daily with instructions to dispense a 30-day supply. Insulin glargine is available commercially as 100 units/mL in 10-mL vials. How many vials should be dispensed for a 30-day supply?

    (A) 1 vial
    (B) 2 vials
    (C) 3 vials
    (D) 4 vials
    (E) 5 vials

22. You receive a prescription for oxycodone/acetaminophen 5/500 mg 1–2 tablets every 4–6 hours PRN pain. Based upon a maximum daily acetaminophen dose of 4 grams, how many tablets should be dispensed for a 30-day supply?

(A) 60 tablets
(B) 120 tablets
(C) 240 tablets
(D) 360 tablets
(E) 480 tablets

23. An elixir contains 250 mg of active ingredient per 5 mL. You receive a prescription for 500 mg PO twice daily with instructions to dispense 120 mL of the elixir. How many days would the elixir last if taken as prescribed?

(A) 4 days
(B) 6 days
(C) 8 days
(D) 10 days
(E) 12 days

24. A pediatric ferrous sulfate suspension contains 75 mg/1.5 mL (20% elemental). How many milliliters would provide the patient with 30 mg of elemental iron?

(A) 0.3 mL
(B) 0.6 mL
(C) 1.5 mL
(D) 3 mL
(E) 6 mL

25. You are asked to compound a prescription for 120 mL of the following lotion:

Rx	Calamine	80 g
	Zinc oxide	80 g
	Glycerin	20 g
	Bentonite magma	250 mL
	Calcium hydroxide topical solution to make	1,000 mL

How many grams of calamine should be used to prepare the quantity specified?

(A) 0.96 g
(B) 8 g
(C) 9.6 g
(D) 80 g
(E) 96 g

26. You receive a prescription for 60 g of zinc oxide ointment. The following formula is available:

Rx	Zinc oxide	1 part
	Starch	1 part
	Petrolatum	2 parts

   How many grams of zinc oxide should be used to prepare the quantity specified?

   (A) 1 g
   (B) 10 g
   (C) 15 g
   (D) 30 g
   (E) 45 g

27. Approximately how many liters of a 0.9% (w/v) aqueous solution can be made from 30 grams of sodium chloride?

   (A) 1 L
   (B) 2 L
   (C) 3 L
   (D) 4 L
   (E) 5 L

28. You receive a prescription for 500 mL of a 0.5% w/v solution of drug A. You have on hand 10% w/v solution of drug A. How many milliliters of your available solution should be diluted with water to make the 500 mL prescription?

   (A) 5 mL
   (B) 10 mL
   (C) 15 mL
   (D) 20 mL
   (E) 25 mL

29. A prescription is written for a total quantity of 100 mEq of NaCl. You have normal saline solution on hand. How many milliliters of normal saline solution should be dispensed? (MW NaCl = 58.5)

   (A) 58.5 mL
   (B) 65 mL
   (C) 527 mL
   (D) 585 mL
   (E) 650 mL

30. A medication order calls for 75 mL of a 0.8 mEq potassium/mL solution. How many grams of potassium chloride should be used to prepare the quantity specified? (MW KCl = 74.5)

    (A) 4.5 g
    (B) 7.5 g
    (C) 45 g
    (D) 75 g
    (E) 450 g

31. A medication order calls for 10 mL of a 1% (w/v) tobramycin (E = 0.07) ophthalmic solution. You have on hand tobramycin 40 mg/mL solution. How many milligrams of NaCl should be added to make the solution isotonic with tears?

    (A) 7 mg
    (B) 33 mg
    (C) 83 mg
    (D) 100 mg
    (E) 400 mg

32. You receive a prescription for amoxicillin 100 mg/5 mL. You have on hand amoxicillin 125 mg/5 mL powder for reconstitution. The label calls for the addition of 63 mL of water to make 80 mL of the 125 mg/5 mL suspension. How many milliliters of water should be added to prepare the concentration specified?

    (A) 68 mL
    (B) 70 mL
    (C) 83 mL
    (D) 88 mL
    (E) 100 mL

33. How many milliliters of a 10% w/v stock solution should be diluted with water to make 500 mL of a 0.25% w/v solution?

    (A) 12.5 mL
    (B) 25 mL
    (C) 50 mL
    (D) 125 mL
    (E) 200 mL

34. A prescription for lansoprazole suspension is written as follows:

   Rx   *Lansoprazole*   *3 mg/mL*

             Sodium bicarbonate 8.4% w/v qs   *150 mL*

             Sig. 5 mL BID

   How many lansoprazole 30-mg capsules are needed to compound the prescription?

   (A) 10 capsules
   (B) 15 capsules
   (C) 30 capsules
   (D) 45 capsules
   (E) 60 capsules

35. What is the caloric requirement for a 52-year-old female with a calculated basal energy expenditure of 1,200 Calories and a stress factor of 1.5 due to a fever?

   (A) 1,200 Calories
   (B) 1,400 Calories
   (C) 1,600 Calories
   (D) 1,800 Calories
   (E) 2,000 Calories

36. The daily caloric requirement for a 62-year-old male is 1,950 Calories. If 250 mL of a 10% IV fat emulsion product were to be used daily, how many milliliters of $D_{70}W$ would need to be administered to meet his caloric requirements?

   (A) 493 mL
   (B) 704 mL
   (C) 855 mL
   (D) 1,220 mL
   (E) 1,675 mL

ANSWERS AND EXPLANATIONS

1. **B**

In this problem, the solution of sucrose in water is being diluted. The $Q_1 C_1 = Q_2 C_2$ method can be used to solve the problem. The volume that is solved for x is the amount of the 2.4% solution that would be made.

$$8.5\% \, (240 \, mL) = 60\% \, (x)$$
$$x = 340 \, mL$$

However, the question asks how much water *should be mixed with* the original 240 mL to dilute the concentration of the syrup to 60%. Therefore, this amount (240 mL) must be subtracted from the amount of syrup to be made (340 mL) to determine how much water to add.

340 mL − 240 mL = **100 mL of water to be added**

2. **D**

$$250 \, mL \times \frac{3 \, mEq \, Na^+}{10 \, mL} \times \frac{1 \, mmol \, Na^+}{1 \, mEq \, Na^+} \times \frac{1 \, mmol \, NaCl}{1 \, mmol \, Na^+} \times \frac{58.5 \, mg \, NaCl}{1 \, mmol \, NaCl} \times$$

$$\frac{1 \, g}{1,000 \, mg} \times \frac{1 \, tablet}{1 \, g} = 4.4 \, tabs = \textbf{5 tabs}$$

If you are using a partial tablet, you must always round up. If you use 4.4 tablets, you will actually expend 5 tablets from inventory, use 4.4 for your product, and discard the remainder of the fifth tablet.

3. **C**

Final solution: 1 L of 1:1,470 benzalkonium chloride (BC) solution

$$1,000 \, mL \times \frac{1 \, g \, BC}{1,470 \, mL} = 0.68 \, g \, BC$$

This solution was produced by diluting 20 mL of the solution you made. Therefore, the solution you made has 0.68 g of BC in every 20 mL.

$$500 \, mL \times \frac{0.68 \, g \, BC}{20 \, mL} = 17 \, g \, of \, BC$$

You need 17 g of benzalkonium chloride. How many milliliters of a 17% w/v stock solution will be required to deliver 17 g?

$$17 \, g \times \frac{100 \, mL}{17 \, g} = \textbf{100 mL stock solution}$$

4. **D**

$$75\,\text{g paste} \times \frac{3\,\text{g ZnO}}{100\,\text{g paste}} = 2.25\,\text{g ZnO}$$

$$\frac{(2.25+5)\,\text{g ZnO}}{(75+5)\,\text{g paste}} = \frac{7.25\,\text{g ZnO}}{80\,\text{g paste}} = \frac{9.06\,\text{g ZnO}}{100\,\text{g paste}} = \textbf{9.06\% w/w}$$

5. **E**

Step 1: Determine the weight of all chemicals present in this prescription.

$$\text{Zinc chloride}: \frac{0.2\,\text{g}}{100\,\text{mL}} = \frac{x}{60\,\text{mL}}$$

$$x = 0.12\,\text{g}$$

$$\text{Phenacaine}: \frac{1\,\text{g}}{100\,\text{mL}} = \frac{y}{60\,\text{mL}}$$

$$y = 0.6\,\text{g}$$

Step 2: Multiply each weight by the listed E value of the chemical.

Zinc chloride: $0.12\,\text{g} \times 0.62 = 0.0744\,\text{g}$

Phenacaine: $\quad 0.6\,\text{g} \times 0.17 = 0.102\,\text{g}$

Step 3: Add the weights from step 2. The sum is the amount of NaCl currently present in this prescription.

$0.0744\,\text{g} + 0.102\,\text{g} = 0.1764\,\text{g}$

Step 4: Determine the theoretical amount of NaCl that would be necessary to make this prescription isotonic if no other chemical were present.

$$\frac{0.9\,\text{g}}{100\,\text{mL}} = \frac{p}{60\,\text{mL}}$$

$$p = 0.54\,\text{g}$$

Step 5: Subtract the value in step 3 from the value in step 4 to determine the amount of NaCl that needs to be added to make this prescription isotonic.

$0.54\,\text{g} - 0.1764\,\text{g} = 0.3636\,\text{g}$

Step 6: Determine the amount of boric acid that would be used instead of NaCl to make this prescription isotonic.

$$\frac{0.3636\,\text{g NaCl}}{q} = \frac{0.52\,\text{g NaCl}}{1\,\text{g boric acid}}$$

$$q = 0.699\,\text{g} \times 1{,}000 = \textbf{699 mg}$$

6. **D**

Step 1: Determine the weight of all chemicals present in this prescription.

$$\text{Phenylephrine: } \frac{0.5\,\text{g}}{100\,\text{mL}} = \frac{x}{30\,\text{mL}}$$

$$x = 0.15\,\text{g}$$

Step 2: Multiply each weight by the listed E value of the chemical. The product is the amount of NaCl currently present in this prescription.

Phenylephrine: $0.15\,\text{g} \times 0.32 = 0.048\,\text{g}$

Step 3: Determine the theoretical amount of NaCl that would be necessary to make this prescription isotonic if no other chemical were present.

$$\frac{0.9\,\text{g}}{100\,\text{mL}} = \frac{y}{30\,\text{mL}}$$

$$y = 0.27\,\text{g}$$

Step 4: Subtract the value in step 2 from the value in step 3 to determine the amount of NaCl that needs to be added to make this prescription isotonic.

$$0.27\,\text{g} - 0.048\,\text{g} = 0.222\,\text{g} \times 1{,}000 = \textbf{222 mg}$$

7. **D**

The concentration of the epinephrine solution is presented as a ratio strength. A concentration of 1:500 translates into 1 g/500 mL. The first step in solving this problem is to determine the amount of epinephrine (in grams) that would be contained in 60 mL of the solution.

$$\frac{1\,\text{g}}{500\,\text{mL}} = \frac{x}{60\,\text{mL}}$$

$$x = 0.12\,\text{g epinephrine}$$

Next, set up a ratio-proportion to determine the volume of the 1% epinephrine stock solution needed to obtain the 0.12 grams of epinephrine.

1% stock solution:

$$\frac{1\,\text{g}}{100\,\text{mL}} = \frac{0.12\,\text{g}}{y}$$

$$y = \textbf{12 mL}$$

8. **D**

To determine the percentage of witch hazel, you must calculate the amount of witch hazel in 100 mL of the compound. According to the problem, there are 45 mL of witch hazel in 120 mL of calamine lotion in this prescription. To solve this problem, set up a ratio-proportion.

$$\frac{45\,\text{mL}}{120\,\text{mL}} = \frac{x}{100\,\text{mL}}$$
$$x = \textbf{37.5\%}$$

9. **D**

First, calculate the number of teaspoons to be administered on a daily basis.

1.5 tsp/dose × 3 doses/day = 4.5 tsp/day

Next, set up a ratio-proportion to determine the total volume (in mL) of penicillin suspension to be administered (assuming 1 teaspoon = 5 mL).

$$\frac{4.5\,\text{tsp}}{x} = \frac{1\,\text{tsp}}{5\,\text{mL}}$$
$$x = 22.5\,\text{mL}$$

Finally, multiply this daily volume by 12 days to determine the total volume of suspension (in mL) that should be dispensed.

22.5 mL/day × 12 days = **270 mL**

10. **B**

Using dimensional analysis, multiply the weight-based dose by the weight of the child (being sure to convert the weight into kilograms), then by 2 (since the weight-based dose is being given twice daily), and then by 30 (to account for the 30-day supply). You can see here that all the units cancel out except for mg. The answer in this first step is the total number of milligrams of Dilantin that will be dispensed for this child for a 30-day supply.

$$\frac{2.5\,\text{mg}}{\text{kg dose}} \times 40\,\text{lb} \times \frac{1\,\text{kg}}{2.2\,\text{lb}} \times \frac{2\,\text{doses}}{\text{day}} \times 30\,\text{days} = 2{,}727.27\,\text{mg}$$

Next, using the concentration of Dilantin suspension of 125 mg/5 mL given in the problem, set up a ratio-proportion to determine the volume of this suspension to be dispensed that will contain 2,727.27 mg.

$$\frac{125\,\text{mg}}{5\,\text{mL}} = \frac{2{,}727.27\,\text{mg}}{x}$$
$$x = \textbf{109\,mL}$$

11. **C**

Set up the problem using dimensional analysis: Multiply the weight-based dose by the weight of the patient, being sure to convert into kilograms; convert the units of time to hours; and convert the dose from micrograms to milligrams, since that is what the question is asking. You can see that all the units cancel out except for mg.

$$\frac{2\text{ mcg}}{\text{kg / min}} \times 167\text{ lb} \times \frac{1\text{ kg}}{2.2\text{ lb}} \times \frac{60\text{ min}}{1\text{ hr}} \times 2\text{ hr} \times \frac{1\text{ mg}}{1{,}000\text{ mcg}} = \textbf{18.2 mg}$$

12. **D**

Given that there are 274 mg of levothyroxine in 2,000 tablets, set up a ratio-proportion to determine how many milligrams are in 1 tablet. Then multiply this answer (in milligrams) by 1,000 to arrive at the answer in micrograms.

$$\frac{274\text{ mg}}{2{,}000\text{ tablets}} = \frac{x}{1\text{ tablet}}$$

$$x = 0.137\text{ mg} \times 1{,}000\text{ mcg/mg} = \textbf{137 mcg}$$

13. **B**

The first step is to determine the total amount of the analgesic ointment that will be made given the formula provided.

$$10\text{ g} + 95\text{ g} + 5\text{ g} + 40\text{ g} + 850\text{ g} = 1{,}000\text{ g ointment}$$

Next, convert the total amount of ointment to be prepared, 5 pounds, into grams.

$$5\text{ lb} \times \frac{454\text{ g}}{1\text{ lb}} = 2{,}270\text{ g}$$

Finally, set up a ratio-proportion to determine how much benzocaine is needed to prepare 2,270 g of ointment, given that 95 g of benzocaine is used to prepare 1,000 g of the same ointment.

$$\frac{95\text{ g benzocaine}}{1{,}000\text{ g ointment}} = \frac{x}{2{,}270\text{ g ointment}}$$

$$x = \textbf{215.7 g}$$

14. **B**

In this problem, the solution of iodine in chloroform is being concentrated (rather than diluted). The $Q_1C_1 = Q_2C_2$ method can be used to solve the problem. The volume that is solved for x is the amount of the 2.4% solution that would be made.

$$(1.4\%)(180\,mL) = (2.4\%)\,x$$

$$x = 105\text{ mL (this is the amount of 2.4\% solution)}$$

However, the question asks how much chloroform *must be evaporated from* the original 180 mL to adjust the iodine concentration to 2.4%. Therefore, this amount (105 mL) must be subtracted from the original amount (180 mL) to determine how much solution must be evaporated.

180 mL − 105 mL = **75 mL must be evaporated**

15. **A**

Alligation:

High Concentration [A]		Parts of High Concentration Ingredient [D]
	Desired Concentration [C]	
Low Concentration [B]		Parts of Low Concentration Ingredient [E]

Parts of high-concentration ingredient [D] = [C] − [B]

Parts of low-concentration ingredient [E] = [A] − [C]

Zinc Oxide Ointment:

Assume pure zinc oxide = 100%

100%		12 − 8 = 4 parts
	12%	
8%		100 − 12 = 88 parts
		Total = 92 parts

Quantity of 100% zinc oxide ointment needed:

$$\frac{4\,\text{parts}}{92\,\text{parts}} = \frac{x}{250\,\text{g}}$$
$$x = \mathbf{10.9\,g}$$

16. **D**

The first step is to multiply the weight-based dose by the weight of the patient using dimensional analysis, being sure to convert the weight into kilograms.

$$\frac{186\,\cancel{lb}}{1} \times \frac{1\,\cancel{kg}}{2.2\,\cancel{lb}} \times \frac{2\,\text{mEq}}{\cancel{kg}} = 169.1\,\text{mEq}$$

At this point, the following milliequivalent formula can be used to determine the weight of sodium chloride (in mg) present in 169.1 mEq. Remember that the valence of sodium chloride (NaCl) is 1. The molecular weight of sodium chloride was given to you in the problem (58.5).

$$mEq = \frac{amount\,(mg)}{molecular\,weight} \times Valence$$

$$169.1 = \frac{x}{58.5} \times 1$$

$$x = 9{,}891.8\,mg / 1{,}000 = 9.89\,g$$

Once the weight of sodium chloride is known, a ratio-proportion can be used to determine the volume of 0.9% sodium chloride solution to be administered. Remember that a 0.9% solution of sodium chloride contains 0.9 g of sodium chloride in 100 mL of solution.

Volume of 0.9% NaCl needed:

$$\frac{0.9\,g}{100\,mL} = \frac{9.89\,g}{x}$$

$$x = \mathbf{1{,}099\,mL}$$

17. **D**

The first step is to determine how much calcium chloride (in grams) is contained in 200 mL of a 10% (w/v) solution. Set up a ratio-proportion to solve this step.

$$\frac{10\,g}{100\,mL} = \frac{x}{200\,mL}$$

$$x = 20\,g\,CaCl_2$$

At this point, the milliosmole formula can be used to determine how many milliosmoles are represented by 20 grams of calcium chloride. Remember that calcium chloride dissociates into 3 species. The molecular weight of calcium chloride was given to you in the problem (147).

$$mOsm = \frac{amount\,(mg)}{molecular\,weight} \times \begin{array}{c} Theoretical\,number\,of\,particles \\ (or\,dissociation\,constant) \end{array}$$

$$mOsm = \frac{20{,}000\,mg}{147} \times 3$$

$$mOsm = \mathbf{408\,mOsm}$$

18. **D**

The first step is to determine how much of the polyethylene glycol 400 would be needed to prepare 1 kg (or 1,000 g) of ointment, starting with a 60% (w/w) polyethylene glycol 400 ointment. A ratio-proportion can be set up to solve this problem.

$$\frac{60\,g}{100\,g} = \frac{x}{1,000\,g}$$
$$x = 600\,g\,of\,polyethylene\,glycol\,400\,needed$$

Next, set up a ratio-proportion with this information to determine the volume of polyethylene glycol solution needed to prepare this compound. Remember that the specific gravity of a substance represents weight/volume in grams per milliliters.

Specific gravity (SG) = wt/vol

$$\frac{1.13\,g}{1\,mL} = \frac{600\,g}{y}$$
$$y = \mathbf{531\,mL}$$

19. **D**

This is a dilution problem that involves ratio strengths. The first step is to determine how much zephiran chloride (in grams) is contained in 50 mL of a 1:750 solution. This can be determined by setting up a ratio-proportion.

$$\frac{1\,g}{750\,mL} = \frac{x}{50\,mL}$$
$$x = 0.067\,g$$

Since the solution will be diluted to a 1:10,000 solution, the next step is to determine what volume of this solution would contain 0.067 g of zephiran chloride. Again, this can be determined by setting up a ratio-proportion.

$$\frac{1\,g}{10,000\,mL} = \frac{0.067\,g}{y}$$
$$y = 666.67\,mL$$

This dilution process involved going from 50 mL of a 1:750 solution to 666.67 mL of a 1:10,000 solution. However, 666.67 mL is not the final answer, as the question asked how many milliliters of water *should be added* to arrive at this amount. Thus, the final step of the problem is to subtract the initial volume from the total volume to arrive at the answer.

666.67 mL − 50 mL = 616.67 mL = **617 mL of water needs to be added**

20.   **C**

Solve this problem using dimensional analysis: Multiply the number of doses per day (2) by the strength of each prescribed dose (440 mcg); by the strength per metered dose (220 mcg/dose) and the number of doses per inhaler (120) to factor in the available dosage form; and by the number of days needed (90). Each fraction should be set up such that all the units cancel out except for inhalers.

$$2 \times \frac{440 \text{ mcg}}{1 \text{ day}} \times \frac{1 \text{ dose}}{220 \text{ mcg}} \times \frac{1 \text{ inhaler}}{120 \text{ doses}} \times 90 \text{ days} = \textbf{3 inhalers}$$

21.   **B**

Solve this problem using dimensional analysis: Multiply the number of units the patient will need each day (65) by the number of units in each milliliter of insulin (100); by the number of milliliters per vial (10); and by the number of days needed (30). Each fraction should be set up such that all the units cancel out except for vials.

$$\frac{65 \text{ units}}{1 \text{ day}} \times \frac{1 \text{ mL}}{100 \text{ units}} \times \frac{1 \text{ vial}}{10 \text{ mL}} \times 30 \text{ days} = \textbf{1.95 vials}$$

Therefore, **2 vials** should be dispensed.

22.   **C**

Solve this problem using dimensional analysis: Convert the maximum daily dose (4 g/day) to milligrams, and multiply by the strength of each tablet (500 mg) and the number of days needed (30). Each fraction should be set up such that all the units cancel out except for tablets.

$$\frac{4 \text{ g}}{1 \text{ day}} \times \frac{1{,}000 \text{ mg}}{1 \text{ g}} \times \frac{1 \text{ tablet}}{500 \text{ mg}} \times 30 \text{ days} = \textbf{240 tablets}$$

23.   **B**

Solve this problem using dimensional analysis: Multiply the strength of the elixir (250 mg/5 mL) by the desired dose (500 mg); by the number of doses per day (2); and by the quantity dispensed (120 mL). Each fraction should be set up such that all units cancel out except for days.

$$\frac{250 \text{ mg}}{5 \text{ mL}} \times \frac{1 \text{ dose}}{500 \text{ mg}} \times \frac{1 \text{ day}}{2 \text{ doses}} \times 120 \text{ mL} = \textbf{6 days}$$

24. **D**

First, use dimensional analysis to determine the amount of elemental iron per milliliter. Multiply the strength of the available suspension (75 mg/1.5 mL) by the percent of elemental iron (20%).

$$\frac{75 \text{ mg ferrous sulfate}}{1.5 \text{ mL suspension}} \times \frac{20 \text{ mg elemental iron}}{100 \text{ mg ferrous sulfate}} = 10 \text{ mg elemental iron/mL}$$

Then, set up a ratio-proportion to calculate the volume of the suspension needed to obtain the 30 mg of elemental iron, and cross-multiply to solve the problem.

$$\frac{10 \text{ mg elemental iron}}{1 \text{ mL}} = \frac{30 \text{ mg elemental iron}}{x}$$

$$10x = 30 \text{ mL}$$

$$x = 30 / 10 = \textbf{3 mL}$$

25. **C**

One approach to solving this problem is to identify the factor that represents the relationship between the desired quantity (120 mL) and the quantity specified in the compounding recipe (1,000 mL), then multiply by this factor to determine the appropriate amount of each ingredient. In this case, the relationship can be expressed by dividing 120 mL by 1,000 mL, yielding a factor of 0.12.

$$\frac{120 \text{ mL}}{1,000 \text{ mL}} = 0.12 \text{ (factor)}$$

Next, multiply the relevant ingredient—in this case, 80 g of calamine—by this factor to calculate the appropriate amount.

$$80 \text{ g calamine} \times 0.12 = \textbf{9.6 g}$$

26. **C**

First, determine the ratio of zinc oxide to the total recipe by finding the sum of the parts: 1 part + 1 part + 2 parts = 4 parts. So the ratio of parts zinc oxide to total parts is 1:4. Next, set up a ratio-proportion to calculate how much zinc oxide is contained in a total weight of 60 grams, and cross-multiply to solve.

$$\frac{1 \text{ part zinc oxide}}{4 \text{ parts total}} = \frac{x \text{ g zinc oxide}}{60 \text{ g total}}$$

$$4x = 60$$

$$x = \frac{60}{4} = 15 \text{ g}$$

27. **C**

The first step in solving this problem is to set up a ratio-proportion representing the relationship between the desired % w/v (0.9%) and the available weight of the product (30 g).

$$\frac{0.9\,g}{100\,mL} = \frac{30\,g}{x}$$

$$x = 3{,}333\,mL$$

The problem asks for liters, so convert from milliliters to liters to solve the problem.

$$3{,}333\,mL \times \frac{1\,L}{1{,}000\,mL} = \textbf{3.33\,L}$$

28. **E**

In this problem, the 10% solution is being diluted to a 0.5% solution. The $Q_1C_1 = Q_2C_2$ method can be used to solve the problem. The volume that is solved for x is the amount of the 10% solution that you would need to start with.

$$10\%\,(x\;mL) = 0.5\%\,(500\;mL)$$

$$x = \textbf{25 mL}$$

29. **E**

Sodium and chloride are monovalent ions, so 1 mol = 1 equivalent. The first step in solving this problem is to determine the number of grams of NaCl per mEq. Because there is 1 mol per equivalent, this is a simple calculation: Divide the molecular weight (which is equal to the EqW) by 1,000 to determine g/mEq.

$$MW\;NaCl = 58.5$$

$$EqW = \frac{58.5\,g}{1}$$

$$1\,mEq = \frac{58.5}{1{,}000} = 0.0585\,g$$

Next, multiply the weight by the desired number of mEq (100) to determine the total weight needed.

$$100\;mEq = 0.0585\;g \times 100 = 5.85\;g\;NaCl\;needed$$

Finally, set up a ratio-proportion indicating the relationship between the available concentration (0.9% for normal saline) and the desired weight of NaCl (5.85 g), and cross-multiply to solve the problem.

$$\frac{0.9\,g}{100\,mL} = \frac{5.85\,g}{x}$$

$$0.9x = 585$$

$$x = 585\,/\,0.9 = \textbf{650\,mL}$$

30. **A**

Because KCl is made up of monovalent ions, the molecular weight is equal to the EqW. Divide the number by 1,000 to determine the weight/mEq.

$$MW\,KCl\ =\ 74.5$$

$$EqW\ =\ \frac{74.5\,g}{1}$$

$$1\,mEq\ =\ \frac{74.5}{1,000}\ =\ 0.0745\,g$$

From here, the problem can be solved using dimensional analysis: Multiply the desired concentration (0.8 mEq/mL) by the weight/mEq (74.5 g/mEq) and by the total quantity desired (75 mL). Each fraction should be set up such that units cancel out except for grams.

$$\frac{0.8\,\cancel{mEq}}{1\,\cancel{mL}}\times\frac{0.0745\,g}{1\,\cancel{mEq}}\times 75\,\cancel{mL}=\textbf{4.5g}$$

31. **C**

First, calculate the total amount of tobramycin in the desired product by multiplying the % w/v by the given volume.

$$\frac{1\,g\,tobramycin}{100\,mL}\times 10\,mL = 0.1\,g\,tobramycin$$

Then, multiply the weight of the active ingredient by the E value of the active ingredient (0.07) to determine the weight of NaCl required to exert the tonic effect represented in the solution.

$$0.1\,g\,tobramycin \times \frac{0.07\,g\,NaCl(eq)}{1\,g\,tobramycin} = 0.007\,g\,NaCl(eq)$$

Next, use the % w/v of normal saline (0.9%) to calculate the total amount of NaCl needed to make the solution isotonic if this were the sole tonicity agent.

$$\frac{0.9\,g\,NaCl}{100\,mL}\times 10\,mL = 0.09\,g\,NaCl$$

Finally, subtract the amount of NaCl already present in the tobramycin (0.007 g) from this total amount (0.09 g) to determine how much should be added.

$$0.09\,g - 0.007\,g = 0.083\,g\,NaCl \times \frac{1,000\,mg}{1\,g} = \textbf{83 mg}$$

32. **C**

First, set up a ratio-proportion to calculate the total weight of medication in the bottle.

$$\frac{125\,mg}{5\,mL} = \frac{x}{80\,mL}$$

$$x = 2{,}000\,mg\,amoxicillin$$

Then, set up another ratio-proportion to determine the total volume needed to provide the desired concentration.

$$\frac{100\,mg}{5\,mL} = \frac{2{,}000\,mg}{y}$$

$$y = 100\,mL$$

Next, calculate the volume of the dry powder to be used in this prescription by subtracting the amount of water added from the total end volume.

volume of dry powder = 80 mL – 63 mL = 17 mL

Finally, determine the amount of water to add for reconstitution by subtracting the volume of dry powder calculated in the previous step from the total volume needed.

100 mL – volume of dry powder (17 mL) = water to add = **83 mL**

33. **A**

In this problem, the 10% solution is being diluted to a 0.25% solution. The $Q_1C_1 = Q_2C_2$ method can be used to solve the problem. The volume that is solved for x is the amount of the 10% solution that you would need to start with.

$$10\%\,(x\,mL) = 0.25\%\,(500\,mL)$$

$$x = \mathbf{12.5\ mL}$$

34. **B**

First, determine the total weight of drug needed by multiplying the concentration (3 mg/mL) by the given volume (150 mL).

$$\frac{3\,mg}{1\,mL} \times 150\,mL = 450\,mg\,lansoprazole\,needed$$

Next, divide the total weight needed by the available capsule strength (30 mg) to determine the number of capsules needed.

450 mg / 30 mg capsules = total number of capsules needed = **15 capsules**

35. **D**

The patient's total caloric requirement can be calculated by multiplying the patient's estimated basal energy expenditure by the stress factor. The patient has an estimated basal energy expenditure of 1,200 and a stress factor of 1.5.

$$1,200 \times 1.5 = \textbf{1,800 Calories}$$

36. **B**

The fat emulsion and dextrose are used in the TPN to meet the patient's caloric requirement. To calculate the amount of dextrose that is needed to meet the caloric requirement, first calculate the calories obtained from the fat emulsion. The fatty acid emulsion contains 1.1 Cal/mL.

Therefore,

$$\frac{1.1\,\text{Calorie}}{1\,\text{mL}} = \frac{x\,\text{Calorie}}{250\,\text{mL}}$$
$$x = 275\,\text{Calories from the fat emulsion}$$

Next, calculate the calories needed from the dextrose solution by subtracting the fat emulsion calories from the total caloric need. The number of calories required from dextrose would be:

$$1,950 - 275 = 1,675\,\text{Calories}$$

Then, calculate the amount of dextrose needed to meet the requirements.

$$\frac{3.4\,\text{Calories}}{1\,\text{g}} = \frac{1,675\,\text{Calories}}{x\,\text{g}}$$
$$x = 493\,\text{g of dextrose}$$

Finally, convert the amount of dextrose into milliliters of solution.

$$\frac{70\,\text{g dextrose}}{100\,\text{mL}} = \frac{493\,\text{g}}{x\,\text{mL}}$$
$$x = \textbf{704\,mL of D}_{70}\textbf{W}$$

Biostatistics

This chapter contains the following:

- **Descriptive statistics: Summarizing the data**
- **Inferential statistics: Predicting outcomes**
- **Statistical test selection**

DESCRIPTIVE STATISTICS: SUMMARIZING THE DATA

Central Tendency

Central tendency is a general term used to describe the distribution of a set of values or measurements and the simplification to a single value near a point in the dataset that represents where the largest portion of data are located. The following are the most commonly used central tendency measures.

Median (*m*): The median is the value directly in the middle of the ranked values in a dataset; that is, 50% of all ranked values are smaller than the median and the other 50% of ranked values are larger. The median is **not** influenced by extreme values (outliers). The median is useful in situations in which there are unusually low or high values that would render the mean unrepresentative of the data.

Mean ($\overline{X}$ or μ): The mean is the average of all observations in a dataset. The mean is the most commonly used measure of central tendency because it has properties that make it useful for statistical analyses. It is influenced by extreme values (outliers) and is most useful when the data are symmetrically distributed without outliers (i.e., normal distribution).

Mode: The mode is the value with the greatest frequency of occurrence. It is not generally used because it is often not representative of the data, particularly when the dataset is small.

Variability

An additional measure that describes the variability in a dataset is, therefore, generally provided with a central tendency measure to better describe the dataset. The following are the most commonly used measures of variability.

Standard Deviation (SD or σ): The standard deviation is the most common measure of the variability around the mean. It is used with a mean because it is most informative when the dataset is normally distributed, as described below. The mean and standard deviation are commonly used together as the most informative measures of central tendency and variability of a dataset, respectively.

Standard Error of the Mean (SEM): The standard error of the mean is defined as the variability of the sample means. It is calculated as the SD divided by the square root of the sample size. This will always be smaller than the sample SD. It is sometimes reported in the scientific and medical literature and is an intermediary step in calculating confidence intervals.

Absolute Range: The absolute range is simply the difference between the largest and smallest observation in a dataset. A disadvantage is that the range is based solely on two observations and is likely not representative of the whole dataset. Absolute range is particularly susceptible to outliers.

Interquartile Range (IQR): Quartiles are calculated in a way similar to the median, which splits a dataset into two equally sized groups. Quartiles split the data into four approximately equal sized groups. The interquartile range is the range between the lower and upper quartiles. Like the median, the interquartile range is not influenced by unusually high or low values and is particularly useful when data are not symmetrically distributed.

- The lower Quartile (Q_L or Q_1) is the 25th percentile; that is, 25% of the data are below the value of Q_1.
- The upper Quartile (Q_U or Q_3) is the 75th percentile; that is, 75% of the data are below the value of Q_3.

Boxplots are one-dimensional graphs that can be drawn from the range, IQR, and median, as displayed here.

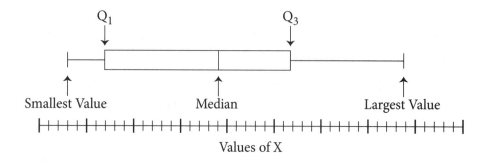

Distributions

Statistical test selection relies heavily on the distribution of data. These distributions can be summarized by a central tendency and variation around that center. The most important distribution is the normal or Gaussian curve. This "bell-shaped" curve is symmetric, with one side the mirror image of the other.

The distribution of any dataset can be assessed visually using a **histogram**. The *x*-axis represents the actual values in the dataset which, for pharmacy, are usually measures made of patients enrolled in a clinical trial (e.g., systolic blood pressure, creatinine clearance, low-density lipoprotein cholesterol concentrations). The *y*-axis represents the frequency of the value or the number of patients who had a value within a defined range. An example of a histogram is displayed here.

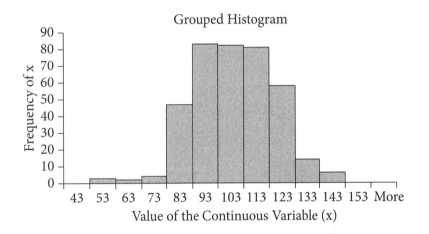

As the sample size (*n*) displayed in the histogram here approaches the population size (*N*), the lines on the graph become smooth and look more like following graph for normally distributed data:

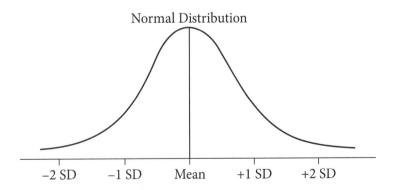

There are important attributes of the Normal Distribution shown in the preceding graph that can be useful in a number of problems on the NAPLEX. Importantly, the data is symmetric about the mean, as shown by the vertical line in the graph. This means that 50% of the values will be greater than the mean and 50% of the values will be less than the mean. Because this is the definition of a median, the mean and median are equal values in a normal distribution. The informative power of the normal distribution comes from the value of the standard deviation:

- The mean ± 1 SD contains 68% of the values in the dataset (or population)
- The mean ± 2 SD contains 95% of the values in the dataset (or population)
- The mean ± 3 SD contains 99.7% of the values in the dataset (or population)

The following graph displays two normal curves with the same means but different standard deviations:

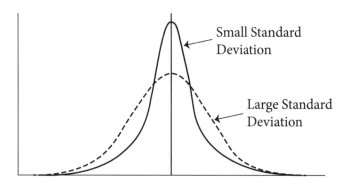

Example:

Patients ($n = 100$) enrolled in a clinical trial have a mean ± SD creatinine clearance of 110 ± 20 mL/min. Approximately how many patients have creatinine clearance values between 70 and 110 mL/min?

Answer: The value of 70 mL/min is 2 SD away from the mean in the negative direction, and the value of 110 mL/min is the value of the mean. Approximately 95% of the values will be ± 2 SD away from the mean. Because the question is asking for only 2 SD in the negative direction and the normal distribution is symmetrical, it will be half the value of 95%. Half of 95% is 47.5%. Therefore, approximately 47.5% of the sample size of $n = 100$ patients will have values in this range. The answer would be approximately 48 patients have creatinine clearance values in this range.

Not all curves are normally distributed. Sometimes the curve is skewed either positively or negatively. For skewed distributions, the median is a better representation of central tendency than is the mean, and the IQR is a better measure of the variability than is the SD.

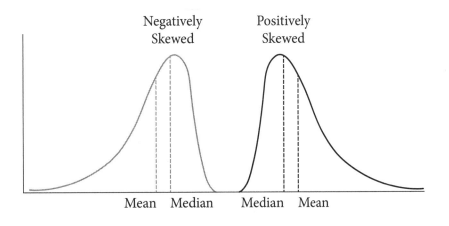

INFERENTIAL STATISTICS: PREDICTING OUTCOMES

The main goal of several studies in the pharmacy literature is to compare measurements from two groups of study patients: a group that receives a standard drug (i.e., control) and a group that receives an investigational drug. Even if both groups are administered placebo, it is highly unlikely that an identical mean and standard deviation of any value will be obtained for both groups. This is due to inherent variability in humans, among other sources, and is termed sampling error. The purpose of inferential statistics is to determine if the observed differences in the measures between the two groups of patients is due to chance (i.e., sampling error) or if one drug is really better than the other.

The following table summarizes important definitions regarding statistical inference.

General Statistical Definitions

Hypotheses	Hypothesis	Theoretical statement that the study is intended to test.
	Null hypothesis	States that there is no difference between the study and control groups.
	Alternative hypothesis	States that the null hypothesis is incorrect; there is a difference between the study and control groups.
Variables	Independent variable	Known variable(s).
	Dependent variable	Variable with a value dependent upon the value of an independent variable.
	Qualitative variable	Variable that yields observations by which individuals can be categorized according to some characteristic or quality.
	Quantitative variable	Variables that yield numerical observations that can be measured through statistical analysis. Qualitative variables can be transformed to quantitative variables by assigning numerical values to the observations.

General Statistical Definitions   *(cont'd)*

Error	Type I error	Rejecting a true null hypothesis: Finding a difference between the study and control groups that does not exist.
	Type II error	Accepting a false null hypothesis: Failing to detect a difference between the study and control groups when a difference truly exists.
Tests	Parametric	Requires prior knowledge of the nature of the data under examination; data must fall under a normal (Gaussian) distribution and be measured on an interval or a ratio scale.
	Nonparametric	Does not require prior knowledge of the distribution of the observations; data need not follow a normal or Gaussian distribution.
Miscellaneous definitions	Accuracy	Measure of how close a measured value is to the expected value.
	Precision	Measure of how close a particular measured value is to the other values in a set of measurements; does not imply proximity between measured values and the expected value.
	Sample	Data set taken under homogeneous conditions; a subset of a population.
	Population	Entire group from which a sample is taken.
	Gaussian (or normal) distribution	A bell-shaped distribution. Given a large enough sample size, the Central Limit Theorem states that the distribution of means will follow this type of distribution even if the population is not Gaussian. • 68% of values fall within $\pm$ 1 SD of the mean • 95% of values fall within $\pm$ 2 SD of the mean • 99.7% of values fall within $\pm$ 3 SD of the mean

Several additional statistical concepts follow, in slightly greater detail. Many of these concepts apply regardless of the statistical test chosen.

Confidence Intervals

Statistical decisions are made based on sampling from a larger population. The true values for the population may be above or below the sample values. For example, the sample mean is unlikely to be the same value as the actual mean of the entire population. Therefore, confidence intervals are calculated from the sample to provide a range of values that is likely to contain the actual population value. The most common confidence interval used is the 95% confidence interval. This interval implies that you are 95% confident that the actual mean value of the population lies within this range of values. The 5% of uncertainty is the same concept as described with the p-value discussed later in this chapter. Therefore, 95% confidence intervals can be used to determine statistical significance with a Type I error rate of 5%, as demonstrated next.

Example:

The following graph displays the 95% confidence intervals for blood pressure measurements following the administration of three drugs. The closed circle represents the sample mean estimate in each group, and the error bars encompass the values of the 95% confidence interval. Which drugs are statistically different from each other?

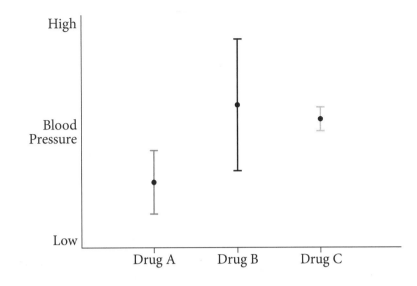

Answer:

When comparing two groups, any overlap of confidence intervals indicates that the groups would have a p-value > 0.05 and are not significantly different. Therefore, if the graph represents 95% confidence intervals and each drug is compared with the others, Drugs B and C are no different in their effects, and Drug B is no different from Drug A. Drug A lowers blood pressure to a greater statistically significant extent than Drug C. Of note, comparing these drugs individually to one another as in this example would increase the Type I error rate >5%, as will be discussed (see ANOVA).

Relative Risk and Odds Ratios

A relative risk (RR) is the ratio of the probability of an event occurring in a treatment (i.e., exposed) group to the probability of the event occurring in a control (i.e., nonexposed) group, as displayed in the following equation:

$$RR = \frac{p(\text{exposure group})}{p(\text{nonexposed group})}$$

Example:

In a local hospital over the last year, the frequency of patients with heart failure developing myopathy among those taking statins was 5 out of 100, and among patients not taking statins, it was 2 out of 100 patients. Calculate the relative risk.

Answer:

$$RR = \frac{5/100}{2/100} = 2.5$$

This implies that patients with heart failure who are taking statins were 2.5 times more likely to develop myopathy than patients who were not taking statins. Clearly, there are many variables in a study that could affect the relative risk beyond that of the statin use. Multivariate regression is commonly used in these types of analyses to account for variables beyond the exposure itself.

Similar to the relative risk, an **odds ratio** (OR) is also a measure of association between an exposure and an outcome. An odds ratio will provide a similar estimate to that of a relative risk, but the calculation is not as intuitive. However, the odds ratio has a mathematical advantage and is commonly reported because it is used in logistic regression to account for study variables beyond the exposure.

It is important to be able to make statistical determinations when provided with confidence intervals for relative risks and odds ratios. Simply put, if the 95% confidence interval contains 1, there is no statistically significant effect of the treatment (i.e., exposure). This is demonstrated in the following table for three hypothetical measures:

Relative Risk or Odds Ratio	Confidence Interval	Interpretation
1.98	(1.45–2.53)	Statistically significant (increased risk)
1.25	(0.78–1.53)	No statistical difference (risk the same)
0.45	(0.22–0.68)	Statistically significant (decreased risk)

Number Needed to Treat or Harm

The **number needed to treat (NNT)** is the number of patients receiving a specific treatment or intervention required to prevent one additional outcome (e.g., MI, stroke). The **number needed to harm (NNH)** indicates how many patients must be exposed to a risk factor to cause harm in one patient who otherwise would not have been harmed. To calculate the NNT or NNH, first calculate the **absolute risk reduction (ARR)** or **absolute risk increase (ARI)** of the exposure, respectively. The ARR and ARI are calculated as the difference between the event rates in the control group and the comparative group. The NNT is calculated as the inverse of the ARR, and the NNH is calculated as the inverse of the ARI, as shown in the equations:

$$NNT = \frac{1}{ARR}$$

$$NNH = \frac{1}{ARI}$$

Example:

In a local hospital over the last year, the frequency of patients with heart failure developing myopathy among those taking statins was 5 out of 100, and among patients not taking statins, it was 2 out of 100 patients. Calculate the relative risk.

In the preceding example, the event rate of myopathy in patients taking statins is 5 out of 100, or 5%. The event rate of myopathy in patients not exposed to statins is 2 out of 100, or 2%. In this case, the treatment is increasing the undesirable outcome of myopathy. Taking a statin increases the probability of myopathy from 2% to 5%. Therefore, instead of NNT, we are interested in calculating the NNH. To calculate NNH, first calculate ARI, and then take the inverse.

$$ARI = 5\% - 2\% = 3\%$$

$$NNH = \frac{1}{0.03} = 33$$

This implies that 33 patients exposed to statins would result in one extra case of myopathy that would not have happened under control conditions. These calculations and concepts are very similar for NNT.

p-Value and Statistical Significance

The p-value is the probability that the difference measured between your study group and the control group is the result of random chance rather than a true difference. The p-value is expressed as a value between 0 and 1; therefore, the higher the p-value, the more likely it is that a difference in sample means was due to chance and that a drug had no effect. When the p-value is low (e.g., <5%), it indicates that it was unlikely that the difference was due to chance; therefore, the drug had a statistically significant effect.

The null hypothesis may be rejected if there is a sufficiently small probability that it is true. A significance level (or α) of 0.05 is most commonly chosen, although it should be chosen based on the relative consequences of making a Type I or Type II error in the particular study setting. When a 0.05 significance level is chosen, if $p \leq 0.05$, a statistically significant difference in treatment effect exists between the control and treatment groups. If $p > 0.05$, the results of the study are considered to be not statistically significant, meaning no difference exists between the treatment and control groups. Choosing a larger significance level, like $p = 0.1$, gives a higher probability of rejecting a true null hypothesis (Type I error, or false positive test).

Types of Statistical Error

As defined in the table at the beginning of this chapter, there are two types of error that can be made at the end of a statistical test. The significance level (i.e., alpha, α) is commonly set to 0.05. This means that there is a 5% chance that a **Type I error (α error)** will be made during hypothesis testing. A Type I error is the conclusion that there is a statistical difference when in reality there is not one. Of course, you cannot know from a given experiment if you made a Type I error or not. You can only know the rate at which they occur (i.e., 5%).

The other type of error is **Type II error (β error)**, which is the conclusion that there is not a difference between groups when, in reality, there is a difference. A Type II error can only be made when the p-value is > 0.05 and the conclusion is made that there is no statistical difference between groups. As in a Type I error, one cannot know from a single experiment if a Type II error has been made, but can only calculate the frequency of the error. The Type I error rate is set at 5%, but the Type II error rate varies depending on the variable being measured and the study itself (see "Power and Sample Size"). Type II error rates are commonly designed to be <10% or 20%. The factors that affect Type II error are the same that affect study power.

Power and Sample Size

The power of a study is the ability to detect a difference between study groups if one actually exists. Study power is indirectly related to the likelihood of making a Type II (β) error. Therefore, as study power increases, the likelihood of concluding that there is not a difference when one actually does exist decreases. Therefore, as power increases, Type II error rate decreases. The following factors affect the power of a study:

- **Sample size (*n*):** The closer the sample size is to the actual population size, the easier it is to detect a difference.
- **Difference between the actual population means:** It will be easier to detect a difference between drugs with large effects versus the control or comparator. For example, it is much easier to show that a β-blocker will lower blood pressure compared to a placebo than it would be compared to an angiotensin-converting enzyme (ACE) inhibitor.
- **Variability around the population means (and sample means):** The more variable effect there is, the harder it is to show a difference. For example, if a drug only works in a small percentage of the population, it will be difficult to show statistical significance in a sample from the entire population.
- **Significance level, α:** The Type I error rate directly alters the Type II error rate. This is one reason why the significance level is traditionally set at 5%. If one wanted to decrease the Type I error rate and set it at 1%, it would increase the Type II error rate and, thereby, decrease the power of the study.

Of the factors just listed, the only way to decrease Type II error (increase power) without increasing Type I error is to increase the sample size.

At the conclusion of a study, if the p-value is > 0.05, the actual study power can be calculated. This is done by simply using the actual values of the factors listed about the study (e.g., the sample size, variability, and mean difference). Of course, it would only make sense to calculate the power of a study if the p-value was > 0.05. If the p-value is < 0.05, it is impossible to make a Type II error. Only a Type I error could have been made with a p-value < 0.05, and the power of the study would be irrelevant.

Correlation

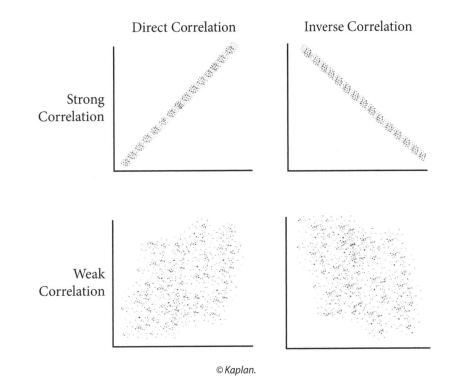

© Kaplan.

A key point to remember is that an observed correlation between two variables does not imply that there is a causal link between the two variables. For example, warm weather causes an increase in both the crime rate and the incidence of sunburn. Crime rate and sunburn incidence will therefore be positively correlated; however, crime does not cause sunburn and sunburn does not cause crime.

STATISTICAL TEST SELECTION

The first thing that must be done when determining what statistical test should be employed is to identify the dependent variable and the scale of measurement that will be used for this variable. These scales are described in the table.

Types of Variables

Qualitative	Nominal	Characteristics that do not have numerical value and do not have order (e.g., gender or race).
	Ordinal	Characteristics that do not have numerical value but have an underlying order to their observations and can be ranked from highest to lowest (e.g., disagree, indifferent, agree, strongly agree).
Quantitative	Interval	Ordered set of categories, similar to an ordinal scale, with the additional requirement that the categories form a series of intervals that are identically spaced. An example is time as read on a clock, 10 A.M., 11 A.M., 12 P.M., 1 P.M., 2 P.M., etc.
	Ratio	Same qualities as an interval scale but with an absolute zero point to indicate a complete absence of the variable being measured. This is the most common type of numerical data in the biomedical and pharmaceutical sciences.
	Ranked	A group of numerical observations that can be arranged according to magnitude, such as in ordinal data. Ordinal data can be transformed into quantitative/ranked data by being assigned values that correspond to each observation's place in the sequence.
	Grouped	Quantitative variables that are categorized, particularly for presentation of data. Nominal variables can be changed to quantitative variables by being placed in groups and assigned numbers. For example, a clinical study could quantify gender by assigning females a value of 1 and males a value of 2.

Tests Appropriate for Numerical Scales of Measurement

Numeric scales (predominantly interval or ratio scales) of measurement are used when the measured values are numbers. Examples include height, weight, or blood pressure level. When the data follows a Gaussian distribution, parametric statistical tests should be used.

- Two independent groups: ***t-test***
- Two dependent groups: ***Paired t-test***
- Three or more independent groups: ***ANOVA***
- Three or more dependent groups: ***Repeated measures ANOVA***

t-Test

The *t*-test is one of the most commonly used statistical tests. It compares means obtained from the numeric data of two groups that are independent of each other. This statistical test is commonly used in the pharmacy literature to compare the outcomes of numeric data (e.g., clinical measures, drug concentrations). In a sample of patients who received an experimental drug versus a different (i.e., independent) sample of patients who received a control drug.

Paired *t*-Test

A paired *t*-test is used when the same sample is being used to compare the experimental and the control drug; that is, this test is appropriate when numeric data is being compared between two dependent groups. This is commonly referred to as a crossover design. A paired *t*-test is the appropriate statistical test for numeric or interval data.

ANOVA

When a third group (or more) is added to a study design for comparison, it is not appropriate to perform multiple t-tests. For example, an experimental drug to lower blood pressure is being compared to a group of patients taking β-blockers and another group of patients taking ACE inhibitors. In this study design, one cannot perform a t-test to compare the experimental drug to the β-blocker group and then perform another t-test to compare the ACE inhibitor group. Each time a t-test is performed there is a 5% chance of a Type I error; thus, multiple comparisons increase this rate of Type I error greater than 5%. Therefore, if three or more groups are being compared, it is appropriate to use an analysis of variance (ANOVA). An ANOVA will generate one p-value from the three groups. If the p-value is < 0.05, it states that at least one drug was different than another at lowering blood pressure. Importantly, the Type I error rate is maintained at 5% for an ANOVA.

To determine which drug has a statistically significant effect, additional tests are needed. These statistical tests are referred to as *post-hoc tests*. The most commonly used post-hoc test is Tukey's test. The Bonferroni and Scheffe's tests are also post-hoc tests that can be used to determine which groups were statistically different if an overall p-value from the ANOVA was less than 0.05. If a p-value is > 0.05 following an ANOVA, no further tests are needed.

Repeated Measures ANOVA

The repeated measures ANOVA is the equivalent of using a paired t-test instead of a t-test. It, therefore, can be used in crossover studies when there are three or more study periods following appropriate wash-out of the drug between each period. This test is referred to as *repeated measures* because it is commonly used when the same measures are being made in patients throughout a study. For example, in many statin clinical trials, the low-density lipoprotein cholesterol (LDL-C) lowering ability of the statins is not determined at only one point but at several points (e.g., 1, 3, 6, 12, 18, and 24 months). To determine if significant LDL-C lowering occurred in patients during these time intervals, a repeated measures ANOVA must be used. The Dunnett's test is the post-hoc test that should be used if an overall p-value < 0.05 is obtained.

When the data does not follow a Gaussian distribution, the same tests used for ordinal data should be employed.

Tests Appropriate for Ordinal Scales of Measurement

Ordinal scales of measurement are used when characteristics have an underlying order to their values but the numbers used are arbitrary (e.g., Likert scales). Various non-parametric tests (e.g., Mann-Whitney U and Wilcoxon Signed-Rank) are used for analyzing such data. Ordinal scales also are used for numeric data that are not distributed normally and that have a small sample size. The following are situations in which a nonparametric test should be considered:

- The outcome is ordinal and the sample is clearly not normally distributed.

- There are values that are too high or too low to obtain accurate measures. It is impossible to analyze such data with a parametric test because the exact value is not determined.

- The sample size is small and the sample is not approximately normally distributed. Data transformation can be done by taking the logarithm of the values. This is common for biological data, which often has outliers in the positive direction (i.e., skewed to the right).

The following table lists parametric tests for normally distributed data and the corresponding nonparametric test for ordinal or non-normally distributed data.

Parametric Versus Nonparametric Statistics

Parametric Tests	Nonparametric Equivalent
t-Test $\longrightarrow$	Wilcoxon-Rank Sum (Mann Whitney U)
Paired t-test $\longrightarrow$	Wilcoxon Sign Rank (Sign Test)
ANOVA $\longrightarrow$	Kruskal-Wallis Test
Repeated measures ANOVA $\longrightarrow$	Friedman Test
Note: The Wilcoxon-Rank Sum is the post-hoc test for the Kruskal-Wallis Test	

Tests Appropriate for Nominal Scales of Measurement

Nominal scales are used for characteristics that do not have numerical value (such as gender or race). The Chi-square test and its variants are used to test the null hypothesis that proportions are equal, or that factors or characteristics are not associated with each other.

PRACTICE QUESTIONS

1. The median value of a data set is the

    (A) mathematical average of all the values in the data set.
    (B) value equidistant from the extremes of a distribution.
    (C) average of the difference between each value in the set and the mean.
    (D) most commonly occurring value in the data set.
    (E) distance between the smallest and largest values in the data set.

Questions 2–3 refer to the following graph.

Total serum cholesterol concentrations were measured in 175 patients with coronary artery disease. The measured serum cholesterol concentrations are displayed in the grouped frequency distribution histogram using 10 equal intervals, shown below.

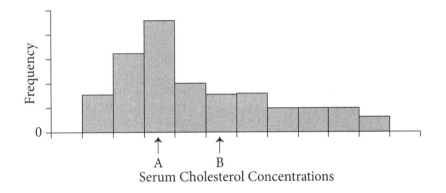

2. The class interval as indicated by "B" in the above histogram MOST likely contains which of the following measures for this dataset?

    (A) Median
    (B) Mean
    (C) Mode
    (D) Standard deviation
    (E) Range

3. Which of the following is the BEST description of the distribution of this sample dataset?

    (A) Normal
    (B) Positively skewed
    (C) Negatively skewed
    (D) Gaussian
    (E) None of the above

4. A study reports that the mean $\pm$ SD peak plasma concentration of a drug is 1.0 ± 0.1 mg/dL in a study consisting of 1,000 patients. Approximately how many patients had values >1.1 mg/dL?

    (A) 840
    (B) 680
    (C) 320
    (D) 160
    (E) 16

5. A clinical study was performed and serum glucose concentrations were measured in 14 diabetic patients following 1 week of an investigational treatment to directly compare it to the decrease following glipizide treatment in a crossover trial. Statistics were performed and a p-value of 0.45 was obtained. Which of the following is (are) the most likely form of statistical error that the researchers could have made?

    (A) Type I error
    (B) Type II error
    (C) Type I or Type II error
    (D) Neither Type I or II error could be made because the results were NOT significant
    (E) Neither Type I or II error could be made because the results were significant

6. In most clinical studies, the Type I error rate is set to 0.05 before the study is performed. This indicates that the research group has a 5.0% chance of making a Type I error. If a research group were to set α at 0.01, corresponding to a Type 1 error rate of only 1.0%, which of the following statements would be TRUE?

    (A) A smaller sample size could be used.
    (B) The study power would increase.
    (C) There would be an increased α error rate.
    (D) There would be an increased β error rate.
    (E) None of the above statements are true.

Questions 7–8 refer to the following table.

A clinical study enrolled 70 patients who were randomized to receive either lisinopril or ramipril (n = 35 per drug). The table shows measures obtained at the end of the study period in patients who received lisinopril and ramipril.

After Drug Treatment (End of Study Period)	Lisinopril n = 35	Ramipril n = 35
Disease states	—	—
Diabetes alone	29%	20%
Atherosclerosis alone	23%	31%
Diabetes and atherosclerosis	43%	34%
Neither disease	5%	15%
Mean serum cholesterol concentrations (mg/dL)	118 ± 4.0	116 ± 4.0
Sex (% male)	62%	46%

Data are presented as percentage of mean ± SD.

7. Which of the following statistical tests would be most appropriate to use to compare the serum cholesterol concentrations in the ramipril versus the lisinopril group?

    (A) *t*-Test
    (B) Paired *t*-test
    (C) Chi-square test
    (D) Wilcoxon sign rank test
    (E) ANOVA

8. Which of the following statistical tests would be most appropriate to use to compare the percentage of males in the ramipril versus the lisinopril group?

    (A) *t*-Test
    (B) Paired *t*-test
    (C) Chi-square test
    (D) Wilcoxon sign rank test
    (E) ANOVA

9. What is the number needed to treat if drug A decreases the risk of myocardial infarction by 10% over drug B?

    (A) 1
    (B) 5
    (C) 10
    (D) 100
    (E) 500

ANSWERS AND EXPLANATIONS

1. B

The median value is the value equidistant from the extremes of the data set. The mathematical average of the values in the data set (A) is the mean. The average of the difference between each value and the mean (C) is the standard deviation. The most commonly occurring value in the data set (D) is the mode. The distance between the smallest and largest values in the data set (E) is the range.

2. B

The mean is the most likely measure listed in the position marked by "B" on the graph. The mean is susceptible to outliers, and this dataset is skewed to the right, which means that there are outliers in the positive direction. The mean is pulled from the real central tendency of the data marked by "A" on the graph. The "A," most likely, is represented by the median, which is not susceptible to outliers and is the best measure of central tendency for skewed data.

3. B

The dataset is positively skewed because there are outliers on the graph in the positive direction. This pulls the mean to the right of the central tendency as described in the answer to question number 2.

4. D

1.1 mg/dL is 1 SD away from the mean, and the question is asking for values greater than that. With 68% of the dataset $\pm$ 1 SD away from the mean, the remaining 32% is outside of this range. Because normally distributed data is symmetrical, there is 16% of the dataset on the two sides that encompass data greater or less than 1 SD away from the mean. Thus, 16% of 1,000 patients equals 160, which is the answer.

5. B

The p-value is > 0.05; therefore, the authors would conclude that the differences observed between the investigational drug and glipizide are due to chance and that the investigational drug was not different than glipizide. Because the authors conclude that there is no difference, the only possible type of error is Type II (β) error. A Type II error is a conclusion that there is no difference when one actually exists. Given the small sample size of this study, the likelihood of a Type II error is likely very high. A Type I error cannot be made because there is no conclusion that a difference exists between the investigational drug and glipizide.

6. **D**

Setting the Type I (α) error rate to 0.01 instead of the traditional 0.05 would increase the Type II (β) error rate. The Type II error is inversely related to power; therefore, the study's power to detect a difference would be smaller. This would mean that a larger sample size would be needed to detect a difference if one actually exists.

7. **A**

The ramipril and lisinopril groups are independent of each other because this study is not a crossover design. Cholesterol concentrations are interval data, thus considered numeric; therefore, the most appropriate test for two independent groups with numeric data is a t-test. The sample size is >30, so the data does not have to be normally distributed. If the sample size were small and not normally distributed, the nonparametric Mann–Whitney U test should be used.

8. **C**

The sex of the patients is considered a nominal variable, which is often referred to as *categorical* because the patients can be placed into categories. Each patient is either a male or a female and cannot be classified as both. The fact that the percentages are provided instead of the actual number of males in each group does not change the fact that the data is categorical. The most appropriate statistical test for this type of categorical data is the Chi-square test.

9. **C**

The number needed to treat (NNT) is the inverse of the absolute risk reduction (ARR). In this case, the ARR is given as 10%. Therefore, the inverse of 0.1 is 10.